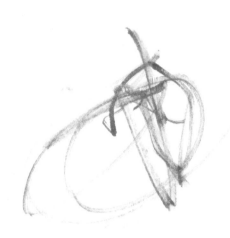

CONTENTS

Contents

INTRODUCTION

Descriptive labels like 'mentally handicapped' or 'mentally retarded' have become widely accepted as preferred ways of referring to people with limited intelligence, instead of terms which they replaced, such as 'idiot', 'imbecile' and 'feeble-minded'. These preferences are culturally determined and reflect our social awareness that some names can be more demeaning for the person named than others. A further change which is currently under way is the growing preference for speaking of 'people with mental handicaps', or 'persons with developmental delay', phrases which give priority to the person and stress that he or she *has* a handicap rather than *is* the handicap.

Even so, the terms 'mental handicap' or 'mental retardation' still suggest a degree of homogeneity about the condition and have an air of finality about them. Why look any further, because the person has irremedial limitations? He or she simply requires humane and considerate care.

In reality, however, 'the mentally handicapped' are a most heterogeneous collection of people who are known to be, or assumed to be, of substantially lower ability. Abilities can be depleted in numerous ways, of which limited cerebral functioning is only one. A brief examination of an institutional population reveals a wide range of genetic, biochemical, sensory and physical handicaps, each of which can limit abilities. The greatest accompanying risk is that the shortfall in ability will be attributed to the wrong handicap. When it is attributed to 'mental handicap', a circular misdiagnosis can occur; thus 'he has low ability because his ability is low'. This tautology invites no further search for remediation. The alternative strategy is to identify the component handicaps from which the delay has arisen, and work to remedy them.

This book is addressed to the many forms of sensory handicap from which mentally handicapped people can suffer; it considers how to assess and treat them, and how to assess, train and equip the people who suffer from them. Readers will find that sensory handicaps occur much more commonly in mentally handicapped people, sometimes from the same congenital source as that which produced the mental retardation, sometimes because mundane limitations on vision or hearing have been ignored or overlooked, and occasionally as a side-effect of the pharmaceutical treatment of other conditions or 'problems'.

It was a great encouragement to find that there were more specialists in various aspects of sensory and mental handicaps than could be included in one volume. Those authors who have contributed have adopted a variety of approaches, from formal academic reviews to discussions of practical helping strategies and comments on the need for further developments of appropriate services. Each orientation has its place here, in our combined bid to stimulate a more constructive and better informed approach to serving sensorily and mentally handicapped people. The work requires multi-disciplinary collaboration between teachers, nurses, social workers, service administrators, speech therapists, doctors, psychologists and research personnel. It is hoped that this book will be of some value to each of these disciplines, and provide a starting-point for further practical or investigative work, as appropriately skilled and specialized resources are usually in short supply.

It is worth making a brief note here of the apparent conflict between meeting the needs of sensorily and mentally handicapped people on one hand, and the principle of normalization on the other. Most approaches to helping sensorily handicapped people require some specialization of staff and professional skills and, to some degree, of service provision. Manual sign vocabularies and mobility techniques are two major areas where specialized staff skills can provide paths to greater independence for deaf or blind people.

Regrettably, the mention of 'specialization' appears to some normalizers to be the very inverse of their guiding principle, in spite of Wolfensberger's (1972) view that 'where the service mainstream excludes persons with special problems and needs, special services must be created' (p. 209). If the particular needs of people with combinations of sensory and mental handicaps are to be met adequately in future, then all of us must develop new skills. We may need to arrange special opportunities to practise and apply such skills, and to support, encourage and maintain contact with like-minded colleagues. It is not bricks and mortar which make institutions, but attitudes, routine work practices, assumptions and often the ignorance of staff like us. Proposals for specialized buildings and services should not be rejected out of hand by normalizers, but should be assessed according to principles like age-appropriateness, proximity to a normal community, opportunities for fostering greater personal independence, and so on. Thus a purpose-built living and training unit for, e.g. deaf and mentally handicapped institutional inmates *may* be the best first step on the path to normalized living, if it encourages staff to develop skills appropriate to the needs of these clients and if the clients feel too threatened by a move directly into the local community. The normalization principle should be used as the means of achieving greater independence for clients, not as an end to be waved like a banner at a great parade.

In conclusion I wish to thank the many contributors to this book for their effort and enthusiasm which have made its publication possible; and Mr David Bond, Dr John Corbett, Mr Paul Ennals, Dr James Hogg and Professor Chris Kiernan for their advice, recommendations and help in identifying and recruiting several of the present contributors.

David Ellis

Reference

Wolfensberger, W. (1972) *The Principle of Normalization in Human Services*, National Institute on Mental Retardation, Toronto

This book is dedicated to the late Oscar Myers, formerly
Principal of Condover Hall School, Shropshire, and first
Chairman of the Committee on the Multi-handicapped Blind,
in recognition of his efforts to raise awareness of the
unmet needs of multiply handicapped blind children in Britain.

LIST OF CONTRIBUTORS

Feriha Anwar, Medical Research Council Developmental Psychology Project, University of London Institute of Education, 2 Taviton Street, London WC1, England.

Janette Atkinson, Visual Developmental Unit, Kenneth Craik Laboratory, Department of Experimental Psychology, University of Cambridge, Cambridge, England.

Christy W. Battle, Program in Communication Disorders, University of Texas at Dallas, Callier Center for Communication Disorders, 1966 Inwood Road, Dallas, Texas 75235, USA.

Anthony B. Best, Lecturer, Department of Special Education, Faculty of Education, University of Birmingham, PO Box 363, Birmingham B15 2TT, England.

Christine Best, Educational Psychologist, City of Birmingham Education Department, Child Advisory and Psychological Services, 29 George Road, Edgbaston, Birmingham 15, England.

David E. Bond, Specialist Educational Psychologist, Royal School for Deaf Children, Victoria Road, Margate, Kent CT9 1NB, England.

Robert Dantona, 139 Riverside Street, Watertown, Massachusetts 02172, USA.

David Ellis, Principal Clinical Psychologist, Turner Village Hospital, Turner Road, Colchester, Essex CO4 5JP, England.

Robert J. Fletcher, Professor, Department of Optometry and Visual Science, The City University, Dame Alice Owen Building, 311-21 Goswell Road, London EC1, England.

Randall K. Harley, Professor of Special Education, George Peabody College for Teachers, Vanderbilt University, Nashville, Tennessee 37203, USA.

Beate Hermelin, Medical Research Council Developmental Psychology Project, University of London Institute of Education, 2 Taviton Street, London WC1, England.

Mary-Maureen Hill, Orientation and Mobility Specialist, Tennessee Rehabilitation Center for the Blind, Nashville, Tennessee, USA.

Anthony Holland, Lecturer, Genetics Unit, Institute of Psychiatry, University of London, De Crespigny Park, Denmark Hill, London SE5 8AF, England.

George R. Karlan, Special Education, Purdue University, South Campus Courts, Building E, West Lafayette, Indiana 47907, USA.

List of Contributors

Barbara I. Kropka, Clinical Psychologist, Bristol and Weston Health Authority, Barrow Hospital, Barrow Gurney, Bristol BS19 3SG, England.

M. Beth Langley, Co-ordinator, Diagnostic Prescriptive Project for the Severely Handicapped, Pinellas County Schools, Pinellas, Florida, USA.

Lyle L. Lloyd, Special Education, Purdue University, South Campus Courts, Building E, West Lafayette, Indiana 47907, USA.

Michael Nolan, Department of Audiology and Education of the Deaf, University of Manchester, Oxford Road, Manchester M13 9PL, England.

Neil O'Connor, Medical Research Council Developmental Psychology Project, University of London Institute of Education, 2 Taviton Street, London WC1, England.

Gwendolyn Pennington Special Education, Purdue University, South Campus Courts, Building E, West Lafayette, Indiana 47907, USA.

Robert D. Stillman, Program in Communication Disorders, University of Texas at Dallas, Callier Center for Communication Disorders, 1966 Inwood Road, Dallas, Texas 75235, USA.

Ivan Tucker, Department of Audiology and Education of the Deaf, University of Manchester, Oxford Road, Manchester M13 9PL, England.

Jan van Dijk, Institute for the Deaf, Theerestraat 42, 5271 GD Sint-Michielsgestel, The Netherlands.

Mette Warburg, Consultant Ophthalmologist, Eye Clinic for the Mentally Handicapped, 40 Sognevej, 2820 Gentofte, Denmark.

Chris Williams, Director of Psychological Services (Mental Handicap and Behaviour Disorders), Exeter Health Authority, Royal Western Counties Hospital, Starcross, Devon EX6 8PU, England.

Sybil Yeates, formerly Honorary Consultant Developmental Paediatrician, Newcomen Centre, Guy's Hospital, London SE1, England.

PART ONE

EPIDEMIOLOGY

1 THE EPIDEMIOLOGY OF VISUAL IMPAIRMENT IN PEOPLE WITH A MENTAL HANDICAP

David Ellis

Introduction

Epidemiology, the study of the distribution of particular medical, social and other characteristics in a given human population, has become an important branch of the medical and social sciences in this century, because it offers to social campaigners and policy-makers alike, the means of specifying more precisely the size and nature of given problems. In many respects any estimate more precise than a guess offers an advantage in helping to determine whether to allocate funds and skills to meet a need, and if so how much, or of what kind.

This chapter reviews available data on visual handicap; also results of a recent national survey in England and Wales will be examined to show the diverse range of visual impairments which have been reported among mentally handicapped people. Firstly, however, we should define two key epidemiological terms, 'incidence' and 'prevalence' to help overcome the confusion between them which arises occasionally. 'Incidence' concerns the number of *new* cases occurring in a given population in a *period* of time, e.g. the number of live births in a definable community in a year. 'Prevalence' is the number of cases present at a given *point* of time, e.g. all people with Down's syndrome on 30 June. Various practical limitations usually mean that all but the most well-controlled studies can only approximate these definitions, and often compromises are struck by researchers or clinicians in order to make data accessible.

VISUAL IMPAIRMENT IN THE GENERAL POPULATION

In Britain, the most important recent prevalence study of visual disability is that of Cullinan (1977; 1978). He found that about 520 in every 100,000 adults functioned as visually disabled, i.e. they had a measured visual acuity of less than 6/18 Snellen in their own homes. This level of acuity was proposed by the World Health Organization (WHO 1973) as an international definition of visual disability. The fractional score indicates that the subject can see, at 6 metres, what a person with normal vision can see at 18 metres. This may appear more like a measure of impairment than of disability, but identification of cases depended on self-selection or identification by another family member in response to questions concerning ability to read ordinary print, or to recognize an acquaintance across the street. Existing registration as blind or partially sighted also guaranteed inclusion.

3

Cullinan's research also found that visually disabled people saw worse at home than when reassessed at hospital, and that the difference was probably due to environmental conditions such as lighting levels. If hospital conditions existed at home, the adult prevalence rate for visual disability would fall from 520 to about 300 per 100,000. Clearly environmental conditions are almost as important as the clinical source of the visual impairment in determining the prevalence of visual *disability*. Comparable data from US sources have been reported in a series of articles (Kirchner and Lowman 1978; Peterson, Lowman and Kirchner 1978; Lowman and Kirchner 1979; Kirchner and Peterson 1979a, 1979b, 1980; Kirchner, Peterson and Suhr 1979). Using provisional results from the 1977 Health Interview Survey (HIS) conducted by the National Centre for Health Statistics (NCHS), Kirchner and Peterson (1979a) reported a general prevalence rate of 6.6 per 1,000 for visual *disability* based on inability to read ordinary newsprint. No supporting information on measured visual acuity was available from this source.

Data from these sources are summarized for comparison in Table 1.1. Considering the substantial difference in sources, the prevalence rates and age/sex distributions are remarkably similar. The most obvious difference occurs in age distribution: in the US data there are more younger, and fewer older males than in the UK. The reason for this difference is not readily apparent. Both reports show clearly that visual disability is mainly a problem of old age.

Registration

Many countries use some form of registration as the basis for providing aid and services to visually handicapped people. In the UK, for example, registration depends on an occupational definition, as interpreted by the ophthalmologist, who completes the registration form. Registerable blindness is defined as 'so blind as to be unable to do any work for which eye-

Table 1.1: Comparative Summary of UK and US Data on Visual Disability

	UK	US			
Prevalence: All	5.2/1000	6.6/1000			
Male		5.4/1000			
Female		7.6/1000			

Age Distribution (Sample Percentages)

Age	M	F	All	Age	M	F	All
-49	5.6	7.3	6.7	-44	15.2	6.8	10.1
50-64	27.8	13.0	18.1	45-64	22.8	15.8	18.6
65+	66.7	79.7	75.2	65+	61.7	77.3	71.1

Sources: Cullinan (1977) (UK) and Kirchner and Peterson (1979a) (US).

sight is essential'. In terms of acuity this usually means less than 3/60 Snellen, or up to 6/60 Snellen where the visual field is also restricted. Partial sight is broadly defined as not blind but substantially and permanently handicapped by visual loss. In this case, the commonly accepted standard of visual acuity is less than 6/18 Snellen. In reviewing world literature on registration practices and results, Cullinan (1977) noted that registers routinely underestimate the numbers of blind or partially sighted people in the population; his own national survey suggested a shortfall of 30-35 per cent on grounds of acuity alone. He estimated a prevalence rate of registered blind and partially sighted people of 2.9 per 1,000. Consequently registers do not measure adequately the prevalence of visual impairments. Reasons for the underestimations appear to include the preferences of patients, e.g. in terms of fear of stigmatization, and variations in the conduct of professional workers involved in registration, such as doctors and social workers.

Multiple Impairments

Both Cullinan (1977) and Kirchner and Peterson (1980) reported a breakdown of their data in terms of additional disabilities, but few of the subdivisions used allow a comparison between the two sets of data. Cullinan reported that 21 per cent had no other disability (HIS: 41 per cent) and 41 per cent were deaf (HIS: Deaf plus hard of hearing = 38.7 per cent). Clearly the personal limitations experienced by visually impaired people were not attributable to their visual impairment alone. Only the HIS reported data on 'Learning Disability and Mental Retardation' and this category accounted for 1.27 per cent of non-institutional severely visually impaired people. Expressed in this way, mentally handicapped people appear to be an insignificant minority. A very different perspective can be taken, however, when we examine data on visual impairment within the mentally handicapped population.

VISUAL IMPAIRMENTS AND MENTAL HANDICAP

Several studies have been reported of mental handicap surveys, or descriptions of institutional populations, which include details on visual impairment. A selection of these is summarized in Table 1.2 and the wide variation in prevalence reported is obvious. If we combine the percentages for blindness and partial sight into a 'visual impairment' prevalence figure, most studies fall into the range of 12-15 per cent. Some explanations for variations between studies can be deduced by considering the various survey characteristics. Firstly, all but one survey (Warburg 1970) used interview schedules or questionnaires to elicit information from parents or

Table 1 2: Summary of Prevalence Data on Visual Impairments Drawn from a Selection of Published Studies

Source	Sample size	Blind %	Partial sight %	Age range (years)	Male/Female ratio	Other
Bernsen (1981)	154	28.6*		4-22	1.3	City cohort (home + hospital)
Richardson et al (1979)	191	0.52	4.7	22	–	City cohort (5 yr)
Mitchell and Woodthorpe (1981)	282	5.38	9.6	15-20	1.47	Administrative prevalence 3 London boroughs (home + hospital)
Humphreys (1976)	472	1.9	11.0	5+	1.36	Community survey of home-based people
Mittler and Preddy (1981)	2,421	4.6	11.0	5-16+	1.32	Home-based schoolchildren
Grunewald (1973)	34,924	2.7*		All	–	National data
Warburg (1970)	706	5	7-8	All	0.72	Two hospital groups Adult & child
Ellis (1982)	30,020	3.6	4.4	All	1.12	National survey of mental handicap hospitals
Community data (Appendix to Part one, this volume)	2,788	1.8	8.7	All	–	Straw poll of British mental handicap registers

* = Blind and Partial sight.

care-givers. The Wessex register questionnaire used by Mitchell and Wood-thorpe (1981) employed a simple three-part classification of vision (1. Blind; 2. Poor; 3. Normal) and this system was used by several of the mental handicap registers summarized in the Appendix to Part One of this volume. Similarly Mittler and Preddy (1981) rated in terms of degree of visual *handicap* (i.e. None; Some; Little Usable Vision). Unfortunately, the Wessex register has less than adequate inter-rater reliability for its sensory handicap ratings (Palmer and Jenkins 1982) and this may limit the value of results obtained.

While 'false positive' errors may occur (i.e. reporting a visual impair-ment which does not exist), it seems more likely that non-expert respond-ents may misclassify a more extreme condition as a less extreme one, using common-sense judgements; thus opaque lenses will be obvious as a case of blindness, while blindness due to extreme myopia (short-sight) and/or narrowed visual fields may be overlooked or scored as 'partial sight' or 'eye problems'. A questionnaire heading like 'eye problems', without further definition, may lead to the inclusion of cases with one eye or with squint. Vision should also be rated with spectacles on, if usually worn. This point is noted on the Wessex questionnaire and on that used by Ellis (1982).

Variations in type of survey and type of population surveyed are also noteworthy. Most studies in Table 1.2 surveyed a range of characteristics of which vision was only one, and this will have imposed some limitations on the specificity of enquiries made about any one characteristic. Intellectual level is another possible source of variation. The studies of Bernsen (1981) and Mittler and Preddy (1981) specified ESN(S) or IQ less than 50, but those of Richardson, Katz, Koller, McLaren and Rubenstein (1979), and Humphreys (1976) used an administrative definition (e.g. use of mental handicap services) implying a wider range of mental ability, while Mitchell and Woodthorpe (1981) used a combination of both definitions. Lastly, studies differed in terms of the home base (hospital or community) and age range of the population examined (see Table 1.2).

In view of all these possible sources of variation, the relative consistency of these results seems remarkably good. There is additional encouragement to accept the prevalence suggested in Table 1.2 when we examine two studies directed particularly at visual impairment in hospital-based popula-tions.

Ellis (1982) surveyed all National Health Service (NHS) residences in England and Wales using a questionnaire which included more specific definitions: 'Blindness' was defined as 'cannot recognize by *vision* a familiar object 3-4 feet away', while 'Partial Sight' was defined as those with '*visual* impairments which are less severe than blindness but who are still substantially and permanently handicapped by *defective vision*'. An additional note indicated that these handicaps should be 'those due to VISUAL impairment rather than to *mental* subnormality'.

These more extensive definitions may explain the more conservative prevalence rates found. They could certainly be expected to help exclude cases with one eye, or mild loss of acuity. When compared to Warburg's (1970) survey, however, there may be reason to suspect a tendency to under-include cases in the NHS study. In 1963 Warburg used a preliminary screening survey to identify visually impaired residents and found rates for blindness and partial sight of 3.6 per cent and 1.5 per cent respectively. She noted also that attendants often did not recognize whether clients were severely retarded or severely visually handicapped. Consequently she examined ophthalmologically adult and child residents at two institutions for mentally retarded people. This expert examination produced the prevalence rates noted in Table 1.2 and suggests the degree to which the NHS survey may have underestimated the true prevalences.

If misclassifications are made to questionnaires, it is likely that care and treatment of mentally handicapped people may be equally inappropriate as care staff are most often the source of information entered on questionnaires. Moreover, the terms 'blind' and 'partially sighted' tend to give an overly simple impression of visual impairments as easily classified into one or two diagnostic boxes. Several additional parameters are worthy of consideration when examining the needs of mentally handicapped people who have visual impairments. Warburg has commented on the prevalence of various clinical and ophthalmological conditions found in mentally handicapped people in Chapter 5, this volume, while Holland has noted the incidence of a number of genetic anomalies involving visual impairments (Chapter 7, this volume). Other sources which provide insights on groups of mentally handicapped people at risk of visual impairments and about the range of impairments which may be sustained, are discussed below. (Summary: Table 1.3.)

Visual Acuity

This general term includes three main types of refractive error, i.e. optical variations which impair the capacity of the eye to focus a sharp visual image on the retina. Firstly in *myopia* (short-sight) the visual image is formed in front of the retina. This can be overcome by moving the object in view closer to the eye. Secondly, *hyperopia* (long-sight) arises when the image of a distant object is focused behind the retina. The subject may bring the object into focus with effort but at the cost of eye strain and sometimes headaches. The third type, *astigmatism*, arises due to asymmetry in the eyes' optical elements, e.g. the image may be in focus in the eyes' horizontal plane but not in its vertical plane. Consequently there is never a wholly sharp retinal image. Hyperopia is reported more often than myopia in mentally handicapped people; Manley and Schuldt's (1970) study confirmed this tendency and discussed some possible reasons for its occurrence.

Table 1.3: Prevalences of Eye Abnormalities Affecting Vision in Mentally Handicapped People: A Summary of Surveys

Source	Age range (years)	Sample size	Untestable or uncooperative %	Range of normal vision (dioptres)	Errors of refraction %	Astigmatism %	Subjects with or given spectacles	Strabismus
Bader and Woodruff (1980)	0-18+	287	—	—	45.6	—	26.1	—
Burstyn (1971)	3-19	115	43.5	−0.50 +1.50	22.6	31.3	—	31.3
Woodruff (1977)	5-18	168	—	−0.5 +2.0	54.1	20.01	—	21.4
Courtney (1977)	9-90	765	—	>1D	—	25.5	—	—
Edwards et al. (1972)	M=6.4 yrs	728	—	—	18.3	—	—	16.9
Evans et al. (1972)	17-65	202	24.3	—	38.1	—	—	—
Warburg (1970)	Adult	257	15.6	−1.0 +2.0	34.2	—	33.1	—
Fletcher and Thompson (1961)	Child	102	—	—	28.4	25	—	37.2
Markovits (1975)	Child	92	—	—	52.2	—	15.2	12.0

Several studies have reported evidence of a raised prevalence of refractive errors in mentally handicapped people. Some of these studies are summarized in Table 1.3 and the large proportions of refractive errors are evident, in spite of considerable variation between studies. There are several limitations to be borne in mind when evaluating these data. The samples used are small for prevalence purposes, and drawn from sources like training centres, clinics and institutions, which make it difficult to meet adequate sampling criteria. Myopia and astigmatism vary with age and the various age ranges used in these studies make direct comparison difficult. A further complication concerns the refraction criteria used to determine whether a visual error exists. Only two studies make their criteria explicit and these are different. Variations of 0.50 dioptres between studies could be expected to change significantly the proportions of errors identified.

In all but two studies (Fletcher and Thompson 1961; Burstyn 1971) it was not made clear whether astigmatism was included among the refractive errors; moreover, it appears likely that some astigmatics were listed also in the data on myopia and hyperopia. This distinction was not overlooked by Woodruff (1977) who also reported the extent of drug use by his subjects. This is an important issue as several drugs given commonly to mentally handicapped people have side-effects on visual function. These include Mysoline (double vision; nystagmus), Largactil (photosensitivity; altered visual accommodation), Valium (blurred vision; double vision) and Melleril (blurred vision). Future prevalence studies should take into account this type of influence on visual function. Finally, in the large sample of Edwards, Price and Weisskopf (1972) only half were mentally handicapped people. The lower prevalence of refractive errors found in this study is consistent with other evidence that more mentally handicapped people have such errors.

Astigmatism

The study by Courtney (1977) into the prevalence of astigmatism is well designed and deserves particular mention. He compared institutional with non-institutional. retardates and with Sorsby, Sheridan, Leary and Benjamin's (1960) study of normal males. A comparison was also made between mildly retarded, and moderately to profoundly retarded inmates. Each retarded group has a significantly higher frequency of astigmatism than the 9.8 per cent reported for the normal sample. The moderately to profoundly retarded group showed a greater likelihood of severe astigmatism than the mildly retarded inmates. No significant differences were found between institutional and community-based retardates of similar ability. Courtney found also that the serious astigmatism of the institutional group was accounted for mainly by white inmates; black inmates' astigmatism was less severe and the reason for this racial difference was not clear. Woodruff's (1977) detailed study of Canadian retarded schoolchildren found broadly similar results on astigmatism to Courtney's and thus tends to confirm the probability of a raised prevalence in the mentally retarded population.

Spectacles

Many refractive errors can be corrected by providing appropriate spectacles. Some uncorrected errors will render the subject blind, while, if defective vision remains uncorrected for too long, *amblyopia* (irreversible loss of visual function or acuity) can result. Few of the studies in Table 1.3 give much data on the extent to which spectacles are prescribed or used, but two produced information of great significance both epidemiologically and clinically. Warburg (1970) reported that, in 257 adult retardates, 88 had refractive errors; of these, 85 could be corrected with spectacles. She found that 51 clients were still using the spectacles two years after they were prescribed. Warburg also drew attention to the often overlooked risk of presbyopia (loss of ability to focus on near objects with age). She reported that, of 215 retardates aged 40 and over, 115 needed spectacles for near vision and 75 of these were still using the spectacles after two years (see also Chapter 5, this volume).

Bader and Woodruff (1980) studied the effects of corrective lenses, using three control groups and across three age levels. They found significant improvements in the group given new spectacles, across a range of behaviours. These included social behaviours such as sociability, eye contact and frequency of temper tantrums, gross motor skills like posture when eating and walking ability, and fine motor skills like reaching for and grasping objects, stacking blocks and quality of work. The sophisticated, well-controlled design of this investigation allows these changes to be attributed directly to the newly supplied spectacles. One of the control groups was equipped with placebo spectacles (i.e. glass with no corrective power). After eight weeks, use of the placebos had fallen by 20 per cent compared to no fall in the number using the 'real' spectacles.

These results are worth remembering when considering the subjects of the studies in Table 1.3 who were excluded from assessment for various reasons. Evans, Wachs and Borger (1972) advised that '49 were judged completely non-testable', without further explanation. Markovits (1975) gave no data but noted that 'some children could barely be examined because of fear, squeezing, lack of co-operation etc.' Burstyn (1971) reported that 31 per cent of his sample failed all assessment criteria but were judged unable to benefit from care because of mental level or handicaps, while a further 14 were untestable because of hyperactivity. Clearly in some of these cases the condition of the eye will have made assessment of refraction impossible or irrelevant, but some could have been excluded because of behavioural difficulties which may have been overcome or reduced if adequate optical correction had been achieved. Adequate assessment of acuity by subjective methods may be difficult for many mentally handicapped people and objective methods may offer some advantage in these cases (see Atkinson, Chapter 10, this volume). We can conclude that up to half the mentally handicapped population need optical corrections and that most of these will benefit from such correction.

Physical Handicaps and Vision

While physical handicaps are not always accompanied by retardation, the two general types of impairment are often found together. In their community study of 282 retardates Mitchell and Woodthorpe (1981) found 4.3 per cent had cerebral palsy and 1.8 per cent had hydrocephaly. The ocular consequences of physical handicap are the focus of our present interest, and several studies (e.g. Walsh 1963; Warburg in Falbe-Hansen 1968; Bankes 1974) of people with visual and mental handicaps reported a raised prevalence for hydrocephalus of between 5 and 9 per cent, while Bankes (1974) found about 10 per cent of his subjects suffered cerebral palsy.

Hydrocephalus

Rabinowicz's (1974) valuable review of this condition described the ocular problems which accompany it. He reported an incidence of 1 in 400 live births and described a series of associated ocular problems. In the 'setting sun phenomenon' the eyes are displaced downwards due to raised intra-cranial pressure. Ten per cent of hydrocephalics have some history of this phenomenon and half those with a positive history showed the presence of optic atrophy. Strabismus (squint) was found in 54 per cent of cases, mainly convergent in form, while nystagmus (rapid jerky movements of the eyes) was found in 30 per cent of cases. Visual acuity was normal in only 37 per cent of cases while 7 per cent had an acuity poor enough for registration as blind. Visual field defects were present in 9 per cent of cases while 31 per cent had optic atrophy.

Cerebral Palsy

Several interesting reviews and discussions of this condition have appeared in recent years. Paneth, Kiely, Stein and Susser (1981) summarized many hospital studies showing mortality and follow-up data for infants of 1,500 g or less. These showed a fourfold reduction in the rate of cerebral palsy (from 24.6 per cent to 5.9 per cent) between the 1950s and 1960s, but with no change in mortality. A small rise (to 8.1 per cent) was found during the 1970s combined with a sharp reduction in mortality rates following great advances in our ability to save the lives of low-birthweight infants. Consequently the prevalence rate for cerebral palsy doubled between the 1960s and the 1970s to 4.6 per 1,000 live births, although this figure is still substantially lower than the 1950s rate. The authors' projections from a New York City 1976 birth cohort led them to conclude that the *morbidity* rate (i.e. proportions showing specified damage) among low-birthweight children must decline at least as fast as the mortality rate if an increased prevalence for conditions like mental retardation and cerebral palsy is to be avoided. Their limited evidence suggests this is not being achieved and thus there may be a modest increase in the prevalence of these handicaps.

Pharoah (1981) also examined epidemiological data for cerebral palsy from various sources in England and Wales. He noted the relevance of a national policy on use of oxygen in incubators during the 1950s to the high infant mortality rates during that period. His discussion of infant mortality trends was broadly in agreement with that of Paneth *et al.*, but he described with healthy scepticism the possible methodological limitations on the validity of available data and concluded that we lack adequate morbidity data on cerebral palsy for monitoring the effectiveness of special and intensive care of neonates.

Cerebral palsy is a collection of syndromes which are, in Perlstein's (1962) definition, 'characterised by chronic motor dysfunction due to involvement of the motor control areas of the brain', while MacKeith, MacKenzie and Polani (1959) described it as 'a persistent but not unchanging disorder of movement and posture, appearing in the early years of life, and due to a non-progressive disorder of the brain, the result of interference during its development'. The central theme in both definitions is the impairment of motor function and this includes impairments in the motor functioning of their visual system. Hiles, Wallar and McFarlane (1975) listed the following conditions drawn from several surveys: strabismus (squint), optic atrophy, nystagmus, refractive errors, visual field defects, retinal dysplasias, cataracts, choroiditis, colobomas of the macula or iris, ptosis, spastic eyelids, corneal leukoma, abnormal head postures and retrolental fibroplasia. Hiles *et al.* (1975) summarized prevalence data on ocular problems which show that these occur in from 56 per cent to 92 per cent of cerebral palsy cases surveyed. Strabismus is perhaps the most common disorder reported in from 15 per cent to 62 per cent of cases seen, and these authors described the use of standard strabismus management procedures in a series of 234 children. Their results indicated cosmetic and functional improvement in the majority of children, most of whom were mentally retarded. A brief review of similar data was also reported by Duckman (1979), who also described (1980) a small sample of children for whom functional improvements were achieved in ocular motility and accommodative control.

A similarly high proportion of visual problems was found in Black's (1982) survey of 120 cerebrally palsied children in an English ESN(S) school. Only 20 per cent had normal eyes while 52 per cent had strabismus and 50 per cent had significant refractive errors. Both Black and Hiles *et al.* noted the increased likelihood of ocular problems in subjects with spasticity, the most common form of cerebral palsy. Black recommended that such children should be given a full ophthalmological assessment routinely to ensure early identification of treatable ocular defects. Finally Gardiner's (1983) brief report of physically handicapped schoolchildren showed that refractive errors are far more common than among normal children, and that low-birthweight infants with cerebral palsy appear to be particularly at risk for refractive errors.

Down's Syndrome

Down's syndrome (DS) is thought to have an incidence of about 1 in 600–800 live births. Various surveys of mental handicap populations, both community and institutional, report a prevalence of between 16.6 and 27 per cent (Kushlick and Cox 1973; Bernsen 1981; Mitchell and Woodthorpe 1981; Mittler and Preddy 1981; Einfeld 1984). Consequently, people with Down's syndrome form a substantial minority in the mentally handicapped population. The prominence of eye problems in DS has long been recognized in the specialist literature and one or two contributions serve to illustrate the types of ocular issues which have been examined. Lowe's (1949) extensive discussion examined many of the clinical features including the physiology of the skull and eyes, an illustrated typology of cataracts and risk of infection within and around the eyes. He concluded: 'The visual acuity of mongoloids is frequently poor because of myopia, nystagmus, strabismus, lens opacities, and failure to reinforce conditioned reflexes during development.' The report is of limited value epidemiologically, and one must turn to other sources for relevant data. Gardiner (1967) examined 60 retarded children, aged 5 to 16 years, of whom 22 had Down's syndrome. By comparing these with the remaining 38 retarded children he showed that the DS group was more likely to have refractive errors and that those children with errors were more likely to be myopic (50 per cent) than the non-DS children (3 per cent). He found that DS children were also more likely to have strabismus and astigmatism. He speculated that the myopic trend in DS, which is contrary to the tendency in mentally handicapped people to be hyperopic, may be related to the presence of congenital heart lesions.

Other reports have not always confirmed this raised prevalence of myopia. Pesch and Nagy (1978) reported a study of 41 people aged 8½ to 23 years, of whom 24 were hyperopic and only 10 myopic. Selection procedures used would exclude cases who were *severely* mentally or physically handicapped (Gardiner reported IQs in the range 30–50). Nine subjects were less than +1 dioptre hyperopic (Gardiner did not state the thresholds he used). Both these features may have influenced the number of errors found by each author. Warshowsky's (1981) screening of 55 DS children aged 2 to 8½ years produced a distribution of refractive scores which appears positively skewed towards hyperopia. He advised, however, that statistical analysis demonstrated negative skewness, suggesting greater prevalence of myopia (although his graph shows less than one-third of cases are myopic). He noted that several other studies showed a raised myopic prevalence and the possibility deserves close consideration in future research.

Walsh (1981) examined 91 DS children and adults and compared them with 357 non-DS inmates of a Swedish institution to demonstrate the raised prevalence of keratoconus (conical cornea) in DS. She found 8 per cent of DS subjects and only one non-DS subject with keratoconus. Keratoconus also accounted for two-thirds of the blind DS subjects, and so its presence deserves serious attention.

Walsh also found raised prevalences for strabismus, nystagmus and cataract compared to those in the non-DS group, although the rate for strabismus (23 per cent) is within the range listed in Table 1.3 for mental handicap populations. Lowe (1949) commented that one-third of the cases he studied had strabismus, often due to high myopia, while 13 per cent had nystagmus, and lens opacities (cataracts) were described by him as 'very common' although rarely required surgery. Congenital cataract was investigated by McDonald (1966) and, although the survey was not restricted to mentally handicapped people, five of the 68 children in her sample with moderate to large opacities had DS. It is worth interpreting the various ocular data from these reports in the light of the increasing longevity of people with DS. Thase (1982) concluded that the life span of people with DS has increased gradually since the 1920s. Their average life expectancy is about 35 years, while 25 per cent survive to age 50. But middle age brings an increased risk of Alzheimer-type dementia, and there is a risk that the consequences of deteriorating vision may be misinterpreted as early signs of a dementing process.

DISABILITIES RESULTING FROM VISUAL IMPAIRMENTS

Some functional disabilities and limitations can result from severe visual impairments in general. The severity of these disabilities will depend on whether or not the visual impairment was present at birth, and on the degree of usable residual vision which may remain.

Motor Development

This general topic is reviewed in detail by Anwar in Chapter 8, this volume, but it is worth summarizing here the observations of Jan, Freeman and Scott (1977) regarding visually handicapped people. Some stages of motor development are prolonged, while acquisition of others will be delayed. A blind baby needs to be taught to roll to the prone position and later to sit up. Crawling may be elicited by providing non-visual sensory cues to motivate the infant. Sitting or standing can be achieved at a normal age but crawling or walking are likely to be delayed and may need help and initiation. Poor motor development can result in hypotonia, poor co-ordination, walking with a plano-valgus deformity on an insecure wide base with feet externally rotated. Misconstrual of such developmental delays may contribute to a diagnosis of mental retardation.

Mobility

The ability to move around without help is, for a blind person, one of the most valuable means of experiencing and demonstrating personal independence. Harley and Hill (Chapter 20, this volume) have reviewed the literature in relation to the needs of mentally handicapped people. Jan *et al.* (1977) confirmed the importance of mobility skills for visually impaired people of normal intelligence. They stressed the need for individually tailored training in a range of mobility skills including posture and balance, and in use of residual vision. They concluded that conceptualization of space is very different for people without vision.

Communication

Development of language and speech for a blind child is subject to several risks. Absence of a physical referent for the words used encourages 'verbalisms' and poor concept formation because the meaning of so many words depends on vision. The non-verbal precursors of language such as imitation, turn-taking and facial expressions also depend largely on visual experience. These processes are reviewed briefly by Ellis (1984). The risks of language delays in visually handicapped infants are illustrated by Reynell's (1978) study which found developmental delays of around one year in verbal comprehension and expression, by the age of five years. Jan *et al.* (1977) also reminded us that blind people can develop a 'broadcasting' form of speech in attempting to keep in contact with others.

Blindisms

Jan *et al.* (1977) provided a good review of these routines, which are behavioural mannerisms like eye pressing and rocking, found among blind people. These routines are not uncommon among mentally retarded people but have been given a special name among visually handicapped people which appears to imply a causal relationship.

Specific Effects of Blindness

The chapter devoted to this topic by Jan *et al.* (1977) drew attention to several physiological differences found in visually handicapped people. These included the absence of alpha rhythms on the EEG records of congenitally blind people, and the earlier age of menarche in visually handicapped girls.

THE NATIONAL (NHS) SURVEY

A questionnaire survey of visual handicaps among mentally handicapped residents of National Health Service (NHS) institutions in England and Wales was conducted between 1978 and 1980. All NHS institutions listed in the Hospitals and Health Services Yearbook (1978) as mental handicap residences were contacted by post. Of 262 contacted 14 were found to be 'holiday homes' (i.e. not permanent residences) or 'not mental handicap'. Of the remaining 248 addresses, 180 (72.5 per cent) returned completed questionnaires (referred to below as 'cases'), providing data on 30,020 inmates. Official statistics for 1979 (Welsh Office 1979; DHSS 1984b) show that the total mentally handicapped NHS residential population was 47,688 inmates so the questionnaire survey produced a 63 per cent sample of the NHS population in England and Wales. The questionnaire collected information on age, sex and degree of mental handicap for all residents. The following data were also sought on blind and partially sighted residents: mobility, self-care skills (washing, feeding, dressing and toileting), language skills, occupation or training opportunities, and behaviour problems (aggression, self-injury, damage to surroundings, stereotyped behaviour, and social withdrawal). Apart from 'behaviour problems' all questions used two-to-four point rating scales. For example, 'dressing' used a three-point scale as follows: 'How many (a) dress and undress themselves? (b) dress and undress with help? (c) are dressed/undressed by staff (or others)?' These data were collected on institutional *populations* rather than on individuals.

The main results (Ellis 1982) showed that an enlarged proportion of the youngest children were visually handicapped while the oldest age group was far smaller than expected. The latter result may reflect poor recognition of visual deterioration in older inmates. Independence in self-care skills, mobility and language was less common among blind residents than among partially sighted residents. Data were reported on behaviour problems and occupational opportunities, and the possibility was noted that limited access to occupation may be related to the presence of behaviour problems. Registration of visual impairment in the UK is a relatively effective means of bringing blind and partially sighted people to the attention of statutory social services. Among the blind people identified by the survey, however, only about 27 per cent had been registered, with an even lower proportion (5.4 per cent) for partially sighted inmates.

Accuracy of Data

An accuracy estimate was built into the questionnaire. All respondents were asked to complete a simple three-point rating for each question, indicating whether the data supplied were 'current figures'; 'estimates' from incomplete or out-of-date figures; or 'a guess' in the absence of available statistics. Between 51 and 63 per cent of institutions responded (responses to some questions were omitted in a few cases), covering between 63 and 65 per cent of the sample. For all questions *except* 'level of mental handicap' (reported separately in parentheses) the response ranges were as follows: 'current figures' 81-94 per cent (54 per cent); 'estimates' 6-15 per cent (34 per cent); 'a guess' 1-3 per cent (13 per cent). It seems likely from these ratings that most data received were reasonably accurate. The exception, 'level of mental handicap', suggests a degree of uncertainty about how to evaluate the intellectual level of residents. The three-part rating scale employed for this question (i.e. 'Not Subnormal'; 'Subnormal'; 'Severely Subnormal') used terminology which was assumed to be well known by mental handicap nursing staff as it had been in use for some years. No respondents indicated difficulty in understanding this terminology. The possible implications of the lower 'accuracy' rating of this question are discussed later.

Further Analysis of Data

The NHS survey data have been analysed further in an attempt to define more clearly some of the characteristics of visually and mentally handicapped inmates. A major limitation has been that the data described *groups* of residents (i.e. each 'case' is a hospital) rather than individuals. Consequently the extent of co-occurrence of two variables cannot be identified at an individual level but only in terms of their frequencies across several *groups* of individuals. Co-occurrence on this level could be present by chance and this introduces some uncertainty when interpreting any correlations found between variables.

The data were edited using the Minitab computer programme (Ryan, Joiner and Ryan 1981) to create a series of 'files' which included only those cases reporting data on the chosen variable. Thus a 'blind' (BL) file was created by deleting all cases which reported no blind residents. A similar file was created of partially sighted residents (PS). BL and PS constituted the core files from which a series of sub-files could be drawn, each based on a given variable, by deleting all cases which reported no residents for that variable. Each resulting sub-file contained the data for *all* cases reporting one or more residents on that variable. These sub-files fell into three categories. Firstly, five 'behaviour-problem' files — each focused on one of the behaviour problems noted above: Aggression (AGR), Self-Injury (SIB), Damage to Surroundings (DAM), Stereotyped Behaviour (STER) and Social Withdrawal (SOC) — were created from both BL and PS, and resulted in an increased frequency of the relevant behaviour problem, of between 15 and 44 per cent. Consequently it is reasonable to expect that frequencies of other variables related to the given problem or characteristic will also be raised, when compared with the core files.

Secondly, four 'special' files were created in the same way, based on these variables: Registration of Visual Handicap (REG); an occupation making Special Provision for Visual Handicap (SPOC); No Behaviour Problems (NOP), and Severe Subnormality (MH3). The first two files, REG and SPOC, raised the frequency of the key variables by between 70 and 200 per cent relative to the core files. The NOP and MH3 files included all clients in all cases on the chosen variable, by excluding all cases with behaviour problems (NOP), or other levels of mental handicap (MH3). Finally three 'size' files were created, based on the *total* resident population of each hospital: up to 100 residents (MIN), 101 to 720 (MED) and 721 upwards (MAX).

From these files, totals were computed for each variable and these were compared to totals for those variables on each core file using a simple chi-square test for goodness of fit. This allowed identification of significant differences in the frequencies reported between the core data file and one of its sub-files in which the occurrence of a given characteristic was maximized. The raw data were then transformed into percentages to make clear the direction of the differences thus identified. These percentages are summarized in Tables 1.4 and 1.5 for most variables, together with the probability values of the chi-squares which produced significant differences.

BL and PS

These two core files are compared in Table 1.4 and several variations between blind and partially sighted inmates are revealed to be statistically significant. Blind inmates are more likely to be registered, and younger; more of the blind are reported to be severely subnormal, more are dependent in self-care skills, more have poorer speech skills. The blind are more likely to have special forms of occupation to suit their visual handicap but more are also without any routine occupation or training opportunities. Lastly, blind people are more likely to self-injure, engage in stereotypies (regular rhythmic movements like rocking to and fro) and to be socially withdrawn.

If the main difference between blind and partially sighted residents is the degree of visual input they receive, then the greater dependency and more limited style of life for the blind suggested by the above summary may be the direct consequence of the greater visual loss. Clearly this interpretation is too simple, as a substantial minority of blind people are reported to be independent in various respects. In addition, the literature reviewed earlier shows that blindness is often accompanied by a range of genetic, neurological, physical and mental limitations. Warburg (1982) showed that the raised prevalence of profound mental retardation among blind children is a consequence of a mixture of cerebral damage, less favourable education, inadequate assessment techniques and additional handicaps. She stressed the relevance of poor motor development to the interaction of these other factors.

Table 1.4: NHS Survey — Blind Residents: Percentage Distributions and Chi Square Probability Values

	BL	AGR		SIB		DAM		STER		SOC	
	%	%	p<	%	p<	%	p<	%	p<	%	p<
All residents (nos.)	(27526)	(20713)		(21787)		(18420)		(22787)		(19874)	
Blind residents	3.96	3.98	ns	4.1	.01	4.2	.025	4.1	.001	4.1	ns
Registered	27.6	22.1	.001	22.8	.001	23.8	.001	25.3	.001	21.5	.001
MALES	50.9	52.9	.025	52.6	.025	52.5	ns	51.5	ns	51.6	ns
0-16 years	17.0	13.4	.001	14.8	.001	14.7	.005	16.9	ns	12.8	.001
60+ years	20.0	19.4	ns	19.5	ns	18.8	ns	18.6	.005	19.8	ns
MENTAL HANDICAP (3)*											
Not subnormal	0.8	0.97	ns	0.89	ns	0.78	ns	0.84	ns	0.99	ns
Severely subnormal	84.7	84.2	ns	86.1	.005	85.7	ns	85.3	ns	84.5	ns
MOBILITY											
Walks normally	52.9	53.8	ns	52.4	ns	56.0	.005	52.9	ns	54.2	ns
Walks with support	21.0	20.6	ns	21.9	ns	20.4	ns	20.2	ns	20.8	ns
Needs wheelchair	13.4	14.1	ns	14.5	.025	11.6	.01	14.1	ns	13.6	ns
Bedridden	12.7	11.5	.05	11.9	ns	12.0	ns	12.8	ns	11.4	.05
SELF-CARE SKILLS											
Washing (3)*											
Washes self	19.2	18.0	ns	17.0	.001	17.1	.01	17.4	.001	18.6	ns
Washed by staff	57.4	60.0	.005	60.6	.001	59.2	ns	59.7	.001	59.7	.01
Feeding (2)*											
Feeds self	56.8	53.8	.001	54.9	.005	55.9	ns	55.3	.01	55.6	ns
Dressing (3)*											
Dress/undress self	24.3	23.5	ns	22.7	.01	22.4	.025	22.8	.005	23.9	ns
Dress/undress by staff	47.5	49.4	.05	49.3	.01	47.4	ns	49.0	.025	48.5	ns
Toileting (3)*											
Toilet-trained	41.8	39.7	.025	38.9	.001	38.9	.005	40.2	.01	40.7	ns
Routinely incontinent	33.8	35.7	.025	35.5	.01	34.1	ns	34.9	.05	33.4	ns
LANGUAGE (3)*											
Normal speech	33.7	32.2	ns	30.9	.001	30.6	.001	30.8	.001	31.7	.025
No speech	42.3	42.5	ns	44.0	0.25	42.5	ns	43.4	ns	42.3	ns
OCCUPATION											
Regularly in ward/Hostel	29.4	28.2	ns	27.7	.01	26.0	.001	27.6	.005	26.0	.001
Regularly outside ward/Hostel	29.3	26.8	.005	28.1	ns	30.7	ns	29.7	ns	28.8	ns
Usually inactive	41.4	45.0	.001	44.2	.001	43.2	ns	42.7	.025	45.2	.001
Special provision for visual handicap	15.2	11.8	.001	13.0	.001	14.5	ns	15.0	ns	12.4	.001
BEHAVIOUR PROBLEMS											
Aggression	15.0	19.9	—	17.1	.001	18.9	.001	15.9	.05	16.6	.025
Self-injury	20.9	24.0	.001	25.3	—	23.4	.005	22.1	.025	23.0	.005
Damage surroundings	11.7	14.7	.001	13.4	.001	16.7	—	12.9	.005	13.4	.005
Stereotypy	22.7	24.9	.005	24.5	.005	25.3	.005	26.1	—	24.6	.01
Socially withdrawn	17.7	19.9	.001	20.8	.001	20.7	.001	19.2	.001	23.9	—

	'Special' Files								'Size' Files						BL/PS	
REG		SPOC		NOP		MH3		MIN		MED		MAX		BL/PS	
%	p<	%	p<	%	p<	%	p<	%	p<	%	p<	%	p<	%	p<
(16042)		(12548)		(2274)		(9308)		(2685)		(16828)		(8013)			
4.0	ns	4.1	ns	2.6	.001	4.1	ns	6.6	.001	3.5	.001	4.0	ns		
47.6	—	33.8	.001	48.3	.001	32.0	.025	50.6	.001	28.3	ns	13.9	.001	15.4	.001
51.3	ns	52.5	ns	31.0	.005	50.5	ns	45.5	ns	51.8	ns	51.2	ns	50.3	ns
19.1	.05	16.9	ns	22.4	ns	32.0	.001	45.5	.001	15.1	ns	4.9	.001	13.7	.001
17.8	ns	17.9	ns	36.2	.005	17.2	ns	12.4	.01	21.3	ns	21.6	ns	22.7	.005
0.31	.05	0.39	ns	0	ns	—	—	0	ns	0.51	ns	1.85	.025	1.11	ns
86.8	.05	89.6	.001	81.0	ns	100	—	92.1	.005	80.2	.001	88.9	.025	80.5	.001
59.7	.001	58.2	.005	56.9	ns	49.5	ns	50.6	ns	48.3	.001	62.4	.001	58.8	.001
18.6	0.25	20.2	ns	20.7	ns	19.5	ns	15.7	ns	22.0	ns	22.5	ns	19.9	ns
11.8	ns	12.2	ns	1.7	.01	13.3	ns	9.6	ns	15.9	.01	10.8	ns	11.0	.001
9.9	.005	9.4	.005	20.7	ns	17.7	.001	24.2	.001	13.9	ns	4.3	.001	10.2	.001
20.2	ns	19.1	ns	41.4	.001	12.8	.001	16.3	ns	18.6	.001	21.3	ns	25.8	.001
53.2	.005	54.0	.05	32.8	.001	62.5	.025	58.4	ns	58.7	ns	56.2	ns	46.3	.001
64.9	.001	64.1	.001	72.4	.025	52.9	ns	53.4	ns	55.3	ns	61.7	.05	60.0	.005
25.5	ns	24.4	ns	41.4	.005	22.1	ns	18.5	.05	25.2	ns	27.2	ns	32.0	.001
42.8	.001	43.2	.01	37.9	ns	54.2	.005	52.3	ns	50.3	ns	42.0	.025	39.7	.001
45.2	.01	42.6	ns	56.9	.025	36.2	.01	33.7	.025	44.2	ns	42.9	ns	49.3	.001
29.6	.001	28.1	.001	24.1	ns	39.1	.01	41.0	.05	35.4	ns	27.8	.01	31.2	.025
33.2	ns	29.3	.01	56.9	.001	27.6	.005	25.8	.025	35.0	ns	37.7	ns	39.2	.001
40.6	ns	36.9	.001	34.5	ns	53.1	.001	59.6	.001	43.2	ns	32.1	.001	36.5	.001
35.0	.001	31.2	ns	41.4	.05	30.5	ns	42.7	.001	27.4	ns	25.6	ns	31.9	.025
34.7	.001	35.8	.001	31.0	ns	34.9	.005	32.0	ns	29.8	ns	26.9	ns	31.7	.025
30.4	.001	33.0	.001	27.6	.05	34.6	.001	25.3	.001	42.8	ns	47.5	.01	36.5	.001
21.1	.001	32.6	—	25.9	.025	18.8	.025	33.2	.001	11.7	.001	11.7	.05	11.4	.001
12.6	.01	11.8	.01	—	—	12.0	.05	5.6	.001	17.9	.005	14.8	ns	16.3	ns
18.9	ns	19.3	ns	—	—	22.9	ns	15.7	ns	25.4	.001	15.4	.005	16.3	.001
11.3	ns	12.4	ns	—	—	13.5	ns	5.1	.005	14.0	.01	11.1	ns	10.6	ns
21.7	ns	24.0	ns	—	—	29.2	.001	26.4	ns	23.7	ns	18.8	.05	18.4	.001
15.3	.025	16.1	ns	—	—	18.5	ns	9.6	.005	21.2	.005	15.7	ns	14.1	.001

Notes: ns = non-significant difference.

* = number, in parentheses, of ratings for each variable; each of the variables has one rating omitted.

Table 1.5: NHS Survey — Partially Sighted Residents: Percentage Distributions and Chi Square Probability Values

	PS	AGR		SIB		DAM		STER		SOC	
Behaviour Problem Files											
	%	%	p <	%	p <	%	p <	%	p <	%	p <
All residents (nos.)	(27997)	(21339)		(18656)		(17455)		(18864)		(17555)	
Partially sighted	4.8	5.2	.001	5.6	.001	5.6	.001	5.2	.001	5.3	.001
Registered	5.4	5.1	ns	4.0	.001	4.6	.05	3.9	.001	4.3	.025
MALES	49.8	39.5	ns	50.5	ns	51.0	ns	49.9	ns	51.4	ns
0-16 years	11.0	10.7	ns	12.3	.01	11.0	ns	11.0	ns	10.2	ns
60+ years	24.9	23.5	.01	21.7	.001	23.4	.05	21.8	.001	22.3	.001
MENTAL HANDICAP (3)*											
Not subnormal	1.34	0.9	.005	0.95	.025	0.9	.025	1.1	ns	0.9	.025
Severely subnormal	77.1	78.4	.025	80.0	.001	78.9	.01	78.6	.05	78.8	.05
MOBILITY											
Walks normally	63.7	63.0	ns	60.4	.001	62.8	ns	60.9	.001	61.8	.05
Walks without support	19.0	20.3	.01	20.6	.01	20.9	ns	20.8	.01	20.7	.025
Needs wheelchair	9.1	9.2	ns	9.8	ns	9.3	ns	9.6	ns	9.3	ns
Bedridden	8.2	7.5	.05	9.2	.01	6.9	.005	8.7	ns	8.2	ns
SELF-CARE SKILLS											
Washing (3)*											
Washes self	31.1	30.5	ns	27.8	.001	28.4	.001	27.7	.001	28.5	.005
Washed by staff	37.3	36.7	ns	39.0	.025	37.0	ns	38.8	ns	37.7	ns
Feeding (2)*											
Feeds self	62.5	60.4	.001	56.9	.001	58.8	.001	56.5	.001	56.9	.001
Dressing (3)*											
Dress/undress self	38.3	36.7	.05	34.0	.001	35.4	.001	34.8	.001	35.4	.001
Dress/undress by staff	33.4	33.0	ns	36.3	.001	33.1	ns	36.4	.001	34.9	ns
Toileting (3)*											
Toilet-trained	55.4	55.3	ns	52.7	.001	54.2	ns	52.1	.001	52.7	.005
Routinely incontinent	29.0	29.1	ns	31.8	.001	30.8	.025	31.4	.005	30.9	.025
LANGUAGE (3)*											
Normal speech	43.7	43.6	ns	39.9	.001	42.4	ns	39.7	.001	41.3	.01
No speech	31.7	30.9	ns	33.9	.001	41.9	ns	34.2	.005	32.3	ns
OCCUPATION											
Regularly in Ward/Hostel	33.9	33.0	ns	31.2	.001	26.7	.005	29.3	.001	27.7	.001
Regularly outside Ward/Hostel	33.6	32.9	ns	34.2	ns	32.8	ns	35.6	.025	35.5	.05
Usually inactive	32.5	34.1	.01	34.6	.005	35.6	.001	35.1	.001	36.9	.001
Special provision for visual handicap	8.3	9.0	.05	8.9	ns	9.4	.025	9.7	.005	7.9	ns
BEHAVIOUR PROBLEMS											
Aggression	17.3	21.0	—	19.3	.001	19.5	.001	19.0	.01	20.1	.001
Self-injury	12.5	13.9	.005	16.0	—	14.1	.005	14.1	.005	13.7	.05
Damage surroundings	9.7	11.0	.001	11.3	.001	13.2	—	11.5	.001	11.2	.005
Stereotypy	14.8	.16.1	.005	17.0	.001	17.1	.001	20.4	—	16.2	.05
Socially withdrawn	11.2	12.6	.001	12.5	.005	12.4	.025	13.4	.001	16.2	—

'Special' Files								'Size' Files					
REG		SPOC		NOP		MH3		MIN		MED		MAX	
%	p<	%	p<	%	p<	%	p<	%	p<	%	p<	%	p<
(9336)		(9974)		(2970)		(6867)		(3078)		(16906)		(8013)	
4.7	ns	4.5	ns	3.5	.001	3.3	.001	5.9	.005	4.2	.001	5.6	.001
16.6	—	5.3	ns	7.7	ns	7.0	ns	13.3	.001	6.2	ns	0.9	.001
48.1	ns	50.7	ns	40.4	.05	41.9	.01	35.0	.001	52.7	.05	51.7	ns
8.5	.05	11.1	ns	5.8	ns	22.3	.001	18.9	.001	12.1	ns	6.2	.001
20.5	.01	16.2	.001	45.2	.001	21.0	.001	34.4	.005	23.0	ns	25.1	ns
0.7	ns	0.4	.05	5.8	.001	—	—	3.9	.005	0.7	.05	1.3	ns
83.0	.001	87.3	.001	61.5	.001	100	—	66.7	.001	73.9	.005	86.0	.001
62.5	ns	59.3	.05	76.9	.005	65.1	ns	73.3	.005	66.1	ns	55.9	.001
27.4	.001	26.2	.001	14.4	ns	14.0	.05	10.6	.005	14.7	.001	28.8	.001
5.8	.005	6.2	.01	4.0	ns	7.9	ns	8.9	ns	11.0	.025	6.9	.05
4.4	.001	8.2	ns	3.9	.05	13.1	.005	7.2	ns	8.3	ns	8.4	ns
27.8	ns	20.4	.001	51.0	.001	24.5	.025	39.4	.01	33.2	ns	22.6	.001
28.5	.001	36.7	ns	22.1	.001	48.0	.001	33.3	ns	39.2	ns	37.0	ns
63.9	ns	61.1	ns	83.7	.001	73.8	.001	85.6	.001	69.6	.001	42.4	.001
34.0	.05	27.8	.001	60.6	.001	38.0	ns	49.4	.001	39.9	ns	29.3	.001
32.9	ns	38.4	.01	20.2	.005	35.4	ns	28.3	ns	33.0	ns	37.3	.05
55.6	ns	49.3	.005	69.2	.005	55.9	ns	62.2	.05	58.5	.025	46.8	.001
30.8	ns	34.4	.005	15.4	.005	27.1	ns	19.4	.005	25.4	.005	39.7	.001
42.8	ns	33.6	.001	62.5	.001	32.8	.001	49.4	ns	42.7	ns	41.2	ns
26.4	.005	33.1	ns	17.3	.005	42.8	.001	28.9	ns	37.0	.001	25.7	.001
33.1	ns	26.2	.001	38.5	ns	42.4	.005	58.3	.001	33.9	ns	22.0	.001
36.6	ns	40.9	.001	35.6	ns	38.0	ns	26.1	.025	32.5	ns	38.1	.025
30.3	ns	32.9	ns	26.0	ns	19.7	.001	10.0	.001	33.5	ns	39.9	.001
12.6	.001	24.7	—	5.8	ns	13.5	.005	12.8	.025	8.2	ns	6.7	ns
17.0	ns	16.4	ns	—	—	15.7	ns	15.0	ns	18.3	ns	16.6	ns
12.4	ns	12.4	ns	—	—	17.0	.025	13.3	ns	12.7	ns	12.0	ns
11.7	ns	12.0	.05	—	—	10.0	ns	7.8	ns	9.0	ns	11.5	ns
16.3	ns	19.1	.005	—	—	16.6	ns	10.6	ns	15.8	ns	15.0	ns
12.9	ns	12.7	ns	—	—	13.5	ns	7.2	ns	12.3	ns	11.1	ns

Notes: ns = non-significant difference.

* = number, in parentheses, of ratings for each variable; each of the variables has one rating omitted.

Size

The comparisons by hospital size are in some ways the most revealing. The MIN files contain small hospitals and hostels and the prevalence of both blindness and partial sight is relatively high in these units. They are more likely to register their visually handicapped residents, and opportunities for occupation are better, including special provisions to take account of the visual handicaps of residents. There are more young residents in these units, particularly those who are blind, while only partially sighted residents are likely to be older. Partially sighted residents are brighter (nearly 4 per cent are not mentally handicapped), more skilled in daily living, and more mobile. More of them are also female. By contrast the blind residents are more severely handicapped, less skilful, less mobile and have substantially less good speech. They are less likely to be aggressive, to cause damage or to be socially withdrawn.

In summary, blind people living in smaller hospitals tend to be younger, more severely handicapped physically and mentally, and more dependent, while of partially sighted people there are more in both the youngest and the oldest age groups in smaller hospitals, and they are more able and more independent in daily living skills.

The MED files show that prevalence of visual handicap is lower in hospitals of between 101 and 720 beds. Severe subnormality is less common than in the core files, but the distribution of self-care skills and occupational opportunities is broadly similar to that shown in the core files, although blind people are less often given special consideration occupationally. Mobility seems to be marginally poorer in these hospitals. There are more males among partially sighted people, while blind people are more likely to present all behaviour problems except stereotypy. The major anomaly is that, while visually handicapped residents are described as more mildly mentally handicapped, there is no parallel reduction in the proportions with poor self-help skills.

Both MAX files contain the same seven largest hospitals and are thus more directly comparable between the blind and partially sighted populations than in MIN and MED files, in which not all the hospitals reported both blind and partially sighted residents. The clients in the MAX files are less likely to be children, less likely to *lack* speech, less likely to be registered, more likely to be unoccupied and more likely to be severely subnormal. In other respects, however, blind and partially sighted tend to diverge. More of the blind are reported to be not mentally handicapped and more are fully mobile, while fewer of the partially sighted are fully mobile. Partially sighted inmates are generally less independent in self-care but have more occupational opportunities, while blind inmates are more independent but have fewer special occupational opportunities. The blind are also less likely to exhibit self-injurious or stereotypic behaviours. The divergence is more apparent than real; the functional differences noted earlier between BL and PS are reduced, but not reversed in the MAX files.

It is ironic that large hospitals appear to meet the particular needs of visually handicapped residents so poorly, as one might expect that large organizations would be the most able to provide resources for this large subgroup. The relatively large proportion who are not mentally handicapped may indicate a paucity of suitable community placements for visually handicapped people. Such placement opportunities are still in short supply in Britain, some five years after these data were collected.

'Special' Files

The REG, SPOC and NOP files contain relatively independent, mobile residents who enjoy better occupational opportunities and marginally reduced proportions of behaviour problems. These trends are less clear in the partially sighted data, however, probably because REG and SPOC are variables with low frequencies among the partially sighted. The files are differentiated by the age and sex variables. Blind REG are more often younger, while more partially sighted REG are adults. NOP clearly favours females and older people. The interpretation of MH3 results presents a problem in view of the poor accuracy ratings given for this variable by questionnaire respondents. The present analysis shows that these files contain significantly more young, high-dependency residents with poorer mobility and speech skills, but they also enjoy more specialized occupations and are more likely to be registered. Some of this pattern may arise because MH3 cases are more often in smaller hospitals and hostels in which high-dependency young residents and better service provisions are more common. It has been reported elsewhere (Ellis 1982) that blind residents were more likely to be rated as severely mentally handicapped than their sighted co-residents. In view of the limited accuracy reported for this data, it is important to question to what extent this lower ability rating is due to the behavioural consequences of the visual handicap rather than the mental impairment. It is interesting that the proportions of partially sighted MH3 residents reported to be independent in self-care skills, mobility and speech were greater than among the blind MH3 residents. Could this variation result from the difference in degree of visual loss? We should define more precisely the criteria by which we estimate the extent of mental impairment, to limit the risk of lowered expectations for blind inmates.

Behaviour Problems

The major features from these data were described in Ellis (1982); self-injury was most common in blind residents and aggression was most common in partially sighted residents, while a large proportion engaged in stereotypies in both groups. Direction of aggression thus tended to discriminate between blind and partially sighted residents and this might be due simply to the difference in the degree of visual loss. The reality must be more complex and there are many published studies of the possible causes and treatments of these behaviour problems.

SIB. The extensive review by Baumeister and Rollings (1976) found reported prevalences for mentally handicapped people in the range 8-14 per cent. A more recent review (Singh 1981) suggested a range of 5.3-37.1 per cent (although a mean of about 12 per cent can be calculated from the raw data he reported), while Jacobson's (1982) survey of over 30,000 individuals found an overall prevalence of 8.2 per cent. It is interesting, therefore, that the PS data fall within the first range, while the BL data for self-injury are substantially greater. This raised prevalence among blind retardates is consistent with the results of Berkson and Davenport (1962) and Schroeder, Schroeder, Smith and Dalldorf (1978); several theories have been proposed for the occurrence of self-injury but none are wholly adequate. These include the homeostatic, psychodynamic, organic, developmental and learning theories (Baumeister and Rollings 1976). More recently attention has been drawn to the possible relevance of biological responses to stress and isolation, both of which are correlated with self-injury (de Catanzaro 1978), while Cataldo and Harris (1982) discussed the possibility that internally produced opiates may reduce pain arising from self-injury and thus help to maintain the behaviour. Jan (1978) described changes in biological function which can follow blindness, particularly regarding regulation of the circadian rhythmn of the pituitary-adrenal axis. The pituitary-adrenal system is implicated in Cataldo and Harris's (1982) account and it is interesting to speculate whether this common feature provides a means of explaining the raised prevalence of self-injury in blind retardates.

One particular behaviour, eye gouging, is reported among many blind people of normal intelligence; Jan *et al.* (1977) reported a frequency of 16.3 per cent in a sample of blind children. Maisto, Baumeister and Maisto (1978) described a survey of retarded inmates, 14 per cent of whom engaged in self-injury. They noted that, while eye gouging was found in about 10 per cent of self-injurers, it 'was considerably higher for blind SIB subjects'. The NHS Survey asked how many 'inflict injuries on themselves e.g. eye-poking, head-banging, scratching'. Consequently, the raised prevalence of self-injury among the blind may be due to eye gouging. Readers interested in this behaviour are referred also to a recent study by Jan, Freeman, McCormick, Scott, Robertson and Newman (1983).

The SIB file shows lower frequencies of registration, children, all self-care skills and specialised occupations, and a higher frequency of males. The higher frequency of severe subnormality is consistent with other reports (Maisto *et al.* 1978; Schroeder *et al.* 1978; Schroeder, Mulick and Rojahn 1980; Singh 1981). The higher frequency of speech-deprived individuals accords with the results of Schroeder *et al.* (1978) who noted that self-injury may be used as a primitive form of communication. This possibility is especially important in view of delays in language development experienced by visually handicapped children (Reynell 1978).

STER. The foregoing discussion of self-injury fits equally well under this heading because of its usual repetitive nature which is a defining feature of stereotyped behaviour. The same set of causal theories are also applicable here, with equally incomplete success at prediction. Prevalence ranges from 5.8 per cent (Jacobson 1982) to 33 per cent (Tierney, Fraser, McGuire and Walton 1981), although the latter included self-injury as a stereotypy. Berkson and Davenport (1962) found stereotyped movements in two-thirds of 71 retardates; they reported that stereotypy was less frequent when subjects manipulated objects, and more frequent when subjects were in a novel restricted environment. These conclusions encapsulate the homeostatic explanation of stereotypy, i.e. that it serves to regulate the supply of external stimulation. These authors reported that blind subjects were more likely to show stereotyped behaviour than sighted subjects. Berkson (1973) demonstrated that the raised frequency in blind subjects was not due to their blindness, *per se*, but probably to a disordered relationship with the physical and/or social environment during early development. The homeostatic account sometimes has been expressed as either under-arousal *or* over-arousal. These alternatives were reconciled by the experimental evidence of Williams (1978) that stereotypy helped to achieve *optimum* arousal, a notion implicit in the Berkson and Davenport (1962) studies. In this context interest has been rekindled in the use of sensory reinforcement (e.g. flashing or coloured lights, noises and vibrations) to help achieve optimum arousal. Murphy (1982) reviewed this topic, Goodall and Corbett (1982) described its clinical use in reducing stereotypies, while Byrne and Stevens (1980) used vibro-tactile reinforcement in teaching skills to deaf-blind retarded children.

In view of Jan's (1978) comment on the effects of blindness on circadian rhythms, it is worth noting the report of Lewis, McLean, Johnson and Baumeister (1981) that stereotyped and self-injurious behaviours of profoundly retarded people follow a rhythmic daily pattern. They suggested the patterning reflects changes (e.g. mealtimes) in the living routine, and an endogenous rest-activity cycle. Do such cyclical patterns have a particular significance for blind people?

The two STER files show an unremarkable picture of unregistered, poorly occupied inmates with limited self-care skills. Partially sighted inmates are more likely to be severely subnormal on the STER file, while blind inmates show a higher rate of stereotypy on the MH3 file. This correlation between stereotypy and severe retardation was also noted by Berkson and Davenport (1962) and by Jacobson (1982).

AGR, DAM, SOC. The NHS Survey asked how many 'are aggressive to others (residents or staff)?'; 'damage surroundings e.g. break objects, damage furniture, tear clothing?'; 'are usually socially withdrawn i.e. move away from social company whenever possible?' The core file frequencies of these behaviours are broadly consistent with the reports of Jacobson

(1982)* and of Scanlon, Arick and Krug (1982)[†]: i.e. Aggression — 10.9 per cent*/18.1 per cent[†]; Damage — 4.3 per cent*/25 per cent[†]; Social Withdrawal — 12.3 per cent*. Their respective definitions of the behaviours are only broadly consistent with those used in the NHS Survey and this may explain some of the variation in frequencies noted.

These behaviour problems have some relationship with better mobility among blind people, and mobility may be a more important precondition for the performance of these behaviours than for either self-injury or stereotypy. Their relationship with self-care and speech skills is somewhat variable. All but the blind DAM file show a higher frequency with no occupation, while both AGR files indicate greater opportunities for specialised occupations.

Combined Prevalence of Behaviour Problems.   The total proportion of sensorily handicapped inmates who presented behaviour problems could not be determined from the original questionnaire, and to remedy this omission a supplementary question was sent to a proportion of the hospitals contacted. Usable data were supplied by 66 hospitals, and Table 1.6 summarises the results.

A comparison was made between these sample data and those in the core files, for each behaviour problem, using a chi-square analysis. No significant differences were found in the partial sight data, while for blind inmates only SIB and SOC data were significantly under-represented relative to the core file. A comparison of the percentage distributions by hospital size (MIN, MED and MAX) showed that the sample data under-represent medium-size (MED) hospitals and over-represent large (MAX) hospitals, relative to the core files.

Table 1.6 shows that a larger proportion of blind inmates had behaviour problems than those with partial sight, and that of those *with* problem behaviour, blind people present more problems 'per head' than do partially sighted people. In addition, the number of behaviour problems per person increases with size of hospital. Thus, most visually handicapped inmates present no behaviour problems at all; but those who do, are likely to present two or three of the problems described here. This 'clustering' is clearly shown in Tables 1.4 and 1.5, where each problem is significantly related to all other problems.

Table 1.6: Proportions of Visually Handicapped Residents with Behaviour Problems

| | Percentage with behaviour problems | Mean no. of problems per person | | | |
		MIN	MED	MAX	TOTAL
Blind	47.0	1.24	1.76	1.87	1.74
Partial sight	42.4	1.30	1.46	1.83	1.61

Behaviour 'Clusters'

Evidence for clustering of behaviour problems is available from Jacobson (1982) who described groups of between 48 per cent and 68 per cent depending on degree of retardation based on 29 behaviour problems in a sample of 30,000 people. Scanlon *et al.* (1982) also reported that 50 per cent of severely handicapped adults living in state institutions were rated as 'severe management problems' by staff and/or parents.

A survey by Shah, Holmes and Wing (1982) of adult mentally handicapped institutional residents related the distribution of a number of personal variables to the quality of social interaction exhibited by inmates. The survey extended the approach used by Wing and Gould (1979) who examined similarities between autistic children and mentally handicapped children. Shah *et al.* used the Disability Assessment Schedule to collect information from nurses in a structured interview. They found 38 per cent of inmates were socially impaired (aloof, passive or odd interactions), including 4 per cent who were autistic. The socially impaired were significantly more likely to have no speech, to be echolalic, to show no symbolic (play or imaginative) activities, to display simple or complex stereotypies and various behaviour problems, and were less likely to engage in constructive activities.

Further significant differences were identified in terms of medical, psychological and demographic variables. The socially impaired group were more likely to be younger and epileptic, and fewer showed expressive or receptive communication skills, or practical skills chosen from self-help, occupational and domestic activities. No difference in sex ratios was found. The authors pointed out the marked tendency for social, communication and symbolic/imaginative impairments to cluster together, forming a 'triad of language and social impairments'. There was also a significant relationship between social impairments and 'disturbed behaviour', including attention-seeking, self-injury, temper tantrums, destructiveness, aggression, stealing and sexual delinquency.

A similar study of the 'triad' was conducted in Sweden by Gillberg (1983) on 112 mentally handicapped children and young adults living in a hostel. Gillberg's results add credence to the notion of a common foundation for social, language and behavioural disorders in severely mentally handicapped people. The major point of concern regarding visually handicapped inmates is that they often show many of the elements making up the 'triad' of impairments.

Shah *et al.* did not indicate the proportion of visually handicapped subjects in their study, but examination of the raw data (Shah 1984, personal communication) showed that blind subjects were more likely to be socially impaired than the sighted (χ = 5.87; p<.025). Gillberg (1983) reported a higher frequency of socially impaired blind subjects but the numbers involved (5 socially impaired; 3 sociable) are small for computation of a reliable chi-square.

The inclusion of blind people within the 'triad' could be interpreted in various ways, if the suggested predominance of social impairment among them proves to be valid. The likely presence of psychosis and/or brain damage among socially impaired inmates is consistent with the raised frequency of severe subnormality among blind people, noted earlier. Alternatively, if visual handicap alone leads the blind person to behave in a socially impaired way *regardless* of level of subnormality, this too could explain why hospital staff rate more blind residents in the 'severe' category. The risk of confusion between the effects of sensory and cognitive impairments should encourage greater attention to this kind of detail in future, to help ensure that the needs of visually and mentally handicapped people are identified more precisely.

CONCLUSIONS

The data reviewed here highlight several major issues regarding mentally handicapped people. The prevalence of visual impairments among them is about ten times higher than in the normal population. They suffer a wide range of additional visual problems, which are particularly common among two clinical subgroups, those with Down's syndrome and those with cerebral palsy.

Some literature carries an implication of a shortage of adequate specialist treatment and training for mentally and visually handicapped people. While the prevalence of visual handicaps in British mental handicap institutions is nearly double that for psychiatric disorders (Wright 1982), there is no consideration of the need to employ ophthalmologists in such institutions. Research into the beliefs and opinions of eye specialists about mentally handicapped people would be welcome in this connection. Adequate service delivery also depends on appropriate specialist training for primary care staff (see Ellis 1983) for which there is very little opportunity in Britain, and the prospect for improvement may depend on political decisions at a regional or national level. A recent government publication which examined special needs in mental handicap (DHSS 1984a) was disappointing in this respect.

While the needs of visually and mentally handicapped people are heterogeneous, it is possible to identify at least four main groupings, which are not mutually exclusive but which serve to highlight major types of need and thus potential areas for future research, and for provision of services.

Firstly, multiply handicapped children are becoming more prevalent following improvements in obstetric skills, and visual impairment appears to be prominent in this group. They appear to be more frequent in smaller hospitals and will require considerable and continuing remedial help to an extent which has not been necessary in mental handicap services so far. Secondly, available data show a *shortfall* of older visually handicapped people relative to the normal population. This is not due to earlier mortality and may reflect some neglect of the visual needs of old people.

A third group is more the subject of conjecture than of hard evidence. The NHS Survey identified a minority of visually handicapped inmates who were *not* mentally handicapped and, because of the poor accuracy of the subnormality ratings used, it seems likely that many more may have been cast into institutions because of the debilitating effects of their visual handicaps. Finally, the remaining large core of people with visual *and* mental handicaps also have particular needs for more specialized help with living and training, if they are to have the same opportunities as their sighted contemporaries. Level of dependency in self-care skills, and engagement in various behaviour problems are key indicators of the need for specialized help. Improvements in communication and mobility skills would probably provide good foundations for improving the functional independence of visually handicapped clients. Hospital managers who invest in specialist staff training could protect their investment by planning to relocate trained staff along with visually handicapped residents into community-based residential settings, as large institutions are run down.

Acknowledgement

I am indebted to Mrs. Phyl McKenzie of Leybourne Grange Library for her help in obtaining most of the literature from which this chapter is constructed; and for moral support.

References

Bader, D. and Woodruff, M.E. (1980) 'The Effects of Corrective Lenses on Various Behaviours of Mentally Retarded Persons', *American Journal of Optometry & Physiological Optics, 57*(7), 447-59

Bankes, J.L.K. (1974) 'Eye Defects of Mentally Handicapped Children', *British Medical Journal, 2,* 533-5

Baumeister, A.A. and Rollings, J.P. (1976) 'Self-Injurious Behaviour', in N.R. Ellis, (ed.), *International Review of Research in Mental Retardation,* Vol. 8, Academic Press, New York

Berkson, G. (1973) 'Visual Defect does not produce Stereotyped Movements', *American Journal of Mental Deficiency, 78,* (1), 81-94

Berkson, G. and Davenport, R.K. (1962) 'Stereotyped Movements of mental defectives: I. Initial Survey', *American Journal of Mental Deficiency, 66,* 849-52

Bernsen, A.H. (1981) 'Severe mental retardation among children in a Danish urban area: assessment and etiology' in P. Mittler, (1981), *Frontiers of Knowledge in Mental Retardation. Volume II Biomedical Aspects,* University Park Press, Baltimore

Black, P. (1982) 'Visual disorders associated with Cerebral Palsy', *British Journal of Ophthalmology 66,* 46-52

Burstyn, R. (1971) 'A Vision survey of 115 Trainable and Educable Mentally Retarded Boys', *American Journal of Optometry and Physiological Optics, 18,* 1021-4

Byrne, D.J. and Stevens, C.P. (1980) 'Mentally handicapped children's responses to Vibro-Tactile and other Stimuli as evidence for the existence of a Sensory Hierarchy',

Apex: Journal British Institute of Mental Handicap, 8 (3), 96-8

Cataldo, M.F. and Harris, J. (1982) 'The Biological Basis for Self-Injury in the Mentally Retarded', *Analysis and Intervention in Developmental Disabilities, 2,* 21-39

Courtney, G.R. (1977) 'Astigmatism among Institutionalized and Non-institutionalized Mentally Retarded', *American Journal of Optometry and Physiological Optics, 54* (6), 347-50

Cullinan, T.R. (1977) *Visually Disabled People in the Community,* Health Services Research Unit Report No. 28, University of Kent at Canterbury

—— (1978) 'Epidemiology of Visual Disability', *Trans. Ophthalm. Soc. U.K., 98,* 267

de Catanzaro, D.A. (1978) 'Self-Injurious Behaviour: A Biological Analysis', *Motivation and Emotion, 2* (1), 45-65

DHSS (1984a) *Helping Mentally Handicapped People with Special Needs: Report of a DHSS Study Team,* DHSS, London

—— (1984b) *In-patient statistics from the mental health enquiry for England, 1979. Statistical and research report series No. 25,* HMSO, London

Duckman, R. (1979) 'The incidence of visual anomalies in a population of cerebral palsied children', *J. Optometric Association, 50* (9), 1013-16

—— (1980) 'Effectiveness of visual training on a population of cerebral palsied children', *Journal American Optometric Association, 51* (6), 607-14

Edwards, W., Price, W. and Weisskopf, B. (1972) 'Ocular Findings in Developmentally Handicapped Children', *Journal of Paediatric Ophthalmology, 9* (3), 162-7

Einfield, S.L. (1984) 'Clinical Assessment of 4500 Developmentally Delayed Individuals', *J. Mental Deficiency Research, 28,* 129-42

Ellis, D. (1982) 'Visually and mentally handicapped people in institutions. Part 1: Their numbers and needs', *Mental Handicap, 10* (4), 135-7

—— (1983) 'Visually and mentally handicapped people in institutions. Part 2. Segregation or Specialization?', *Mental Handicap, 11* (1), 8, 9 and 29

—— (1984) 'Communication Difficulties and Visually Handicapped People', in T. Culhane, R. McKibben and J. Roberts (eds.), *Communication problems of the Mentally Handicapped. Occasional Paper No. 28,* Dept. Language and Linguistics, University of Essex

Evans, J., Wachs, H. and Borger, J.M. (1972) 'A Survey of Visual Skills of Institutionalized Retarded Patients', *American Journal of Mental Deficiency, 76* (5), 555-60

Falbe-Hansen, I. (1968) 'Congenital Ocular Anomalies in 800 Mentally Deficient Patients', *Acta Ophthalmologica, 46,* 391-7

Fletcher, M.C. and Thompson, M. (1961) 'Eye Abnormalities in the Mentally Defective', *American Journal of Mental Deficiency, 66,* 242-4

Gardiner, P.A. (1967) 'Visual Defects in cases of Down's Syndrome and in other mentally handicapped children', *British Journal of Ophthalmology, 51,* 469–74

Gillberg, C. (1983) 'Psychotic behaviour in children and young adults in a mental handicap hostel', *Acta Psychiatr. Scand., 68,* 351-8

Goodall, E. and Corbett, J. (1982) 'Relationships between Sensory Stimulation and Stereotyped Behaviour in Severely Mentally Retarded and Autistic Children', *Journal of Mental Deficiency Research, 26,* 163-75

Grunewald, K. (1973) *Blind, Deaf and Physically Handicapped mentally retarded. An epidemiological study as a base for action.* Proceeding of 3rd Congress, International Association for the Scientific Study of Mental Deficiency, *1,* 349–352

Hiles, D.A., Wallar, P.H. and McFarlane, F. (1975) 'Current Concepts in the Management of Strabismus in Children with Cerebral Palsy', *Annals of Ophthalmology, 7* (6), 789-98

Holmes, N., Shah, A. and Wing, L. (1982) 'The Disability Assessment Schedule: a brief screening device for use with the mentally retarded', *Psychological Medicine, 12,* 879–90

Hospitals & Health Service Yearbook (1978), Institute of Health Service Administration, London, ISBN 090 1003166

Humphreys, E.J. (1976) 'Survey of the mentally handicapped in West Devon', *British Journal of Mental Subnormality, 22* (43), 77-85

Jacobson, J.W. (1982) 'Problem Behaviour and Psychiatric Impairment within a Developmentally Disabled Population. 1: Behaviour Frequency', *Applied Research in Mental Retardation, 3,* 121–39

Jan, J.E. (1978) 'Differences in Biological Function between the Blind and the Sighted', *Developmental Medicine and Child Neurology, 20,* 668-78

—— Freeman, R.D., McCormick, A.Q., Scott, E.P., Robertson, W.D. and Newman, D.E. (1983) 'Eye-pressing by Visually Impaired Children', *Developmental Medicine & Child Neurology, 25,* 755-62

——, —— and Scott, E. (1977) *Visual Impairment in Children and Adolescents,* Grune and Stratton, New York

Kirchner, C. and Lowman, C. (1978) 'Sources of Variation in the estimated prevalence of Visual Loss', *Journal Visual Impairment and Blindness, 72* (8), 329

—— and Peterson, R. (1979a) 'The Latest data on visual disability from NCHS', *Journal Visual Impairment and Blindness, 73* (4), 151-3

—— and —— (1979b) 'Employment; Selected characteristics', *Journal Visual Impairment and Blindness, 73* (6), 239-42

—— and —— (1980) 'Multiple Impairments among non-institutionalized blind and visually impaired persons', *Journal Visual Impairment and Blindness, 74,* 40-4

——, —— and Suhr, C. (1979) 'Trends in School Enrollment and Reading methods among legally blind school children 1963-1978', *Journal Visual Impairment & Blindness, 73* (9), 373-9

Kushlick, A. and Cox, G.R. (1973) 'The Epidemiology of Mental Handicap', *Developmental Medicine and Child Neurology, 15,* 748-59

Lewis, M.H., MacLean, W.E., Johnson, W.L. and Baumeister, A.A. (1981) 'Ultradian Rhythms in Stereotyped and Self-Injurious Behaviour', *American Journal of Mental Deficiency, 85* (6), 601-10

Loewer-Sieger, D.H. (1975) 'The prevalence of severe visual impairment in children in the Netherlands', *Child: care, health & development, 1,* 275-82

Lowe, R.F. (1949) 'The eyes in Mongolism', *British Journal of Ophthalmology, 33,* 131-74

Lowman, C. and Kirchner, C. (1979) 'Elderly blind and visually impaired persons: projected numbers in year 2000', *Journal Visual Impairment and Blindness, 73* (2), 69-73

Maisto, C.R., Baumeister, A.A. and Maisto, A.A. (1978) 'An Analysis of Variables Related to Self-Injurious Behaviour among Institutionalized Retarded Persons', *Journal Mental Deficiency Research, 22,* 27-36

Manley, J.N. and Schuldt, W.J. (1970) 'The Refractive State of the Eye and Mental Retardation', *Journal Optometry and Archives. American Acadamy of Optometry, 47* (3), 236-41

Markovits, A.S. (1975) 'Ophthalmic Screening of the Mentally Defective', *Annals of Ophthalmology, 7*(6), 846–8

MacKeith, R.C., MacKenzie, I.C. and Polani, P.E. (1959) 'The Little Club Memorandum on terminology and classification of "cerebral palsy"', *Cerebral Palsy Bulletin, 1,* 23

McDonald, A.D. (1966) 'Congenital Cataract', *Developmental Medicine and Child Neurology, 8,* 301-9

Mitchell, S. and Woodthorpe, J. (1981) 'Young mentally handicapped adults in three London boroughs; prevalence and degree of disability', *Journal Epidemiology and Community Health, 35,* 59-64

Mittler, P. and Preddy, D. (1981) 'Mentally handicapped pupils and school-leavers; a survey in North West England' in B. Cooper (ed.), *Assessing the Handicaps and Needs of Mentally Retarded Children,* Academic Press, London pp. 33–51

Murphy, G. (1982) 'Sensory Reinforcement in the Mentally Handicapped and Autistic Child: a Review', *Journal of Autism and Developmental Disorders, 12*(3), 265-78

Palmer, J. and Jenkins, J. (1982) 'The "Wessex" Behaviour Rating System for Mentally Handicapped People: Reliability Study', *British Journal Mental Subnormality, 28* (55), 88-96

Paneth, N., Kiely, J.L., Stein, Z. and Susser, M. (1981) 'Cerebral Palsy and Newborn Care. III: Estimated Prevalence Rates of Cerebral Palsy under differing Rates of Mortality and Impairment of Low-Birthweight Infants', *Developmental Medicine & Child Neurology, 23,* 801–7

Perlstein, M.A. (1962) 'Cerebral Palsy: Incidence, etiology, pathogenesis', *Archives of Paediatrics, 79,* 289-98

Pesch, R.S. and Nagy, D.K. (1978) 'A Survey of the visual and developmental-perceptual abilities of the Down's Syndrome child', *Journal American Optometric Association, 49* (9), 1031-7

Peterson, R., Lowman, C. and Kirchner, C. (1978) 'Visual Handicap: Statistical data on a Social Process', *Journal Visual Impairment and Blindness, 72* (10), 419

Pharoah, P.O.D. (1981) 'Epidemiology of Cerebral Palsy: a review', *Journal Royal Society of Medicine*, 74, 516-20

Rabinowicz, I.M. (1974) 'Visual Function in children with Hydrocephalus', *Trans. Ophthalm. Soc. U.K.*, 94, 353-66

Reynell, J. (1978) 'Developmental Patterns of Visually Handicapped Children', *Child: care, health & development*, 4, 291-303

Richardson, S., Katz, M., Koller, H., McLaren, J. and Rubinstein, B. (1979) 'Some characteristics of a population of mentally retarded young adults in a British city. A basis for estimating some service needs', *Journal Mental Deficiency Research*, 23, 275-85

Ryan, T.A., Joiner, B.L. and Ryan, B.F. (1981) *Minitab Reference Manual*, Pennsylvania State University

Scanlon, C.A., Arick, J.R. and Krug, D.A. (1982) 'A Matched Sample Investigation of Nonadaptive Behaviour of Severely Handicapped Adults across four Living Situations', *American Journal of Mental Deficiency*, 86 (5), 526-32

Schroeder, S.R., Mulick, J.A. and Rojahn, J. (1980) 'The Definition, Taxonomy, Epidemiology and Ecology of Self-Injurious Behaviour', *Journal of Autism and Developmental Disorders*, 10 (4), 417-32

Schroeder, S.R., Schroeder, C.S., Smith B. and Dalldorf, J. (1978) 'Prevalence of Self-Injurious Behaviours in a Large State Facility for the Retarded: A Three-Year Follow-up Study', *Journal of Autism and Childhood Schizophrenia*, 8 (3), 261-9

Shah, A., Holmes, N. and Wing, L. (1982) 'Prevalence of Autism and related conditions in Adults in a Mental Handicap Hospital', *Applied Research in Mental Retardation*, 3, 303-17

Singh, N.N. (1981) 'Current Trends in the Treatment of Self-Injurious Behaviour', *Advances in Pediatrics*, 28, 377-440

Sorsby, A., Sheridan, M., Leary, G.A. and Benjamin, B. (1960) 'Vision, visual acuity and ocular refraction of young men', *British Medical Journal*, 1, 1394-8

Thase, M.E. (1982) 'Longevity and Mortality in Down's Syndrome', *Journal Mental Deficiency Research*, 26, 177-92

Tierney, I.R., Fraser, W.I., McGuire, R.J. and Walton, H.J. (1981) 'Stereotyped Behaviours — Prevalence, Function and Management in Mental Deficiency Hospitals', *Health Bulletin*, 39 (5), 320-6

Walsh, F.B. (1963) 'Blindness in an Institution for the Feebleminded', *Archives of Ophthalmology*, 69, 165

Walsh, S.Z. (1981) 'Keratoconus and Blindness in 469 Institutionalized Subjects with Down's Syndrome and other causes of Mental Retardation', *Journal Mental Deficiency Research*, 25, 243-51

Warburg, M. (1963) 'Diseases of the Eye among Mental Defectives', *Acta Ophthalmologica*, 41, 157

—— (1970) 'Tracing and Training of Blind and Partially Sighted Patients in Institutions for the Mentally Retarded', *Danish Medical Bulletin*, 17 (5), 148-52

—— (1982) 'Why are the blind and severely visually impaired children with mental retardation much more retarded than the sighted children?', *Acta Ophthalmologica (Copenhagen)*, Supplement 157, pp. 72–81

Warshowsky, J. (1981) 'A vision screening of a Down's Syndrome population', *Journal American Optometric Association*, 52 (7), 605-7

Welsh Office (1979) *Mental Health Statistics for Wales*, HMSO, Cardiff

Williams, C. (1978) *Strategies of intervention with the Profoundly Retarded Visually Handicapped Child: A brief report of a study of stereotypy*, Division of Education and Child Psychology, British Psychological Society, Occasional Papers II No II, 68-72

Wing, L. and Gould, J. (1979) 'Severe impairments of social interaction and associated abnormalities in children: Epidemiology and classification', *Journal Autism and Developmental Disorders*, 9, 11-29

Woodruff, M.E. (1977) 'Prevalence of Visual and Ocular Anomalies in 168 Non-Institutionalized Mentally Retarded Children', *Canadian Journal of Public Health*, 68, 225-32

WHO (1973) *The Prevention of Blindness* WHO Technical Report Series No. 518, World Health Organization, Geneva

Wright, E.C. (1982) 'The Presentation of Mental Illness in Mentally Retarded Adults', *British Journal Psychiatry*, 141, 496-502

THE EPIDEMIOLOGY OF HEARING IMPAIRMENT IN PEOPLE WITH A MENTAL HANDICAP

Barbara I. Kropka and Chris Williams

Introduction

Many of the difficulties inherent in attempting to understand the relationship between hearing impairment and mental handicap arise not only because the resulting multiple handicap is complex, but also because research into the area has confounded the issues with problems of varying definitions and criteria. The result is often confusion for the interested reader faced by the available literature. This chapter will review the information to date with the resulting implications for the individuals affected, and for those professionals working with and for them. Interest in hearing impairment in the mentally handicapped is a fairly recent phenomenon. In their 1963 bibliography of world research into mental handicap from 1940 to 1963, numbering some 16,000 papers, Heber, Simpson, Gibson and Milligan (1963) reported only about 60 papers on topics related to hearing impairment. Most of the available literature dates from the late 1960s, with interest in the area growing steadily ever since.

Key Definitions

This chapter will examine issues such as what kinds of impairment are in question, and why are they important? What epidemiological factors are involved? What should professionals working in the field try to do about the problems?

To begin, definitions of the key phrases 'mental handicap' and 'hearing impairment' are required. Straightaway the problems begin! The definitions of these terms are understandably complex, because the natures of both resulting handicaps are decided by the interplay of a variety of factors.

Mental Handicap

Bensberg and Sigelman (1976) noted that most definitions of mental handicap have emphasized one of three themes:

1   the capacity to learn;
2.   knowledge acquired to date;
3.   the ability to adjust or adapt to the total environment, particularly to novel situations.

They report that Prehm (1974) indicated that definitions of mental handicap have also included the following:

4. that mental handicap originates during the developing period, or before the ages 16 to 18, and excludes conditions caused by trauma and disease that may produce intellectual impairment in adults;
5. that an organic cause must be identifiable;
6. that mental handicap is essentially incurable.

Historically, intelligence tests have been used (and abused) as the sole criterion for deciding whether or not a person should be termed mentally handicapped. Happily, in the present day, determining an IQ score is no longer considered to be of such over-riding importance, and measures of adaptive behaviours play a much greater role in assessment, and subsequently in programming. Bensberg and Sigelman (1976) cite Grossman's definition of adaptive behaviour as 'the effectiveness or degree with which the individual meets the standards of personal independence and social responsibility expected of his age and cultural group'. These standards naturally would vary with different age and cultural groups. Adaptive behaviour includes sensori-motor skills, self-help skills, communication skills, independence and domestic skills, and social skills. The American Association on Mental Deficiency (Heber 1961) produced the following definition which is in current usage: 'Mental retardation refers to significantly subaverage general intellectual functioning existing concurrently with deficits in adaptive behaviour and manifested during the developmental period.' The reference to subaverage intellectual functioning means that no one scoring above the cut-off point of an IQ of 70 on standard tests of intelligence should be labelled as mentally handicapped.

Hearing Impairment

A variety of more or less sophisticated definitions of hearing impairment can be found in the literature. Lloyd's (1973) functional definition is:

> Hearing Impairment refers to a deviation in hearing sufficient to impair normal aural–oral communication. The degree of hearing impairment is the result of the degree of deviation in hearing ... interacting with a number of other factors, such as age of onset, age of detection and intervention, duration, type of pathology and related factors, use of amplification, habilitative programming, family factors, and resilience or adaptive abilities.

Types of Hearing Impairment

There are three basic types of hearing impairment:

1. Conductive — caused by disease which interferes with the conduction of sound from outside in the environment to the middle ear.

2. *Sensori-Neural* — caused by disease to the cochlea and neural auditory pathway.

An important distinction between these two types is created by the efficacy of treatment. Whilst intervention can often alleviate conductive problems, it is unlikely to reduce the degree of hearing loss due to permanent damage to the nerve processes (Taylor 1975).

3. *Mixed* — in which there are defects in both areas.

Hearing Impairment and Mental Handicap

Hearing impairment is multi-causal. Williams (1982) summarized the causes and showed how closely the causes of hearing impairment parallel and at times coincide with the causes of conditions associated with mental handicap; genetic factors, traumatic factors, both pre- and post-natal, disease factors such as Rubella and meningitis and environmental factors such as trauma and toxins, are all features common to the two conditions. Williams concluded that it was not surprising that the two conditions often coexist. The consequences of hearing impairment in terms of the resulting handicap depend on the relationships noted above, particularly between the following: the site of lesion, the aetiology, the age of onset and the degree of impairment.

Yeates (Chapter 6, this volume) discusses the first two factors. The age of onset of the impairment, and the degree of impairment can have serious consequences for language development. The presence of hearing impairment can markedly limit verbal language both in acquisition and expression. Generally, the earlier the age of onset and the greater the degree of impairment, the more serious the effect will be on language development and social competence. Denmark (1978) wrote: 'Deafness is an invisible handicap whose consequences are not apparent to the casual observer.' It is important to stress, because of the role of hearing in language development, that, if hearing impairment is not suspected or diagnosed, the deficit and lack of progress in language development or usage may be wrongly assigned to the presence of mental handicap. Williams (1982) showed how masking of cognitive ability could occur in deaf individuals whose initial presentation suggested mental handicap, in most cases lacking adequate vocal language, but whose major disability was deafness.

Stewart (1978) made the important point that hearing impairment in a mentally handicapped person does not produce a simple additive effect, but one of reciprocal limitations. A hearing-impaired individual would have a more difficult time learning because of hearing loss, which would increase his level of retardation. Increased retardation would further diminish use of auditory input and cause further retardation. The relationship between combined handicaps is, therefore, multiplicative rather than purely additive. The severe potential implications of hearing impairment make its diagnosis and assessment a priority, in order that alleviation and habilitation can be attempted. Kropka (1979) noted:

> In an institutional setting the hearing impaired often represent a 'hidden' minority within the hospital population. These residents may be absorbed into the hospital community and little priority given to this aspect of their handicap even though impaired hearing has serious consequences for everyday living and long-term resident management, affecting assessment, treatment and rehabilitation.

Although researchers have identified the problem, as documented in various papers over the last twenty years (Table 2.1), it is a problem still very much with us. More often than not, knowledge has not been converted into action, and people have no real understanding of the implications of hearing impairment in people with a mental handicap. Diagnosis and assessment of the condition to establish prevalence is often problematic.

Diagnosis and Assessment

Brannan, Sigelman and Bensberg (1975) wrote 'We cannot overemphasise the difficulties which presently plague diagnosis of hearing impairment amongst the mentally retarded and which prohibit accurate assessment of the scope of the problem.' Schein (1979) pointed out that the problems of detection can largely be overcome provided an adequate effort is made.

Birch and Matthews (1951) suggested that audiometrics should become a standard part of the admission procedure into hospital in the interests of adequate diagnosis. Subsequent workers have provided similar recommendations. The National Development Group (1978) recommended that all residents in mental handicap hospitals should be audiologically assessed or screened. In 1979 the National Development Team found that hospital residents are not always screened for auditory defects and that even those with obvious impairments have not always been seen by specialists. Kropka (1979) found that 61 per cent of *known* hearing-impaired people in her study had never had formal audiological assessment. The latest DHSS document (1984) stresses the need for assessment, as a part of good practice in service delivery. For further details on audiology with the mentally handicapped see Fulton and Lloyd (1968), Lloyd (1970), Lloyd and Cox (1972), Lloyd and Moore (1972) and Chapter 11 this volume.

ESTIMATES OF PREVALENCE OF HEARING IMPAIRMENT IN PEOPLE WITH A MENTAL HANDICAP

The outstanding point about estimates of prevalence is the extraordinary range reported, varying from 0 to 80 per cent, (see Table 2.1). There is no doubt that hearing impairment is a relatively common condition, as the majority of research has indicated. Comparison of surveys is made virtually impossible by the variety of criteria and definitions used. Different studies have created variability in the data due to sampling differences. Particular problem include the treatment of difficult-to-test subjects and varying criteria of hearing loss and assessment procedures. Bensberg and Sigelman's (1976) review discussed this issue.

Problems of Data Collection

The studies reviewed in this section are of two types: those involving surveys, relying on staff reports as a measure of hearing impairment, and those basing data on audiological assessment.

The latter are less common on a large scale due to the amount of work involved in their administration, but are obviously more reliable and valid. The former are more common, but have certain inherent problems. Usually with surveys involving staff opinion, it is not known whether the opinions given are based on subjective judgement or on assessment by audiologists. This is a real concern when trying to establish estimates of hearing impairment. Staff may only be detecting more obvious losses and milder (although functionally significant) losses may go undetected, as illustrated later in this section (Jackson and Struthers 1974; Jitts and Keyes 1983).

Questionnaire surveys have also tended to use definitions of hearing impairment that are quite unspecific, usually giving no precise guidelines to

Table 2.1: Summaries of a Selection of Research Studies into Prevalence and Incidence of Hearing Impairment, 1959-72

Kodman, Power, Philip and Weller (1959)	20% of children in special education had losses of 30dB+, in comparison with only 5% of 'normal' children.
Rittmanic (1959)	40% of his sample of mentally handicapped people had losses of 15dB+.
Schlanger (1961)	0-50% of mentally handicapped people in his postal survey of institutions suffered some degree of hearing loss.
Lloyd and Reid (1967)	16% of the population of a residential centre had a loss greater than 15dB in each ear.
Rittmanic (1971)	Prevalence of 8-56% in a review of 27 surveys of the mentally handicapped.
Lloyd and Moore (1972)	15% of children in facilities for the mentally handicapped had a 'significant' hearing impairment.

respondents to define the term 'hearing loss'. Typically, criteria and techniques used by respondents to determine losses are not available to investigators, giving rise to the possibility of wide variation in precision of estimated data.

Mittler and Preddy (1981) made the following points in relation to their own survey, but they apply to most others. With a large survey their methods were necessarily crude and the resulting data of unknown reliability. Not only is accuracy of information doubtful because respondents do not usually have the time to fill out lengthy questionnaires on clients, but respondents often do not have the information required by the investigators.

Often full medical diagnoses have not been carried out or vital information on abilities and disabilities is either unavailable or was not recorded in a way that allows objective analysis and subsequent report. Mittler and Preddy point out the need to establish a comprehensive record-keeping system is something often reported by respondents. These difficulties should be borne in mind when examining the available research. The following section reviews studies of both types in some detail.

Results of Recent Prevalence Studies in Institutions and in the Community

Institutional Studies

Vernon and Kilcullen (1972) presented data on the hearing-impaired mentally handicapped population in State Hospitals for the Retarded in Maryland. A study carried out by Kilcullen in 1968 indicated that 15 per cent of the patients had significant measurable hearing losses as determined by brief audiological screening procedures carried out by hospital nurses. Further analysis of the 461 patients who made up the 15 per cent indicated that about 16 per cent of them could be identified as deaf for practical purposes of communication. Kilcullen also reported IQ figures on 319 people; 9 per cent of them were in the IQ 50-69 range and a further 1 per cent had IQ's above 70.

In the United Kingdom the DHSS (1971) provided figures based on a survey done in Wessex, which had indicated that 1 in 5 severely mentally handicapped children and 1 in 5 adults in hospital had some form of sensory impairment.

Tempowski, Felstead and Simon (1974) reported 13 per cent of referrals to an assessment clinic (145 people, 34 adults and 111 children in 1,049 cases) as being diagnosed with a hearing loss of over 30dB.

Brannan, Sigelman and Bensberg (1975) surveyed US public institutions for the mentally handicapped. The survey was posted to 212 state facilities for the mentally handicapped listed in the 1973 directory. Of 212, 181 responded, of which 158 returned a more or less complete form, a return rate of about 75 per cent. Unfortunately many respondents did not provide complete data and the prevalence figures were based on 111 institutions, 52 per cent of the number surveyed.

These 111 institutions had a total population of 98,034 residents. Of these:

1. 9,343, or 9.5 per cent were classified as hearing impaired;
2. 7,100 or 7.2 per cent were classified as hard of hearing;
3. 2,243 or 2.3 per cent were classified as deaf.

Brannan *et al.* presented a breakdown of the data by age distribution and IQ range, as indicated in Tables 2.2 and 2.3. They found that the hearing-impaired population does not differ from the general institutionalized population with respect to age and degree of retardation. The hearing impaired were mostly over 18 years and severely or profoundly retarded.

Brannan *et al.* concluded that the validity of their prevalence figures was jeopardized by incomplete data, approximate figures and varying definitions of hearing impairment. They found that it is more difficult to estimate the numbers of hard of hearing compared with the numbers of deaf people due to the problem of functional definitions. To define deafness is, in general, easier than to define hearing impairment.

Table 2.2: Age Distribution of Total Mentally Retarded Population, Hard of Hearing and Deaf Population in US Institutions for the Retarded, 1975

Age	Total MR %	HOH %	Deaf %
< 6	1.4	1.3	1.9
6-12	10.7	11.7	15.6
13-18	20.7	11.7	22.1
19-39	41.6	39.3	37.3
40-60	19.8	26.9	18.4
> 60	5.8	3.1	4.7
Total	100	100	100

Source: Brannan *et al.* (1975).

Table 2.3: IQ ranges of Total Mentally Retarded Population, Hard-of-Hearing and Deaf Populations in US Institutions for the Retarded, 1975

IQ range	Total MR %	HOH %	Deaf %
Borderline 70-84	2.9	2.8	4.1
Mild 55-69	10.7	9.9	9.9
Moderate 40-54	19.2	22.3	22.0
Severe 20-39	29.9	30.8	29.5
Profound 0-19	37.3	34.2	34.5
Total	100	100	100 .

Source: Brannan *et al.* (1975).

The National Development Team for the Mentally Handicapped (1979) presented figures for the prevalence of sensory handicap, for the 50,000 people living in residential facilities for mentally handicapped people, based on staff reports. They concluded that one in five of children and one in ten of adults suffered from defects of vision and hearing. This was double the prevalence for adults quoted by the DHSS in 1971.

Kropka, Williams and Clements (1984) have recently undertaken a questionnaire survey of all National Health Service hospitals and hostels for the institutionalized mentally handicapped in England and Wales. All hospitals and hostels in the 1981 Hospital and Health Services Yearbook were circulated a copy of the detailed questionnaire.

Information was received on 18,657 people resident in facilities for the mentally handicapped. This amounted to approximately one-third of the institutionalized mentally handicapped population. Of these, 1,997 people (10.7 per cent) had some degree of hearing impairment; 632 (3.4 per cent) were reported to suffer from a severe impairment and were classified as deaf, while 1,365 people (7.3 per cent) were classified as partially hearing, in accordance with the criteria provided.

Denmark and Adams (1982) carried out a similar postal questionnaire survey into the institutionalized hearing-impaired mentally handicapped population, in England, Scotland and Wales. Their questionnaire was briefer than that of Kropka *et al.* (1984) and consequently received a higher number of returns, gathering information on 37,137 people or over three-quarters of the institutionalized population.

They found that 2,894 (7.8 per cent) suffered from some degree of hearing impairment, somewhat lower than that reported by Kropka *et al.* (1984). Denmark and Adams (1982) found that 3.6 per cent were 'deaf', and the main difference between the two surveys concerned the prevalence for partial hearing; 4.2 per cent from Denmark and Adams and 7.3 per cent from Kropka *et al.* Brannan *et al.* (1975) also found it was more diffi-cult to estimate the numbers of hard-of-hearing people in comparison with the numbers of deaf people and put the problem down to difficulties with functional definitions.

School and Community Studies

Murphy (1978) carried out a survey to discover the percentages of ESN(S) and ESN(M) children who had some degree of hearing loss. He posted 1,039 questionnaires to ESN(S) and (M) schools in England and Wales. Of these, 540 were returned completed, a response rate of 52.4 percent. Tables 2.4 and 2.5 summarize his data of regional variation and of hearing loss in (S) and (M) schools.

Murphy concluded that hearing impairment was evenly distributed by region, ranging from 8.0 to 13.0 per cent. The results were considered to support previous surveys which concluded that 10-15 per cent of educa-tionally subnormal children had some degree of hearing loss. However,

Table 2.4: Percentage of Hearing Loss Reported by Regions in England and Wales in ESN(S) and (M) Schools, 1978

	ESN(S)	ESN(M)
Wales	10.0	11.6
South-west England	13.0	8.6
South-east England	12.0	8.3
Midlands	10.3	9.5
North-east England	11.5	10.6
North-west England	8.0	9.3

Source: Murphy (1978).

Table 2.5: Numbers and Percentages of Children in ESN(S) and (M) Schools in England and Wales Suffering from an (Un)identified Type of Hearing Impairment, 1978

	ESN(S)	ESN(M)
Return N:		
(No. of children in *total*)	18,111	27,982
Total N having:		
(a) Severe unilateral loss	0.6%	0.6%
(b) Mild unilateral loss	1.6%	2.8%
(c) Severe bilateral loss	1.9%	0.8%
(d) Mild bilateral loss	2.2%	1.8%
	= 1,122	= 1,652
+ 'unspecified' impairment:	145	63
	1,267 (7%)	1,715 (6.2%)
Further N of children *suspected* of hearing loss:	681 (3.8%)	712 (2.5%)
Total percentage of known *and* suspected hearing loss:	10.8%	8.7%

Source: Murphy (1978).

incomplete returns were felt to affect the accuracy of the questionnaire, to some extent.

Mittler and Preddy's (1981) large-scale study of mentally handicapped children attending ESN(S) schools in north-west England can be compared to Murphy's study. They found 7 per cent of 2,592 children had some hearing loss, whilst Murphy had reported a figure of 8 per cent for children in the same geographical area. Mittler and Preddy also found hearing impairment in 40 per cent of *school leavers*. However, they suggest their information may be of doubtful validity because they did not know whether sensory functions were expertly assessed. Importantly, they reported that *no* information on hearing handicap was available on 6.6 per cent of all age groups. In contrast, in the school leavers' category, all bar 0.9 per cent had been assessed. Mittler and Preddy also commented that less than half (only 30 of 73) of children who were prescribed hearing aids actually used them.

Further estimates of the prevalence of hearing impairment in people with a mental handicap living *in the community* are provided in the Appendix to Part One of this volume, which summarizes data collected from six mental handicap registers in England and Wales. The data suffer from the usual problems encountered in this kind of information, notably the possibility of incompleteness and identification. The range of hearing impairment in the community data reported by four areas in Table A is from 3.1 per cent to 10.1 per cent, the average being 6.1 per cent. This is lower than prevalences reported earlier in this chapter in NHS populations. Ellis discusses this point further in the Appendix and notes that impairment may be underestimated if the results of other surveys are taken into account.

Jitts and Keyes (1983) studied the prevalence of hearing loss in a population of school-aged intellectually handicapped children in Australia. They believe that work on hearing impairment and mental handicap has been restricted by a number of factors, apart from lack of agreement over criteria or techniques used in assessment. They report concern over the lack of agreement in what is considered hearing within 'normal range limits', over which parameters determine the various types of hearing loss, that the qualifications of personnel conducting assessments were not specified in reports.

In their own study, they detail the equipment used and also precise procedural criteria on which assessment of hearing loss was based. Table 2.6 gives details of the children. They assessed the populations of two schools, using a screening procedure, followed, when appropriate, with either pure-tone audiometry or play audiometry and impedance measures. Those subjects investigated further were assessed for pure-tone sensitivity as far as intellectual capacity allowed, using one or more of four testing techniques. All subjects with hearing loss were tested twice.

Jitts and Keyes found that the prevalence of significant hearing loss (above 30dB) was 16.6 per cent overall, 17.5 per cent in the city school and 15 per cent in the provincial school. The prevalence of slight hearing loss (less than 30dB loss) was also very high, amounting to 32.8 per cent overall, 32.5 per cent in the city and 33.3 per cent in the provincial school. Thus the combined prevalence for hearing impairment of any degree was 50 per cent. Only 21 per cent of those people found to have a hearing loss

Table 2.6: Information Available on Children Attending Two Australian Schools, 1983

	City school	Provincial school
No. of students	90	60
No. of males	56	31
No. of females	34	29
IQ range	20-55	20-55
Average age of all	12 years, 2 mths	12 years, 4 mths

Source: Jitts and Keyes (1983).

had been previously detected so more than three-quarters of those with losses had previously gone undetected. No specific sex differences were reported.

Jitts and Keyes's results matched well the results quoted by Lloyd and Reid (1967), who also found an overall percentage of 16 per cent hearing impairment in either ear in the population of a residential centre, and 10 per cent impairment for loss in both ears. Jitts and Keyes noted that 14.1 per cent of the children assessed had a mild sensori-neural hearing loss. Although they could not find any figures on the prevalence of mild sensori-neural hearing loss in non-intellectually handicapped children, they concluded that a figure of 14 per cent was far in excess of that found in a representative group of the population.

It is obvious that hearing impairment is common in the mentally handicapped, often going undetected. It seems likely that data obtained from staff responses to questionnaires, e.g. the Kropka *et al.* (1984), and Denmark and Adams (1982) surveys, are likely to *underestimate* the prevalence. Only those with major impairments will be readily detected, while people with mild to moderate loss of hearing may be overlooked.

ESTIMATES OF HEARING IMPAIRMENT ASSOCIATED WITH CERTAIN CLINICAL SYNDROMES

This section will review some studies carried out to determine the prevalence and incidence of hearing impairment in association with a number of specific clinical conditions, followed by a discussion of research investigations into the effects of exudative Otitis Media because of its common occurrence in research reports on mentally handicapped people.

Down's Syndrome

It has long been known that people with Down's syndrome are particularly susceptible to hearing loss (Rigrodsky, Prunty and Glovsky 1961). Schwartz and Schwartz (1978) reported studies which indicated Down's syndrome new-borns have an abnormally small auricular length. They believe that the generalized hypotonia characteristic of Down's people may lead to Eustachian tube dysfunction. This condition, combined with the common occurrence of a narrow external auditory meatus, could result in a high prevalence of undetected persistent middle ear pathologic conditions.

Cunningham and McArthur (1981) pointed out that Down's syndrome is characterized by a tendency to upper respiratory tract infection and, combined with anatomical abnormalities, this leads to a high probability of hearing disorders.

Table 2.7 summarizes eight studies of hearing impairment in Down's

Table 2.7: Details of Eight Studies Investigating Hearing Impairment in Down's Syndrome Subjects

Author of study	Number of subjects	Subjects from Institution (I) or or Community (C)	Children (Ch) and/or Adults (Ad)	Detailed investigative procedures reported?	Prevalence of hearing loss found (%)	Type of hearing loss found (%)
1. Fulton and Lloyd (1968)	79	I	Ch + Ad	Yes	39	55 conductive 22 sensori-neural 22 mixed
2. Brooks et al. (1972)	100	I	Ch + Ad	Yes	77	41 conductive 19 mixed 17 sensori-neural
3. Schwartz and Schwartz (1978)	39	C	Ch	Yes	67 had evidence of pathologic middle ear conditions	
4. Balkany et al. (1979)	107	C	Ch	Yes	78	54 conductive 16 sensori-neural 8 mixed
5. Nolan et al. (1980)	13	ATC — residential and day care	Ch + Ad	Yes	69	1. 69 DS had middle ear dysfunction compared to 15 non-DS 2. In Adults: 36 mixed 27 conductive 9 sensori-neural
6. Cunningham and McArthur (1981)	24	C	Ch	Yes	80-85	69 conductive 26 mixed 5 sensori-neural
7. Keiser et al. (1981)	51	74% C 26% I	Ad	Yes	1. at 15dB: 74 2. at 25dB: 38	32 conductive 45 sensori-neural 23 mixed 47 conductive 38 sensori-neutral 15 mixed
8. Oakes (1981)	29	C	Ch	Yes	62	1. majority conductive 2. 55% had susceptibility to ear infection

syndrome people. The percentages of prevalence reported are very high, ranging from 39 to 85 per cent. Six of the eight studies indicated that conductive-type losses were the most common in people with Down's syndrome, whilst the remaining two indicated that the most prevalent were sensori-neural and mixed losses. Both Brooks, Wooley and Kanjilal (1972) and Keiser, Montague, Wold, Maune and Pattison (1981) indicated that the percentage of people with normal hearing decreases with age and, whilst all kinds of hearing impairments increase over age, sensori-neural type losses increase in particular.

Assessment

Nolan, McCartney, McArthur and Rowson (1980) quoted a survey by Whelan and Speake (1977) who had surveyed 305 Adult Training Centres (ATCs) in England and Wales, asking if they would like more contact with a range of professionals thought to be of potential benefit to their clients. The ATC staff proposed an increased contact with speech therapists as a priority, but no mention was made of increased contact with audiologists.

Nolan *et al.* concluded that, although concern was being expressed over the communication difficulties of clients, it was focused on speech difficulties, with the importance of adequate hearing going largely unnoticed. Keiser *et al.* noted that the percentage of hearing loss found depended upon which criteria were used. She used pure-tone air conduction, pure-tone bone conduction, and a measure for speech reception threshold. The speech reception threshold measure indicated the greatest losses while the bone conduction measure indicated the lowest.

Cunningham and McArthur (1981) stressed that assessments should be carried out by qualified people who are familiar with mental handicap. In their study, 50 per cent of those failed by their independent audiologists had been passed by Local Authority screening procedures. Cunningham and McArthur believed this result to be due to Local Authority personnel being unfamiliar with mentally handicapped people and therefore the reliability of investigative procedures was decreased accordingly.

Suggestions for Treatment and Management

Fulton and Lloyd (1968) pointed out that, if otological treatments were more widely available to Down's syndrome people, a decrease in the prevalence of reported hearing impairment would result.

Keiser *et al.* also suggested early intervention procedures with Down's syndrome babies. They suggested Otitis Media and other conductive impairments must be identified and treated. Children should receive frequent screening, followed by otological and audiological management, including a hearing aid, if thought useful.

Keiser *et al.* suggested that parents and other care-givers should be made aware of the problems posed by hearing impairment and the environment arranged to suit accordingly. Cunningham and McArthur further suggested that parents should be alerted to the necessity of keeping the external auditory canal free from wax. Balkany, Downs, Jafek and Krajicek (1979) pointed out that all help was required to remedy hearing loss and that clinicians did not always regard hearing loss as significant in handicap. He felt that not all clinicians believed the handicapped could benefit from amplification.

Cunningham and McArthur recommended that specialist help should be available to the Down's syndrome child locally at his or her neighbourhood clinic rather than in a specialist resource. They felt this provision would have two beneficial effects. Firstly, it would reduce the effects of travel and expense for parents. Also, provision of this kind would be more in line with the principles of normalization (Wolfensberger 1972), the alternative of attending a specialized unit serving to highlight the special needs of the child in an unnecessary way.

Finally, Brooks *et al.* commented that, if Down's syndrome children with a hearing loss were detected early and received appropriate habilitative interventions, a higher communicative ability and higher educational achievement could reasonably be expected.

Viral Infections

Vernon and Hicks (1980) cited the work of Jaffey (1978), Linthicum (1978) and Weinstein (1976), and reported that there are some 16 viruses known to cause hearing loss. The viruses include Rubella, herpes simplex, cytomegaloviruses, adenoviruses and coxsackie. Vernon concluded that some research was so new that the full implications of it were unknown.

Vernon and Rabush (1981) noted that there may be markedly greater numbers of hearing-impaired youth enrolling in education programmes in the US over the next few years, due to changing aetiologies of hearing loss, and to medical advances. Vernon and Rabush reported that the greatest cause of increasing prevalence of deafness in children are sexually transmitted diseases, such as chlamydia trachomatis, B-strep, cytomegalovirus and herpes simplex.

Rubella

Rubella is also known as the three-day measles (Vernon and Hicks 1980) or German measles. It is a relatively harmless rash and fever, unless the disease occurs in a pregnant woman, when the virus attacks the developing foetus. Those parts of the foetus which are developing during the time the virus strikes are frequently damaged. Vernon and Hicks noted that with certain organs, such as the ear, the period of development is fairly specific and hence they will only be severely affected if the virus strikes while they are forming. Conversely, in the nervous system and other organs development occurs throughout gestation and continues through to adulthood

(Buimovici-Klein, Lang, Ziring and Cooper, 1979).

Ziring (1978) reported that Rubella had replaced syphilis as the leading cause of birth defects and mental retardation resulting from maternal infection. Chess and Fernandez (1980 a,b) reported that 42 per cent of their sample of deafened Rubella children were also mentally handicapped indicating the severity of the consequences of maternal infection. Earlier studies had also indicated the connections between Rubella, lower intelligence and hearing handicap. Hardy, Haskins, Hardy and Shimiz (1973) followed an evaluation of the IQ in 171 Rubella children up to the age of 5; while 40 per cent were average or above in intelligence, 31 per cent were borderline to dull normal and 29 per cent were mentally handicapped. Rubella is therefore a major influence in the aetiology of hearing impairment and the mentally handicapped.

Cytomegalovirus

Cytomegalovirus (CMV) is recognised as the leading cause of congenital viral infection, involving 0.5 to 2.4 per cent of all live births in the US (Pass, Stagno, Myers and Alford 1980). Pass *et al.* noted that, although most CMV-infected new-borns are asymptomatic at birth, some do have symptoms of infection. They cited an early study by Weller and Hanshaw (1964) who characterized the problems most common in infected people and found that mental handicap was one of them. McCracken, Shinefield and Cobb (1969) also found hearing impairment in 20 per cent of their CMV-infected patients.

Pass *et al.* studied 34 infants and children ranging from 9 months to 14 years of age. During their study 10 of their patients died. Of the 24 survivors only 2 were normal and 14 were functioning within the mental handicap range (61 per cent). Further, hearing impairment had been diagnosed in 30 per cent of the sample, including 4 people with bilateral profound or severe loss and 3 with unilateral loss. Pass *et al.* concluded that the likelihood of survival with normal intellect and hearing sensitivity following symptomatic congenital CMV infection is very small. They also reported that, although it was impossible to predict central nervous system (CNS) sequelae based on the extent of disease apparent in the new-born period, all clients with an IQ of less than 50 were clearly abnormal by one year of age. Similarly, hearing deficits were apparent by two years of age. On comparing the symptomatic CMV group with those suffering an asymptomatic neonatal period, Pass *et al.* concluded that those who are symptomatic at birth have a significantly higher risk of auditory and other handicaps.

Reynolds *et al.*'s (1974) longitudinal study found that among 267 neonates there were 18 with inapparent CMV infection. It was found that some degree of sensori-neural hearing loss occurred in 9 of the 16 patients tested (56 per cent) compared with 2 of 12 controls (17 per cent). Four of the 16 had definite bilateral or unilateral damage to the sensori-neural hearing mechanism. Reynolds *et al.* felt that, although the evidence for an associated mental handicap was less conclusive, there was a definite trend in this direction and 2 children (10 per cent) manifested 'incapacitating and debilitating mental and behavioural dysfunctions'. Reynolds *et al.* concluded 'that CMV infection probably has an important causal role in mild to moderate auditory and mental dysfunction in children'.

Stagno (1980) has reported the discovery of a simple inexpensive screening test for asymptomatic CMV infection. The test is able to identify two of every five infants with the infection. Although there is no satisfactory way of treating or preventing CMV, early detection of its presence would alert physicians to check for sensori-neural hearing loss and other neurological symptoms, which would make it possible to watch for, and alleviate, developing problems.

Complications of the Rh Factor

Another leading aetiology of deafness and major cause of mental handicap is complication of the Rh factor (Bensberg and Sigelman 1976).

Vernon (1967) established that, of 45 applicants to the California School for the Deaf who had an established erythroblastosis fetalis condition (due to Rh incompatibility between them and their mothers in utero), over 70 per cent were multiply handicapped.

Until recently, Rh factor complications were the leading cause of perinatal deafness, accounting for 3.4 per cent of deafness in children. Vernon and Rabush (1981) cited Wysowski, Flynt, Goldberg and Connell's (1979) study which indicated that complications of Rh factor can now be prevented and in future will cause only 1 per cent deafness in children compared with over 3 per cent previously.

Low Birthweight

It has long been known that there is a link between prematurity and hearing impairment. Campanelli, Pollock and Hennor (1958) reported that 15.9 per cent of low-birthweight infants had some degree of hearing loss. This was attributed to 'immaturity', ototoxic drugs, the ambient noise of the incubators and the presence of perinatal complications, like hypoxia.

Vernon (1967) reported a prevalence rate of 17.4 per cent for premature births among applicants to a school for the deaf. He contrasted this with the 7.6 per cent found in the general population and concluded prematurity was much higher amongst the deaf.

Vernon and Kilcullen (1972) noted that prematurity was a leading aetiology of deafness in children, with an estimated prevalence of 11-17 per cent, and that prematurity was similarly associated with mental handicap.

Anagnostakis, Petmezakis, Papazissis, Messaritakis and Matsaniotis (1982) performed a study into hearing loss in low-birthweight infants (less than 1,800 g). They followed up 98 perinatal intensive care survivors and assessed them at a mean age of $6^1/_2$ years and found 9 per cent with sensori-neural hearing loss. The children with hearing loss had experienced more frequent apnoeic attacks, hyperbilirubinaemia and hypothermia during their neonatal periods, compared with their healthy counterparts. The researchers found no evidence to suggest that the duration of stay in an incubator or the use of ototoxic drugs had any effect on the hearing of their sample. The nine children with impairment had losses ranging from 30dB to 60dB, and five of the children had bilateral losses of which their parents were unaware, prior to the audiological assessment carried out as a part of the study. Of the 98 children, 14 had exudative Otitis Media with a mean hearing loss of 22dB. Following otological treatment, *none* of the children had any problems at follow-up one month later.

The researchers concluded that the combined effects of apnoeic attacks and severe neonatal jaundice may be of some aetiologic importance in sensori-neural hearing loss in low-birthweight infants and that this harmful effect may be accentuated by the presence of hypothermia. Anagnostakis *et al.* suggested that children who suffered from these neonatal complications should be carefully followed up for early detection of hearing impairment.

Hereditary Diseases

Norrie's Disease

In 1927, Norrie described seven cases apparently with the same type of hereditary blindness. Warburg (1966) delineated the disease from other congenital eye diseases and found that hearing and brain functions were also often impaired. She termed the condition Norrie's disease and reported it was characterized by ophthalmological, audiological and mental changes. The ophthalmological changes caused a progressive condition of blindness during infancy. Warburg noted that 'psychotic' symptoms appeared in some patients at any point following the first year of life.

Also, a progressive decline in functioning associated with mental handicap and dementia was to be found in over 30 per cent of sufferers. The disease affects males and is inherited as an x-linked recessive trait. Females are completely unaffected but are carriers of the condition.

The hearing loss associated with Norrie's disease is sensori-neural, appearing in early or middle childhood. Parving and Warburg (1977) reported a study of eleven patients with the condition; ten had some degree of sensori-neural hearing loss, with audiological investigations revealing cochlear damage. Further, six of the eleven patients (54 percent) were mentally handicapped.

Usher's Syndrome

Usher's syndrome is a hereditary condition of retinal degeneration associated with congenital severe hearing loss. Vernon and Kilcullen (1972) reported that 25 per cent of those having the syndrome were also mentally handicapped. (For further information on Usher's syndrome, see Guest's article.)

Otitis Media — 'Glue Ear'

Many of the preceding sections examining hearing impairment in relation to certain clinical conditions have alluded to Otitis Media as a component of the hearing impairment. It is commonly found in the hearing-impaired mentally handicapped. The state described as 'Otitis Media with effusion' (OME) is best regarded as an unresolved middle ear inflammation occurring in the presence of chronic Eustachian tube dysfunction and resulting in the production of inflammatory exudate in the middle ear. It is this which gives rise to a variable degree of hearing loss (Ballantyne 1977; Silva, Kirkland, Simpson, Stewart and Williams 1982).

Otitis Media with effusion has become accepted as a common problem in childhood. Masters and Marsh (1978) commented on the relationship between OME and learning disabilities. They found that in children diagnosed as having specific learning disabilities, 23 per cent were found to have middle ear conditions, compared with 13 per cent of a control group. They concluded that middle ear pathology and learning disabilities deserved research because of a possible causal link.

Paradise (1981) reviewed a number of studies examining relationships between OME and certain conditions, for example, permanent intellectual impairment. He concluded that there was no convincing evidence that adverse developmental outcomes of a lasting nature can arise due to single or multiple episodes of OME, provided that the episodes subside without leaving residual hearing loss.

Silva *et al.* (1982) discussed results from otological and audiological examinations of 879 five year-old children. A group of 47 children were found to suffer from OME and were compared to those who were otologically normal (N = 355). Comparisons noted whether they differed in background characteristics, speech articulation, language or motor development, intelligence or reported behavioural problems. While children with bilateral OME did not differ in terms of background characteristics, they were significantly disadvantaged in speech articulation, verbal competence, motor development and intelligence. They also had significantly more behaviour problems. This finding that OME is associated with developmental and behaviour problems in children suggests an urgent need to identify this problem in children who may be affected.

Interestingly, Silva *et al.* noted that the pattern of developmental test deficits and behavioural problems in OME was similar to that found in children often described as having 'minimal brain dysfunction' or 'specific learning disabilities'. They suggested that, because of the striking similarity of deficits, 'minimal brain dysfunction' in some cases may better be termed 'minimal Eustachian tube dysfunction', and concluded that children exhibiting developmental and behavioural problems should be examined for OME.

IMPLICATIONS OF PREVALENCE STUDIES

The preceding sections of this chapter have indicated that hearing impairment of different types is a common, although often undetected, handicap in the mentally handicapped. Certain clinical conditions, such as Down's syndrome, are particularly susceptible to hearing impairment. Also, the presence of pathologic middle ear conditions, such as Otitis Media with effusion, has been commonly reported, and has been implicated as a factor which can cause developmental and behavioural problems.

Typically, studies of hearing loss by direct audiological assessment have found large percentages of people suffering from hearing impairment who were previously undetected. The implication here is that studies of prevalence by questionnaire relying on staff reports, which are the larger and more common form of study, may underestimate the numbers of people suffering from impairment, particularly those termed 'partially' or 'hard of hearing'.

The presence of hearing impairment can markedly limit verbal language both in terms of acquisition and expression. If hearing impairment is not suspected or diagnosed, the deficit and lack of progress in language development and usage may be wrongly assigned to the presence of mental handicap.

The 'Masquerade'

Kropka (1979) conducted a study of the hearing-impaired population in the mental handicap hospitals of Devon. She found 100 hearing-impaired people, or 10 per cent of the total institutionalized population; of these, 15 people scored above IQ 70 on the WAIS Performance subtests, taking them formally out of the mental handicap range. Williams (1982) noted how masking of cognitive ability had occurred in these deaf individuals whose initial presentation had been that of mentally handicapped people, in most cases lacking adequate vocal language. Their average performance IQ was 80 (dull-normal range), their average score on the Social Training Achievement Record (STAR) was 63 per cent, their mean age was 58 years and they had spent an average of 38 years in a mental handicap hospital.

In most cases, these deaf people had been admitted before the National Health Service had taken over institutions and created services for the mental handicapped. The majority of these people had been sent to institutions for training to learn a trade and somehow had got caught up and left in the system. The following case histories illustrate how three such people came to spend a large part of their lives in a mental handicap hospital before coming to light as part of Kropka's (1979) hearing-impaired project.

Case History 1: AB

Male

D.O.B. 14.8.1903   **Admitted 1921**

Early History   'This patient was backward in the commencement of walking and talking and was observed to be mentally defective in infancy. He attended school but failed to learn at the normal rate and when he left was unable to take up any work and at the age of 18 was sent to R.W.C.I.'

4.3.1921   *From Application for Admission*
'It is very desirable that this lad should be admitted as soon as possible, for had he applied earlier he might have done exceedingly well.'

30.5.1921   Mr B. was admitted to R.W.C.I. on a 'place of safety' order on
31.5.1921   and readmitted under the Mental Deficiency Act (1913) on
He was classed as a feeble-minded individual of medium grade.
From Medical Certificate
'This boy's intelligence is fair if not disturbed by questions put suddenly or in different forms. He is easily disturbed mentally, and his mental age is about 10. He has no ambitions at present and has a childish voice and manner.'
'He is a dull heavy-looking young man of the Mongolian type. Although 18 years old, has the ways of a child, has childish I.Q., learns everything by telling and showing, is fairly intelligent, draws simple sketches fairly well and has some ear for music.'
'Is very childish, obstinate and at times bad tempered, he is much behind his years, likes toys, does not read but learns by being told and shown, habits clean, is not vicious and capable of taking care of himself.'

18.11.1979   *Psychology Report*:
WAIS Performance IQ 98 ('Average' range of intelligence)
STAR rating: 73%

Case History 2: CD

Male

D.O.B. 6.6.1937   **Admitted 1949**

Early History   'The general level of intelligence in the family is low for the patient is deaf and practically dumb, his mother is also deaf, two brothers have been in the Deaf School and another is deaf and dumb.'

1941-1944   Mr D. was at the School for the Deaf.
1944-1949   Report from the Deaf School: 'He is very childish in manner, unable to tell the time or dress or feed himself. On a number of occasions he

stole articles from motor cars. In 1949 he was charged with larceny and an order made under Section 8 of the Mental Deficiency Act sent him to the R.W.C.I.

19.11.1951   *Medical Officer's Notes*

'He is feeble-minded of low grade. He is handicapped by being deaf and he can only make inarticulate sounds; it has been found impossible to teach him anything and he cannot be tested by routine intelligence tests.'

6.7.1980   *Psychology Report*

'His overall score of 70 indicates a borderline mental handicap. This is partly contributed to by his hearing handicap. A pro-rated score of his visual-perceptual items places him at an average ability level. Mr D. is quite capable of benefiting from continued social training with a view to eventual group home or hostel accommodation. He requires continued training in communication and sequencing skills.'

Case History 3: EF

Male

D.O.B. 29.8.1940   **Admitted 1976**

Early History

'At the age of 4 years he was said to be noisy and destructive and beyond his mother's control. He was found to be a defective within the meaning of the Mental Deficiency Acts 1913-1938 and was admitted to a Hospital under Section 6 on

23.8.1944   He was discharged on

12.8.1949   and admitted to a School for Deaf Children. It was reported he made no progress there. At home he was said to be violent towards others including his sisters and grandmother and was admitted to — Hospital on a Place of Safety Order in

April 1950   It was reported at — that communication was difficult as he was deaf and unable to speak. He was violent towards other patients occasionally attacking their eyes. He was transferred to a special hospital.

13.12.1954   'He is classified as suffering from severe subnormality and mental illness under Section 26 of the Mental Health Act 1959. He presents as a neat and tidy person, always happy and smiling, talking in sign language. He is able to wash and dress himself and is little trouble where hygiene is concerned. ... He attends the severely subnormal dances, also the deaf group meetings which are held weekly. He watches TV, attends swimming and enjoys physical education classes. At a recent case conference it was decided that this man no longer requires care and supervision in a Special Hospital and would well be managed in a local hospital caring for the subnormal.'

18.6.1980   *Psychology Report*

Mr F. was admitted to R.W.C.H. under Section 26 in 1976, but his status has been informal since 1978. He is profoundly deaf and does not wear a hearing aid. He is no longer violent but is said to have a low frustration tolerance.

7.7.1980   *Psychology Assessment*

Performance IQ (pro-rated) 76

Schonell Reading Test 6.10 years.

Mr F.'s overall score on the Performance Scale of WAIS was 74 suggesting he is borderline mentally handicapped. He appears to have been profoundly deaf in both ears from an early age if not from birth. In spite of this great handicap he is able to function at a borderline M.H. intellectual level.'

'Mr F. dresses smartly and appears to take pride in his personal grooming. He appears to be profoundly deaf but does not wear a hearing aid. He makes a great effort to communicate using gestures and signs so it is likely that he would make use of a hearing aid if audiological tests indicated that he had sufficient residual hearing for an aid to be of some benefit ... his present intellectual abilities, willingness and ability to learn all suggest he should be able to live outside the hospital in the future possibly in a supervised group, home or hostel. As a step towards this it might be helpful for him to have future social and intellectual training when his progress could be assessed.'

The discovery of people such as those described in the case histories led Williams (1982) to speculate further that, if 1 per cent of institutionalized people in Devon were deaf, but not mentally handicapped, the possibility existed that some 500 people, or 1 per cent of the total institutional population in the country, were also hearing impaired and not mentally handicapped.

The survey carried out by Kropka, Williams and Clements (1984) was set up to investigate this possibility. At the time of writing this chapter, not all the data in the survey have been fully analysed but information from a preliminary analysis has tended to support the notion. In the preliminary analysis summarizing data on a total of 16,759 institutionalized people, 5 per cent of the deaf and 3 per cent of the partially hearing population were classified as being 'not subnormal: IQ above 70' in comparison with only 1.7 per cent of all residents. It is not known whether information on the IQ ranges reported was based on objective test evidence or on subjective judgements, although the latter is more likely.

Thus it would appear that there is a large number of able hearing-impaired people living in institutions and attention should be focused on identifying them and providing habilitation towards community living.

CONCLUSIONS

Apart from the minority of the very able hearing-impaired institutional population 'masquerading' as mentally handicapped, the majority of them do suffer the presence of dual handicaps. The hearing-impaired population in an institution tends to go unnoticed but the serious and severe consequences of the dual impairments warrant the following procedures:

1. Identification

Audiological screening of whole institutionalized populations followed by more thorough audiological assessment, as appropriate, should take place. The target population should be identified and habilitative procedures undertaken, for otological treatment of wax or Otitis Media. The prescription of hearing aids should be considered *together with* training in their use for client *and* care-giver (McCoy and Lloyd 1967).

Psychometric and social competence assessments should be administered as should assessment of physical, emotional and visual needs, prior to placement (Arkell 1981).

2. Provision/Training for Clients

Training programmes should be based on the needs of the target population (Arkell 1981). Typically, training is required in self-help, communication, motor skills, social/emotional, pre-academic/cognitive and leisure skills (Arkell 1981; Kropka, Bamford and Williams 1983).

Training communication skills is a topic of extreme importance. It will not be covered here except to refer the reader on to further reading on Total Communication (Kiernan *et al.* 1982; Chapter 19 this volume).

3. Staff Training

Staff working with hearing-impaired people need in-service training on hearing loss and its implications.

The DHSS (1984) has recently published a document called 'Helping Mentally Handicapped People With Special Needs'. It is a review of current approaches to meeting the needs of mentally handicapped people with special problems, including hearing impairment. It is strongly recommended reading for anyone concerned with services for this common but highly disadvantaged group.

References

Anagnostakis, D., Petmezakis, J., Papazissis, G., Messaritakis, J. and Matsaniotis, N. (1982) 'Hearing Loss in Low Birth-weight Infants', *American Journal of Diseases in Childhood,* 136, 602-4

Arkell, C. (1981) 'Assessment of multiply handicapped deaf students for programme development', *American Annals of the Deaf*, pp. 526-32

Balkany, T.J., Downs, M.P., Jafek, B.W. and Krajicek, M.J. (1979) Hearing loss in Down's syndrome, *Clinical Paediatrics, 18,* 116-18

Ballantyne, J. (1979) *Deafness,* Churchill Livingstone, Edinburgh

Bensberg, G.J. and Sigelman, C.K. (1976) 'Definitions and prevalence' in L.L. Lloyd, (ed.), *Communication Assessment and Intervention Strategies,* University Park Press, Baltimore

Birch, J.W. and Matthews, J. (1951) 'The hearing of mental defectives: its measurement and characteristics', *American Journal of Mental Deficiency, 55,* 384-93

Brannan, C., Sigelman, G.K. and Bensberg, G. (1975) *The hearing impaired/mentally retarded: A summary of state institutions for the retarded,* Research and Training Centre in Mental Retardation, Texas Tech. University

Brooks, D.N., Wooley, H. and Kanjilal, G.C. (1972) 'Hearing loss and middle ear disorders in patients with Down's syndrome', *Journal of Mental Deficiency Research, 16,* 21

Buimovici-Klein, E., Lang, P., Ziring, P. and Cooper, L. (1979) 'Impaired cell-mediated immune response in patients with congenital rubella: correlation with gestational age at time of infection', *Pediatrics, 64,* 620-5.

Campanelli, P.A., Pollock, F.J. and Hennor, R. (1958) 'An otoaudiological evaluation of 44 premature children', *Archives of Otolaryngology, 67,* 609-15

Chess, S. and Fernandez, P. (1980a) 'Do deaf children have a typical personality?', *Journal of American Academy of Child Psychiatry*

—— and —— (1980b) 'Impulsivity in rubella deaf children: a longitudinal study', *American Annals of the Deaf, 125,* 505-9

Clark, A.C. and Bensberg, G.J. (1974) 'Hearing impaired mentally retarded persons in state and private facilities for the retarded', *American Annals of the Deaf, 119,* 71-4

Cunningham, C. and McArthur, K. (1981) 'Hearing loss and treatment in young Down's syndrome children', *Child: Care, Health and Development, 7,* 357-74

Denmark, J.C. (1978) 'Early profound deafness and mental retardation', *British Journal of Mental Subnormality, 24* (2), 81-9

—— and Adams, J. (1982) 'Questionnaire Survey into Hearing Impairment in Institutions in England, Scotland and Wales', personal communication, unpublished data

DHSS (1971) *Better Services for the Mentally Handicapped,* HMSO, London

—— (1984) *Helping Mentally Handicapped People With Special Needs: Report of a DHSS Study Team,* DHSS, London

Fulton, R.T. and Lloyd, L.L. (1968) 'Hearing Impairment in a population with Down's syndrome', *American Journal of Mental Deficiency, 7,* 298–302

Guest, M. *Usher's Syndrome: Hearing Loss and Retinitis Pigmentosa.* NADBRH, Grays Inn Road, London (undated)

Hardy, M.P., Haskins, H.L., Hardy, W.G. and Shimiz, H. (1973) 'Rubella: Audiologic Evaluation and Follow-up', *Archives of Otolaryngology, 98,* 237-45

Heber, R. (1961) *A Manual on Terminology and Classification in Mental Retardation,* 2nd edn, Monograph Supplement, American Journal of Mental Deficiency

—— Simpson, M., Gibson, A., Milligan, G.E. (1963) *Bibliography of World Literature on Mental Retardation January, 1940–March, 1963,* US Dept. of Health, Education and Welfare, Public Health Service, Washington DC

Jackson, S. and Struthers, M. (1974) *A Survey of Scottish Adult Training Centres,* Jordanhill College, Glasgow

Jaffey, B. (1978) 'Viral Causes of Sudden Ear Deafness' *Otolaryngolic Clinics of North America, 11,* 63-9

Jitts, S. and Keyes, C. (1983) 'Incidence of hearing loss in a population of school-aged intellectually handicapped children', *Australian Journal of Audiology, 5,* 71-5

Keiser, H., Montague, J., Wold, D., Maune, S. and Pattison, D. (1981) 'Hearing loss of Down Syndrome Adults', *American Journal of Mental Deficiency, 85*(5), 467-72

Kiernan, C.C., Reid, B.D. and Jones, I.M. (1982) *Signs and Symbols: A Review of the Literature and Survey of Use of Non-vocal Communication Systems,* Heinemann, London

Kodman, R., Power, T.R., Philip, P.P. and Weller, G.M. (1959) 'An investigation of hearing loss in mentally retarded children and adults', *American Journal of Mental Deficiency, 63,* 460-3

Kropka, B.I. (1979) *A Study of the Deaf and Partially Hearing Population in the Mental Handicap Hospitals of Devon,* A Report to the Royal National Institute for the Deaf, London

—— Bamford, J. and Williams, C. (1983) 'From "cabbages" to "kings" in one month: or, with the deaf–blind you never know until you try', *Mental Handicap, 11,* 10-13

—— Williams, C. and Clements, M. (1984) *The Deaf and Partially Hearing in Mental Handicap Hospitals in England & Wales,* A National Questionnaire Survey Sponsored by the British Institute of Mental Handicap (S. Western Division)

Linthicum, F. (1978) 'Viral causes of sensorineural hearing loss', *Otolaryngologic Clinics of North America, 11,* 29-33

Lloyd, L.L. (1970) 'Audiologic aspects of mental retardation' in N.R. Ellis (ed.), *International Review of Research in Mental Retardation,* Vol. 4, Academic Press, New York

—— (1973) 'Mental retardation and hearing impairment' in A.G. Norris (ed.), *PRWAD Deafness annual,* Vol. 3, Professional rehabilitation workers with the Adult Deaf, Washington DC

—— and Cox, B.P. (1972) 'Programming for the audiologic aspects of mental retardation', *Mental Retardation, 10* (2) 22-6

—— and Moore, E.G. (1972) 'Audiology' in J. Wortis (ed.), *Mental Retardation An Annual Review,* Vol. 4, Grune and Stratton, New York

—— and Reid, M.J. (1967) 'The incidence of hearing impairment in an institutionalized mentally retarded population', *American Journal of Mental Deficiency, 71,* 746-63

Masters, L. and March, C.E. (1978) 'Middle ear pathology as a factor in learning disabilities', *Journal of Learning Disabilities, 11,* 54-7

McCoy, D.F. and Lloyd, L.L. (1967) 'A hearing aid orientation program for mentally retarded children', *Training School Bulletin, 64,* 21-30

McCracken, G.H., Shinefield, H.R., Cobb, K. (1969) 'Congenital cytomegalic inclusion disease: A longitudinal study of 20 patients', *American Journal of Diseases in Childhood, 117*, 522

Mittler, P. and Preddy, D. (1981) 'Mentally handicapped pupils and school-leavers: A Survey in North West England' in B. Cooper (ed.) *Assessing the handicaps and needs of mentally retarded children*, Academic Press, London, pp. 33-51

Murphy, K.P. (1978) *Results of a Survey to discover the percentage of ESN(S) and ESN(M) children who have some degree of hearing loss*, Royal National Institute for the Deaf, Gower St., London

National Development Group (1978) *Helping handicapped people in hospital. A report to the secretary of state for social services by the National Development Group for the Mentally Handicapped*, DHSS, London

National Development Team (1979) *Development Team for the mentally handicapped; Second report: 1978-1979*, DHSS, London

Nolan, N., McCartnay, E., McArthur, K. and Rowson, V.J. (1980) 'A study of the hearing and receptive vocabulary of the trainees of an adult training centre', *Journal of Mental Deficiency Research, 24*, 271-86

Oakes, E. (1981) 'The relationship between hearing loss and language development in young Down's syndrome children', thesis, Manchester University, Faculty of Education

Paradise, J.L. (1981) 'Otitis media during early life: How hazardous to development? A critical review of the evidence', *Pediatrics, 68*, 869-73

Parving, A. and Warburg, M. (1977) 'Audiological Findings in Norrie's Disease', *Audiology, 16*, 124-31

Pass, R.F., Stagno, S., Myers, G.J. and Alford, C.A. (1980) 'Outcome of symptomatic congenital cytomegalovirus infection; Results of long-term longitudinal follow-up', *Pediatrics, 66* (5), 758-62

Prehm, H.J. (1974) 'Mental Retardation definition, classification and prevalence', in P.D. Browning (ed.), *Mental retardation, rehabilitation and counselling*, Charles C. Thomas, Springfield. Ill

Rigrodsky, S., Prunty, F. and Glovsky, L. (1961) 'A study of the incidence, types and associated etiologies of hearing loss in an institutionalized mentally retarded population', *The Training School Bulletin, 58*, 30-44

Rittmanic, P.A. (1959) 'Hearing rehabilitation for the institutionalized mentally retarded', *American Journal of Mental Deficiency, 63*, 778-83

—— (1971) 'The Mentally Retarded and the Mentally Ill', in D. Rose (ed.), *Audiological Assessments*, Prentice Hall, Englewood Cliffs; NJ

Reynolds, D.W., Stagno, S., Stubbs, K.G., Dahle, A.J., Livingston, M.M. Saxon, S.S. and Alford, C.A. (1974) 'Inapparent congenital cytomegolovirus infection with elevated cord IgH levels', *The New England Journal of Medicine, 290* (6), 291-6

Schein, J.D. (1979) 'Multiply Handicapped Hearing Impaired Children', in L.J. Bradford and W.G. Hardy (eds.), *Hearing and Hearing Impairment*, Grune and Stratton, New York

Schlanger, B.B. (1961) *The effects of listening training on the auditory thresholds of mentally retarded children*, US Office of Education, Washington DC

Schwartz, D.M. and Schwartz, R.H. (1978) 'Acoustic impedance and otoscopic findings in young children with Down's syndrome', *Archives of Otolaryngology, 104*, 652-6

Silva, P.A., Kirkland, C., Simpson, A., Stewart, Y.A. and Williams, S.M. (1982) 'Some developmental and behavioural problems associated with bilateral otitis media with effusion', *Journal of Learning Disabilities, 15* (7), 417-21

Stagno, S.B. (1980) 'New test spots infants with cytomegalovirus infection', *Medical World News, 21* (7), 39-42

Stewart, L.G. (1978) 'Hearing impaired/developmentally disabled persons in the United States: Definitions, causes, effects and prevalence estimates', *American Annals of the Deaf, 123*, 488-95

Taylor, I.G. (1975) 'What do we mean deaf?' in B. Northwood (ed.), *I See What You Mean*, BBC Publications, London

Tempowski, I., Felstead, H. and Simon, G. (1974) 'Deafness and the Mentally Retarded', *Apex, 2*, 4-5

Vernon, M. (1967) 'Rh. factor and deafness; the problem, its psychological, physical and educational manifestations', *Exceptional Children, 34*, 5-12

—— and Hicks, D. (1980) 'Overview of rubella, herpes simplex, cytomegalovirus and other

viral diseases: their relationship to deafness', *American Annals of the Deaf*, p. 125
—— and Kilcullen, E. (1972) 'Diagnosis, retardation and deafness', *Rehabilitation Record,* *13*, 2, 24-27
—— and Rabush, D. (1981) 'Major developments and trends in deafness', *Exceptional children, 48*, 3, 254-5
Warburg, M. (1966) 'Norrie's disease', *Acta. opthalmologica, supplement, 89*
Weinstein, L. (1976) 'Infectious diseases', *Hospital Practice, 20*, 14-15
Weller, T.H. and Hanshaw, J.B. (1964) 'Virological and clinical observations on cytomegalic inclusion disease', *New England Journal of Medicine, 266*, 1233
Whelan, E. and Speake, B. (1977) *Adult training centres in England — Wales,* Report of the first National Survey, University of Manchester, Hester Adrian Research Centre.
Williams, C. (1982) 'Deaf Not Daft, the deaf in mental subnormality hospitals', *Special Education: Forward Trends, 9* (2), 26-8
Williams, C. (1982) 'STAR: Social Training and Achievement Record', British Institute of Mental Handicap, Kidderminster, Worcs.
Wolfensberger, W. (1972) *Principles of Normalization,* NIMH Toronto
Wysowski, D.K., Flynt, J.W., Goldberg, M.F. and Connell, F.A. (1979) 'Rh hemolytic disease', *Journal of the American Medical Association, 242*, 1376-9
Ziring, P. (1978) 'Psychiatric Sequelae of 1964-65 rubella epidemic', *Psychiatric Annals, 8* (57), 60-1, 64-6

3 THE MULTI-SENSORILY IMPAIRED (DEAF–BLIND) IN THE MENTALLY HANDICAPPED POPULATION — AN UNKNOWN QUANTITY?

Christine Best

Introduction

Researching into available literature on the prevalence of deaf–blindness, i.e. the combination of visual and hearing impairment, one is immediately concerned by the dearth of accurate data. In the UK, in recent years, four studies have attempted to look at the prevalence in part, but there exists no definitive study of multi-sensory impairment in the mental handicap population.

This chapter will aim to look briefly at the data available from the work of Ellis (1982), Kropka and Williams (1982), and Colborne-Brown and Tobin (1982) and focus in detail on the study carried out on behalf of the National Deaf–Blind and Rubella Handicapped Association (NDBRHA) by Best (1983).

Recent Prevalence

Ellis (1982) studied the prevalence of visual impairment in the mentally handicapped population. From his figures of 3.6 per cent blind and 4.4. per cent partially sighted residents in institutions it seems most likely that a small number indeed have additional hearing impairments. Kropka and Williams (1982) indicated in their preliminary results that 'the largest proportions of deaf and partially hearing persons have normal vision. Significant numbers do, however, have visual impairments.'

In the non-hospital setting, Colborne-Brown and Tobin (1982) gave details of the prevalences of additional handicaps in 411 children who were not receiving education in schools for the visually impaired. Of these children, 74 per cent could be described as multiply handicapped; 11 per cent had both visual and mental handicaps, 36 per cent had visual, mental plus another handicap and 27 per cent had visual plus other (excluding mental) handicaps. Although hearing impairment was not specified, it could be predicted that some of this sample were multi-sensorily impaired.

In the Appendix to Part One of this volume, Ellis describes a Case Register Study which provided some details of 40 deaf–blind clients. As he states: 'In spite of the small numbers of clients involved, it is interesting that one-quarter to one-third of clients with hearing handicaps also have visual handicaps.'

The 'Sense' Survey

Thus, given that the available data on this combination of handicaps are limited, the author carried out research on behalf of 'Sense' (National Deaf–Blind and Rubella Handicapped Association) in 1982. The rationale for this research was that during the 1970s a number of units for deaf–blind children (other than Condover Hall School) were established within Schools for the Blind, Schools for the Hearing Impaired, Schools for the Educationally Subnormal (Severe) (now Schools for Severe Learning Difficulties), and hospital schools. These units grew in number and size, and admissions were primarily of children suffering from the effects of maternal Rubella. Within the past two years many heads of units have stated that:

1. the number of Rubella children under ten years of age has decreased, and
2. the number of children who are non-Rubella but have multiple sensory defects plus additional handicaps has increased.

This has resulted in many units changing in character and function. If the apparent change in population is a long-term one, then it has implications for the provision of placements, staffing and the development of appropriate teaching and assessment tools and techniques.

As many children in deaf–blind units are referred for placement from the Schools for Severe Learning Difficulties (SLD), it appeared wise to start any investigation of this population with the SLD schools. However, the greatest problem in gathering statistical data with this population of multi-sensorily impaired is the heterogeneity of the group. The range of impairments is large and complex, with numerous combinations. The multi-sensorily impaired appear on a continuum, from severely deaf and totally blind to partially hearing and partially sighted. There are those who can attempt some manual communication plus speech, and those whose profound difficulties prevent the establishment of all but primitive levels of communication. According to McInnes and Treffry (1982) the multi-sensorily impaired have one of the least understood of all difficulties; they are not just the blind who cannot hear, nor the deaf who cannot see. Rather, they are those who have been denied the effective use of *both* distance senses. The international definition accepted by most agencies is as follows: 'a deaf–blind child is one who has a visual and auditory deficiency to such an extent that he is unable to function satisfactorily in either a school for the deaf or a school for the blind.' In the UK it would appear that this definition has been taken literally — only approximately 110 children are being educated in specialist units; the others are apparently placed in schools for children with Severe Learning Difficulties, and therefore come under the mental handicap 'umbrella'.

In a survey carried out by Hills and Best (1972), 34 out of 71 hospitals contacted said they had discovered children classed as deaf–blind, although none were being taught as such. Several hospitals attempted to group these children together and provide more staff and a ward training programme for each child. Initial results seem to have been encouraging, particularly in basic skill areas such as self-care and toileting. Dantona (1980) referred to educational placements in the United States in which over 2,000 deaf–blind children were being educated in state institutions for the retarded. However, McInnes and Treffry's (1982) contention, that in the past many children who had both a visual and auditory impairment were assumed to be profoundly retarded and institutionalized, may be valid. Faced with a multitude of complex perceptual, psychological and physiological problems and a lack of appropriate assessment tools for the population, it is easy to see how this situation may occur.

Categories of Deaf–Blindness

What then is the extent of multiple sensory impairment to children placed in Schools for Severe Learning Difficulties? For the purpose of the survey four categories of deaf–blindness were used:

A. Severely deaf + totally blind;
B. partially hearing + totally blind;
C. severely deaf + partially sighted;
D. partially hearing + partially sighted.

Although not ideal, it was felt that these categories gave a general description which would provide information concerning the degree of impairment. Certainly they do not tell whether the assessment is clinical or functional, nor is there any indication as to whether the child is functioning 'as if' multi-sensorily impaired.

Survey Results

The 'SENSE' survey was carried out in 1982/3. Head teachers of 481 ESN(S) and hospital schools were sent a postal questionnaire. Of these 278 (58 per cent) replied, of which 124 indicated that they had deaf–blind children on their rolls. This gave a total of 288 deaf–blind children who were detailed on the questionnaire. Table 3.1 shows that the majority of the children fall under Category D — partially hearing-partially sighted. Under 50 per cent are ambulant, only 36 per cent can use a communication system and 69 per cent have additional handicaps.

Table 3.2 gives the causes of the handicaps as detailed by the schools, and shows the largest single grouping is 'no specific diagnosis', followed by 'Rubella' and 'syndromes'. Although 'Rubella' could be grouped under 'syndromes', separation was necessary in order to study those children suffering from the effects of it. Syndromes detailed by schools included

Table 3.1: Details of 288 Deaf–Blind Children Specified by Schools

	Age 2-5 (n=47)	Age 6-11 (n = 112)	Age 12-19 (n=129)
Category A (SD-TB)	7 (15%)	8 (7%)	21 (16%)
Category B (PH-TB)	4 (8%)	17 (15%)	21 (16%)
Category C (SD-PS)	8 (17%)	14 (12%)	26 (20%)
Category D (PH-PS)	28 (62%)	73 (65%)	61 (47%)
Ambulant	10 (21%)	34 (30%)	76 (58%)
Additional handicaps	34 (72%)	83 (74%)	80 (62%)
Rubella	4 (8%)	12 (10%)	47 (36%)
Using communication system	10 (21%)	29 (25%)	65 (50%)
Sex distribution	25m/22f	61m/51f	66m/63f

Table 3.2: Causes of Deaf-Blindness in Children

	Age 2-5 (n=47)	Age 6-11 (n=112)	Age 12-19 (n=129)	Total
No specific diagnosis	17 (36%)	53 (47%)	43 (33%)	113
Rubella	4 (9%)	12 (11%)	47 (36%)	63
Syndrome	9 (19%)	15 (13%)	19 (15%)	43
Birth trauma	6 (13%)	7 (6%)	6 (5%)	19
Accident and NAI	2 (4%)	6 (5%)	4 (3%)	12
Meningitis	1 (2%)	5 (5%)	4 (3%)	10
Encephalitis	2 (4%)	2 (2%)	2 (2%)	6
Other medical diagnosis	6 (13%)	12 (11%)	4 (3%)	18

Down's, Zellweger's, Hurler's, Hallerman-Streif and Usher's. Taking the Rubella children as a separate group, there appears to be a pattern with regard to handicaps and abilities that is not so evident in other causes of deaf–blindness.

In Table 3.3 it is evident that a higher proportion of Rubella children are in Category C (severely deaf–partially sighted) than those in the non-Rubella group, with a high proportion from both groups in the partially hearing–partially sighted category (D). Compared to the other causes of deaf–blindness, the Rubella children are more likely to be able to walk, have a communication system (if limited) and have fewer additional handicaps.

However, it does appear that the majority of Rubella children are over the age of twelve and that the numbers of these children are declining in ESN(S) and hospital schools. The data for those children under five are possibly an underestimation of the problem, as many children will be placed in other settings such as nurseries, child development centres and so on. The twelve Rubella children aged 6-11 certainly suggest a decrease compared to the group of 47 aged 12-19. Excluding the Rubella children, there is a large population of 225 children whose needs are possibly slightly different from those of Rubella children, especially in the areas of ambulation and communication, and it may be that they require specialist teaching techniques of a different nature. Table 3.4 shows the type of additional handicaps in evidence in the 225 non-Rubella children. Children may have more than one of those handicaps described, but the figures give the dominant handicap. The most common additional handicap is that of physical handicap and the survey showed varying types of this, such as spastic quadriplegia and muscle deterioration.

What Help Do These Children Receive?

Of the 124 schools who gave details of deaf–blind children, only 2 had a qualified teacher of the visually handicapped on their staff and 9 employed a teacher of the hearing impaired. However, 74 per cent (88 schools) received advisory help from teachers of the hearing impaired, whereas only 50 per cent (62 schools) received advice from teachers of the visually handicapped. This leaves 62 schools who received no help for their children from any agency for the visually handicapped. This is disturbing, as the children in those schools will receive no help in the development of their residual vision, nor will the teachers receive guidance in the use of the specialist techniques geared to these children.

Eighty-seven schools reported that they required training courses for

Table 3.3: Comparison of Rubella and Non-Rubella Children

	Rubella (n=63)	Non-Rubella children (n=225)
Category A (SD-TB)	8 (13%)	28 (12%)
Category B (PH-TB)	7 (11%)	35 (16%)
Category C (SD-PS)	22 (41%)	26 (12%)
Category D (PH-PS)	26 (45%)	136 (60%)
Ambulant	43 (66%)	77 (34%)
Communication system	41 (65%)	63 (28%)
Additional handicaps	38 (60%)	162 (72%)

Table 3.4: Additional Handicaps in Non-Rubella Children

	Age 2-5 (n=43)	Age 6-11 (n=100)	Age 12-19 (n=82)
Epilepsy	6 (14%)	31 (31%)	20 (24%)
Hydrocephaly	2 (5%)	6 (6%)	3 (3%)
Physical handicap	17 (40%)	36 (36%)	25 (30%)
Other (e.g. behavioural)	5 (12%)	5 (5%)	9 (10%)

their staff: 25 schools requested courses on visual handicap, 22 for teaching techniques, 15 for hearing impairment, 14 for multiple sensory handicaps and 12 for language and communication.

Nearly three-quarters of the children were placed within the special care units in schools, with only 24 children placed in special classes for multi-sensorily impaired. Although the special care unit setting may be suitable for many of the children described by schools, some may be denied adequate education because of the complex nature of their sensory impairments. If more services for the visually handicapped were available to these children, then many might progress to other, more advanced settings within the schools. Communication with the children appeared limited. Only 104 children made use of a communication system and Table 3.5 gives details.

Thus the proportion of 77 per cent with no communication at ages 2-5 falls to 50 per cent with no communication at 12-19 years, so there appears to be an increase in use of communication within the school years. However, this does perhaps distort the true picture as most of the Rubella children are in the age group 12-19 years, and with their higher level of communication the prediction is most likely that only 25 per cent of the children in the schools will develop some form of communication. It is difficult to be sure whether this is due to the abilities of the children or to the lack of suitable education available to them. Kiernan, Reid and Jones (1979) stated that just over half of the ESN(S) schools used non-vocal communication systems and, although this is encouraging in terms of the development of communication in these schools, the methods used to teach communication are not always suitable for children with multiple sensory impairments.

Conclusion

The 'SENSE' Survey identified 288 children with multiple sensory impairments being educated within ESN(S) and hospital schools. However, these children represent a 58 per cent response rate to the postal questionnaire. A projected 100 per cent response suggests a figure of almost 500 children of this type in the schools. This compares to the 110–120 children who are currently educated in specialist deaf–blind units within schools for the visually or hearing impaired and schools for the mentally handicapped, and who were not included in the survey.

Table 3.5: Methods of Communication used by Deaf–Blind Children

	Age 2-5 (n = 47)		Age 6-11 (n = 112)		Age 12-19 (n = 129)	
Speech	3 (6%)	Speech	6 (5%)	Speech	12 (9%)
Makaton	7 (15%)	Makaton	18 (16%)	Makaton	47 (36%)
Touch	1 (2%)	Signal/Gesture	3 (3%)	Paget-Gorman	1 (1%)
None	36 (77%)	RCST Chart	1 (1%)	Touch	4 (3%)
		None	84 (75%)	Signal/Gesture	1 (1%)
				None	64 (50%)

The projected figure of 500 children in schools for the mentally handicapped may not, of course, be accurate, as the return rate may only
indicate schools which have deaf-blind children on their rolls. Nevertheless,
a conservative estimate may be made of between 300 and 400 children.
Several conclusions can be drawn from this and the other studies. Certainly
there are many children with complex sensory and additional difficulties
within the schools for the mentally handicapped and it would seem that
their total special needs are ignored in terms of specialist provision to meet
those needs. Taking van Dijk's (1981) concept of the 'unique' child which
focuses on the pattern of development and functioning rather than on
definitions of vision and hearing, it would appear that these children are
being treated as a sum of their parts rather than as an entity. In other
words, the teacher of the hearing impaired will provide for one element,
the teacher of the visually impaired for another, the physiotherapist for
another, and so on — all often working with minimal or non-existent
contact with each other. Thus the effects of multiple sensory impairments
in combination would seem to be ignored.

Future Developments

Regarding implications for the future, several suggestions can be offered.
Firstly, we should develop teachers training courses to deal with deaf–
blindness. At present SENSE offers training days, workshops and confer-
ences in the UK and is carrying out feasibility studies to establish a course
at postgraduate level in multiple sensory impairment. Often, however,
professionals work in isolation trying to match or modify techniques to
help a particular child achieve his or her potential. To aid them, publications and videos are needed to show the variety of techniques which can be
used with a range of children and adults. Similarly, as the bulk of the
Rubella children are now approaching adulthood, attention must be given
to the development of appropriate activities for occupation and recreation.
Best (1982), in a BIMH/DHSS research project, provided an excellent
start in this area. An extension of this work could be provided to accommodate those with additional physical difficulties.

It is evident from the survey, that children suffering from a variety of
syndromes may be worth further research study, e.g. the development of
Down's children with multiple sensory impairments. Rubella appears to be
well documented in contrast to Zellweger's or Hurler's syndromes.

Assessment appears to be a priority area for further study. The current
mood of dissatisfaction with normative testing and associated questions
regarding test validity and reliability makes curriculum-related assessment
an area of great interest, as this may provide more appropriate information
from which to devise appropriate training programmes. As Galbraith
(1984) stated, methods are needed 1) to establish existing skill levels, 2) to

decide what should be taught next, 3) to establish arrangements for teaching those skills, 4) to evaluate and record progress.

Most professionals will have contact with deaf–blind children only on rare occasions and so inevitably there is a plea for research, evaluation and development in this minority area in order that a true picture of the complex situation be given.

References

Best, A.B. (1981) 'An Investigation into the needs of Blind & Deaf–Blind Mentally Handicapped Adolescents & Young Adults', unpublished, M.Ed. thesis University of Birmingham
—— 1985, in press 'Handbook of Training for Visually/Mentally Handicapped Adolescents & Adults'. BIMH, Kidderminster, UK
Best, C. (1983) 'The "new" deaf–blind?: Results of a national survey of Deaf–Blind children in ESN(S) and hospital schools', *British Journal of Visual Impairment, I* (2), 11–13
Canadian Deaf–Blind and Rubella Association, 'Definition of Deaf–Blindness', CDBRA IAEDB Newsletter 1983
Colborne-Brown, M. and Tobin, M. (1982) 'Integration of the educationally blind', *New Beacon, 66,* 781
Dantona, R. (1980) 'The development of services for deaf–blind persons in the United States' in IAEDB Report on the Hanover Conference, IAEDB Dec. 1980
Ellis, D. (1982) 'Visually and mentally handicapped people in institutions Part I: Their numbers and needs', *Mental Handicap, 10* (4), 135–7
Galbraith, D. (1984) 'Psychological Assessment of Deaf Children', *Journal of the Association of Educational Psychologists, 6* (5)
Hills, J. and Best, A.B. (1973) 'Survey of deaf–blind children in mental handicap hospitals in England and Wales', *Teacher of the Blind, 42,* 3
Kiernan, D., Reid, B. and Jones, L. (1979) 'Signs and Symbols — Who uses What? *Special Education — Forward Trends, 6* (4)
Kropka, B. and Williams, C. (1982) 'The deaf and partially hearing in mental hospitals in England & Wales: preliminary results of a questionnaire survey' (unpublished) BIMH South Western Division, Royal Western Counties Hospital, Starcross, Devon
McInnes, J.M. and Treffry, J.A. (1982) *Deaf–Blind Infants and Children,* Open University Press
van Dijk, J. (1981) *International Presentation on the Provision for the Deaf--Blind — the Netherlands,* Proceedings of the International Conference on Provision for the Deaf–Blind, NADBRH 1981

4 IMPLICATIONS OF DEMOGRAPHIC DATA FOR PLANNING OF SERVICES FOR DEAF–BLIND CHILDREN AND ADULTS

Robert Dantona

Introduction

The Rubella epidemic which struck the United States from 1963 to 1965 focused national attention upon the thousands of deaf–blind children expected to result from that epidemic and the impending educational crisis these children would face when they reached school age.* Prior to the Rubella epidemic there was a dearth of educational programmes for deaf–blind children. By 1968 only 250 of 600 known school-age deaf–blind children benefited from educational programmes scattered about the United States, with fewer than 100 enrolled in just eight specialized Deaf–blind Departments with programmes designed to provide educational services for such children.

The Federal Government responded to concern about the educational needs of these children by developing legislation to authorize the establishment of centres and services for deaf–blind children. On 2 January 1968 this legislation was enacted by President Lyndon B. Johnson (section 609 of Public Law 90-247). On 13 April 1970 Public Law 90-247 was amended by Public Law 91-230 (PL 91-230), Title VI the Education of the Handicapped Act (EHA), of which section 622 provided authority to establish centres for deaf–blind children.

The Federal agency responsible for administering the deaf–blind legislation and for developing and implementing a national programme to provide appropriate educational services was the Bureau of Education for the Handicapped (BEH). In May 1980, a new Department of Education was established (formally the US Office of Education) and the BEH was renamed the Office of Special Education (OSE) under the Office of Special Education and Rehabilitation Services (OSERS) which brought together for the first time under one administration special educational and rehabilitative services. Recently, OSE was renamed as Special Education Program (SEP).

---

*The term 'deaf–blind children', or 'child', is defined as follows in the Federal Register, Vol. 40, No. 35 — Thursday, 20 February 1975: 'The term "deaf–blind children" means children who have auditory and visual handicaps, the combination of which causes such severe communication and other developmental and educational problems that they cannot properly be accommodated in special education programs solely for the hearing handicapped child or for the visually handicapped child.' (Rules and Regulations. Part 121 c — Centers and Services for Deaf–Blind Children.)

Centers for Deaf–Blind Children

Under the direction of BEH, from 1969 to 1980, significant progress was made in the development and growth of educational programmes and services for deaf–blind children throughout the United States. During this period BEH established a number of Centers for deaf–blind children under PL 91-230. In 1969, eight multi-State Centers covering 39 states were established. In 1970, two additional multi-State Centers were funded — these ten multi-State Centers were in operation from 1970 to 1974. From 1974 to 1978 one singe-State Center was established and nine of the original ten multi-State Centers were funded so that all 50 States and Territories were included. From 1978 to 1983 the BEH approved the establishment of eight single-State Centers and eight multi-Centers for a total of 16 Centers for deaf–blind children providing services in all 50 States and Territories. Figure 4.1 shows the areas covered by these 16 Centers.

These Centers worked closely with BEH and carried out national goals and objectives established by the Bureau. The co-ordinators of those

Figure 4.1: Sixteen Centers for Deaf–Blind Children, 1978-83

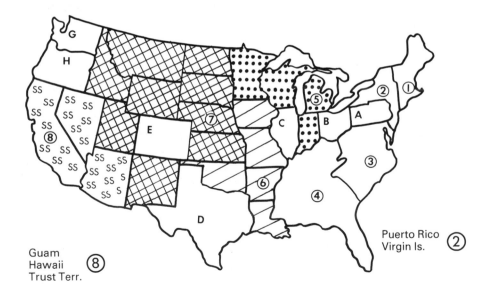

Key:
A-H Single-State Centers

1. New England
2. Mid-Atlantic
3. South Atlantic
4. South-east
5. Midwest
6. South Central
7. Mt. Plains
8. South-west

Centers first funded in 1969, and during the past 14 years, are to be commended for their untiring efforts to co-ordinate resources at the State and local level that would assure a full continuum of services for deaf–blind children and their parents. By 1980 the Centers established more than 300 programmes for deaf–blind children with public and private educational institutions under subcontract agreements to assure delivery of the following services to 5,998 deaf–blind children: comprehensive diagnostic and evaluative services; educational and training programmes including the integration of all necessary professional allied services; continuous in-service training and technical assistance to teachers and others who play direct roles in the lives of these children.

The Centers have also been involved in the development and demonstration of new educational or alternative programmes: in-service training for parents, professionals and allied personnel; dissemination of materials and information about practices found effective in working with deaf–blind children; and child-find activities including the maintenance of a registry.

Significant demographic data were collected by the Centers for the 1979-80 programme year and a summary of that data and its implications for planning educational and long-term rehabilitation services follows. Important questions are raised throughout for consideration by persons at State, local and national levels who are responsible for planning education and rehabilitation services for the deaf–blind population.

Achievements of the Centers in 1979-80

As Table 4.1 indicates, 5,998 children were provided with educational services; 5,022 of these were enrolled in full-time educational programmes which also provided pre-vocational/vocational instruction to 1,185 of them. Another 696 children were enrolled in part-time educational programmes, while 69 of those children received pre-vocational/vocational instruction. And 280 children were provided with itinerant home services until they could be placed in full or part-time educational programmes. During the summer, some 2,136 children benefited from summer service programmes which, for the more severely handicapped deaf–blind child, served as an extended school year programme.

Table 4.2 shows that, of 5,998 children located, 4,958 had received educational reassessments and 1,519 were provided with initial medical and educational evaluations. The total exceeds 5,998 due to double counting of some children. The educational programme placement of the 5,998 children is shown in Table 4.3.

Demographic Data

The geographic distribution of an estimated 6,117 deaf–blind children for 1980-1 is shown in Figure 4.2. The estimated total reflects a modest

Table 4.1: Educational Services for Deaf–Blind Children, 1979-80

Service categories	Single-state centres	Multi-state centres	Total
Educational services			
1. Full-time (not emphasising pre-voc/voc)	833	3,004	3,837
2. Full-time (emphasising pre-voc/voc)	361	824	1,185
3. Part-time (not emphasising pre-voc/voc)	199	428	627
4. Part-time (emphasising pre-voc/voc)	30	39	69
5. Home services	77	203	280
Totals	**1,500**	**4,498**	**5,998**
6. Summer services	431	1,705	2,136

Table 4.2: Medical Diagnostic and Educational Evaluation Services, 1979-80

Service categories	Single-state centres	Multi-state centres	Total
Medical diagnosis and educational evaluation			
1. Identification	246	1,273	1,519
2. Periodic reassessment	1,212	3,746	4,958
Total	**1,458**	**5,019**	**6,477**

Table 4.3: Educational Placements for Deaf–Blind Children, 1979-80

Service categories	Single-state centres	Multi-state centres	Total
A. Residential services			
1. Residential schools	191	913	1,104
2. State institutions for retarded	452	1,672	2,124
3. Group homes	15	169	184
Subtotal	658	2,754	3,412
B. Day schools	—	—	2,586
Total	**658**	**2,754**	**5,998**

increase of the 5,998 children located in 1979-80. The data in Figure 4.2 reveal that 38 per cent of the deaf–blind children (2,341) are located in six States — California (597), New York (536), Texas (522), Ohio (249), New Jersey (223) and Michigan (214). Another 33 per cent (2,039) are located in 14 States with the number in each State ranging from a low of 108 to a high of 199. A total of 4,380 deaf–blind children (71 per cent) reside in only 20 States. The remaining 1,737 children (28 per cent) are distributed among 36 States and Territories as shown in Figure 4.2.

Figure 4.2: Estimated Number of Deaf–Blind Children, 1980-1

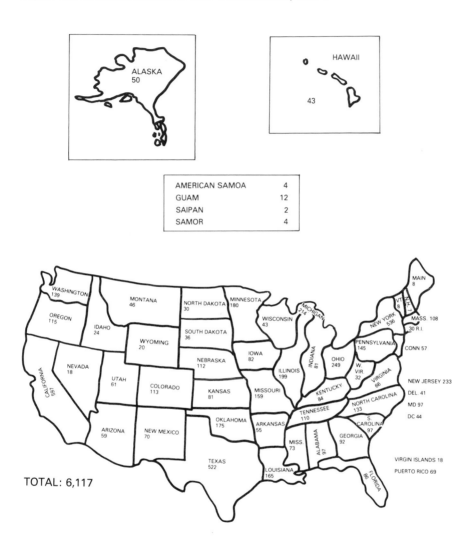

Figure 4.3 shows the age distribution of 5,990 deaf–blind children reported by the Centers in February of 1980. The graph indicates that, of the 5,990 children reported, there are 1,317 children (or 22 per cent) whose age ranges (15–17) coincide with the 1963-5 Rubella epidemic period. The significant number of children indicated as 14 years of age (556) suggests that perhaps many of those children born in 1966 may have been victims of the Rubella epidemic as it ran its course late in 1965. Regardless of aetiology, this graph clearly suggests the amount of time remaining for each of the 5,990 children in the educational system before they reach age 21 and exit into the realm of rehabilitation services.

Figure 4.3: Age Distribution of Deaf–Blind Children Served, February 1980. Total Children: 5,990.

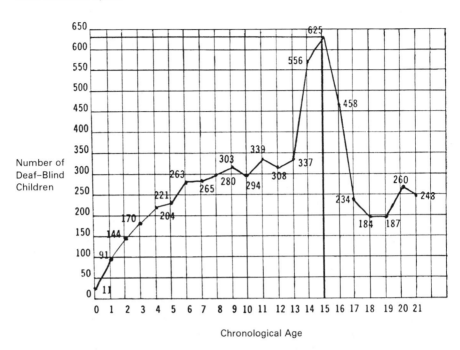

Chronological Age

The graph also reveals that only 620 children between the ages of zero and four had been identified in 1980 suggesting that the child-find efforts of the States mandated by Public Law 94-142 (the Education for all Handicapped Children Act, 1975), as well as the efforts of the Centers, had diminished over the period from 1975 to 1980 resulting in a level number of about 6,000 deaf–blind children reported over those years.

As for the number of children reaching age 21 and exiting from educational programmes, the graph indicates the alarming number of deaf–blind youths who, from 1986 to 1988, will need rehabilitation services, vocational training and job placement services and alternative programmes and settings ranging from independent living centres to total dependence centres which will provide lifelong services for the most severely handicapped deaf–blind person. During this period there will be an average of 546 school-leavers per year, more than twice the number who entered vocational rehabilitation during the period from 1981 to 1985.

The following questions must be asked and answered by responsible officials, educators and rehabilitators at the local, State and Federal levels: Will we be prepared to provide the essential rehabilitative and lifetime services needed for these clients after they reach age 21? If we are not prepared, will they ultimately be placed in State institutions for the retarded for the remainder of their lives? It should be evident that the early and timely linkage between educational service programmes, and State vocational rehabilitation agencies or Commissions for the Blind is critical if the transition from educational services to rehabilitative services is to be successful. To achieve this goal, it is essential for all special educators and rehabilitation counsellors to work together, both in the classroom and in rehabilitation facilities, to develop the multitude of services that may be needed for the lifetime of many deaf–blind persons.

Adult Rehabilitation Services

In recognition of this need to bridge the gap between educational and rehabilitation services, the Bureau, in 1973-4, approved the development of eight pilot projects to be implemented by certain Centers for planning pre-vocational and vocational services for deaf–blind children. In 1974-5, these projects were completed and resulted in the following products: a two-volume 'Pre-Career Curriculum Guide for Deaf–Blind' and a 'Deaf–Blind Pre-Vocational Course', for teachers in training developed by the San Francisco State University and co-ordinated with the pre-vocational training programme of the California School for the Blind; 'A practical Guide to Prevocational Activities for Deaf–Blind Children', developed by Oak Hill School for the Blind, Hartford, Connecticut which introduces the deaf–blind child to experiences a normal child naturally encounters. This guide was also designed to serve as a logical sequel to a previous guide designed by Oak Hill entitled 'A Practical Guide To The Training of Low-Functioning Deaf–Blind Children'. The Mountain-Plains Center developed a comprehensive manual entitled 'A Cognitive Approach to Pre-vocational and Daily Living Skills Training' for deaf–blind children.

In addition, model programmes were established in some Centers such as: a community residence programme for deaf–blind adolescents at Perkins School for the Blind; a pre-vocational training project at the Central Wisconsin Center for Developmental Disabilities which used senior citizens as role models for deaf–blind students to replicate their social and work behaviour patterns; the Southwest Regional Deaf–Blind Center developed an on-the-job training programme with McDonald's fast food franchise, and a video tape entitled 'Earning Our Own Way' was produced and is shown as part of McDonald's training programme for managers and personnel around the country.

Around the nation, as they developed curricula materials, programmes for deaf–blind children also focused on the inclusion of structured task-orientated skills with prescribed goals and objectives in the pre-vocational/vocational area. The goal was to facilitate the transition of children from educational to rehabilitative services. Thus, by 1980 some 1,254 out of 5,998 deaf–blind children were enrolled in educational programmes which emphasized pre-vocational/vocational skills training.

Educators of deaf–blind children have long realized that no single curriculum developed by a particular programme is applicable to every deaf–blind child. As a result, the Bureau established a goal for Centers to develop Individualized Educational Plans (IEP) for each deaf–blind child, unique to the needs of that child. This goal preceded by at least two years the 1975 mandate to the States under Public Law 94-142 to establish IEPs for all handicapped children. Thus, many deaf–blind programmes developed curricula materials to meet the general needs of the children they served and then developed IEP's to meet the specific needs of a particular child. As deaf–blind programmes developed their own curriculum guide, they adopted an eclectic approach and drew from existing curricula and guides from the fields of blind, deaf, retarded, multiple-handicapped, orthopaedically handicapped, and the deaf–blind. Such guides were modified and adapted to meet the needs of the deaf–blind child so that the works and effort of many disciplines may be evidenced in any particular deaf–blind curriculum reviewed by a teacher. One of the Centers compiled more than 60 curricula or guides on a 1975 document entitled 'Curricula For The Deaf–Blind — An Annotated Bibliography of Curriculum Development Materials Relevant to the Education of Deaf–Blind Children'.

Implications of Demographic Data for Planning Educational and Rehabilitative Services

A review of the educational placements of these 5,998 children reveals that they are placed in three types of settings; State residential institutions for the retarded; day school programmes; and residential schools for the deaf, or the blind child. The 300 programmes in these settings may consist of a single deaf–blind child in a day school classroom, to one or more deaf–blind children in a classroom for deaf children or other multi-handicapped children, or a special class designed for deaf–blind children in an institution, or in integrated classrooms in an institutional setting; to specialized programmes or departments in schools for the blind.

The implications of the three types of educational placements for planning services for this population while they are currently served and as they reach age 21 and exit from the educational system are presented for the consideration of service providers at all levels.

State Institutions for the Retarded

With 2,124 deaf–blind children in State institutions, their deinstitutionalization was recognized as a high national priority by Public Law 94-142 in 1975. An intensified effort was made by the Centers from 1977 to 1980 resulting in the deinstitutionalization of more than 300 deaf–blind children to alternative programmes developed in the community. The programme placements included group homes, foster home services, surrogate parents, community residence programmes, and transitional community-based training programmes with home-like settings located on the grounds of a residential school or a State institution.

Service providers at institutions and responsible advocacy organizations, and the parents must persist in their efforts to stimulate State, local and Federal awareness on the need to plan for and provide alternative programmes and services which will permit institutionalized deaf–blind children the opportunity to enter their rightful place in the open community. To achieve this goal we must plan now to develop and train the variety of personnel who will be needed to provide lifetime services and placements for these severely handicapped children and youths. We must also prepare the community, including the multitude of service providers who will have an impact upon the lives of these deaf–blind individuals, in order to increase their acceptance by the community.

Day School Programmes

The placement of 2,586 out of 5,998 deaf–blind children in public or day school programmes by the Centers was a significant achievement which demonstrated long before the 1975 mandate of Public Law 94-142 that such severely handicapped children could be placed in the least restrictive environment. However, this accomplishment should not diminish our concern for those deaf–blind children presently enrolled in day school programmes. For these children, teachers and parents must determine the following: Are the services provided sufficient to meet their changing needs, especially as they enter adolescence? Are essential support services available to parents to help them cope with emotional and behavioural problems as children enter adolescence? Is the education provided based on the assumption that a child's vision and hearing will remain constant throughout the child's lifetime? Will there be a need for certain of these children to be placed in a residential setting?

Residential School Programmes

The same concerns expressed above apply to 1,104 deaf–blind children in residential schools for the deaf or for the blind, and departments for deaf–blind children. Additionally, we must determine what ongoing support services are provided for the parents of these children to assure a continued place for the child with their family — not only for the summer, but also for that moment when educational services terminate at the age of 21. The severity of the handicaps of these children, just as for those in State institutions, may require lifetime care and treatment; will the services, and trained personnel, be there when needed?

Most importantly for all these children, regardless of their educational placement, it is essential there be a linkage between the educational system and rehabilitation system so that the teacher and rehabilitation counsellor can work together to develop a long-term educational/rehabilitative work plan to assure a smooth transition from one service mode to the other; and to match the educational curriculum to the potential work skills and adult-living skills needed by deaf−blind persons so they are more adequately prepared for vocational training/work orientated programmes after the age of 21.

Work Potential of Deaf−Blind Population

The potential in job training opportunities for deaf−blind youths is directly related to the severity of the combined visual and hearing defects and is compounded by the addition of other physical and/or mental handicaps. Therefore, it is important for the teacher and rehabilitator to work together as early as possible. Both should develop an education and rehabilitation work plan for each deaf−blind individual combining the expertise of the two disciplines for the maximum benefit of the student while he or she is still in the educational system. It is too late to become concerned about the rehabilitation future or work potential of a deaf−blind youth after he leaves the educational system.

It has been estimated by teachers of deaf−blind children that perhaps 60 to 75 per cent of the 5,998 deaf−blind children may be trainable for some minimal-type assembly work or the packaging of products in a fully sheltered workshop setting. Such workshops require continuous super-vision and instruction by trained staff. Where will the trained staff come from and will they be available, when needed?

Perhaps another 5 to 15 per cent of this deaf−blind population may have the capacity to work in competitive or semi-sheltered workshops depending on the severity of their dual sensory loss, the level of their communication skills, mobility and daily living skills, and the absence of other debilitating physical or mental conditions. The Centers have clearly demonstrated that some of these deaf−blind youths were able to participate successfully in employment on a competitive basis. But such success does not happen by chance. The needs for training personnel, preparing the community, service providers and other support agencies, are critical factors if the deaf−blind person is to have an equal opportunity for accept-ance in the community and the right to fail or succeed on his own.

Sources of Demographic Data

Demographic data on the deaf−blind children's population are collected by the following: each State education agency is required to maintain a child count on all deaf−blind and other handicapped children under Public Law

94-142 and Title I of Public Law 89-313; so is each Deaf–Blind Center: in 1984 these now number as many as 26, mostly single-State Centers; and the Helen Keller National Center for Deaf–Blind Youths and Adults (HKNC) is responsible for a registry on deaf–blind adults, and in recent years also collected and centralized data for the children in collaboration with the regional and single-State Centers.

These data are available on a State-by-State basis as well as on a programme-by-programme basis within each State. No matter how incomplete the information might be, it is the best available at this time for planning purposes and provides the following minimal information: the number of deaf–blind children aged 5 to 21 enrolled in educational and institutional programmes; the number of children aged 0 to 5 for those States mandated under their own regulations and/or Public Law 94-142 to serve this pre-school age group; the location and type of programmes; the age breakdown for the known population; and, on a programme basis, information based on the Individualized Educational Plan (IEP) for monitoring the progress of each child as required under PL 94-142, and for determining the effectiveness of the child's programme and its components.

This minimal information is sufficient for those responsible agencies at the State, local and Federal levels to plan now in order to assure that the rehabilitative services needed from 1986 to 1988 for some 546 deaf–blind youths per year are in place before the need arises, or reaches a crisis proportion. To achieve this goal, the following additional information is needed for each State:

What existing rehabilitative facilities are available to provide needed services for these deaf–blind youths and adults?

What modifications must be made to the physical plant or to the programme itself to make it possible to include the deaf–blind person in that programme's case load?

What are the manpower needs of these facilities to make it possible for them to serve the deaf–blind client? What kind of training can be provided for existing staff so they can work with the deaf–blind client; or, will we need to train new and more specialized personnel especially where the more severely handicapped deaf–blind person is concerned?

How will the needs of the more severely disabled deaf–blind person be provided for after age 21 and after it is realized they cannot be served by existing rehabilitation facilities or programmes?

What other programme alternatives, facilities and resources must be planned for and developed, before these youths reach age 21 so that they are not automatically placed in State institutions? Do these options consider the need for lifelong services for those individuals who will not have the capacity to 'make it' in the traditional sheltered or semi-sheltered workshop setting?

What agency or agencies at the State level will take the responsibility for co-ordinating the needed resources at the local levels to serve these deaf–blind persons?

What will be the economic cost related to these rehabilitative services and programmes; the training of new and existing manpower to meet the varied needs of this population; and the development and construction of new facilities or modification of existing ones that may be needed for the lifelong programme and services required for many of these persons?

Since the inception of the Centers in 1969, they have worked in co-operation with the Special Education Program (formally BEH and OSE), and the State and local education agencies to resolve the educational crisis for deaf–blind children brought about by the Rubella epidemic. We have learned from this experience that other causes besides Rubella account for more than 70 per cent of the 5,998 children located by the Centers. The 'educational crisis' has always existed for deaf–blind children since there has never been a time when sufficient educational facilities and trained personnel have been available to meet their needs on an ongoing basis.

The Centers have done much to improve the availability of educational programmes for deaf–blind children — with programmes now available for them in every State and the Territories. The right to education has been assured under Public Law 94-142 — the Education for all Handicapped Children Act, which mandates that deaf–blind and all severely handicapped children are entitled to a free and appropriate public education.

The Future of Rehabilitative Services

In 1984, the 'educational crisis' is a 'rehabilitation crisis' as increasing numbers of deaf–blind youngsters reach age 21 and leave the educational system. The availability of timely and relevant rehabilitative services and programmes for these youngsters is uncertain because another 5,000 deaf–blind adults aged 21 and over also need such services.

The use of demographic data currently available on the deaf–blind children's population as well as data being collected for deaf–blind adults by the HKNC is essential if this nation's resources are to be developed in time to meet the rehabilitative needs and lifetime needs of many deaf–blind adults. The use of such data must be an ongoing process in the planning and development of special education and rehabilitative services for deaf–blind people — whether it be for a single programme to be developed or for a national effort.

Leadership must come from the Federal level and in particular from the Office of Special Education and Rehabilitative Services (OSERS) administrators of both Federal programme efforts on behalf of deaf–blind children and youths under the newly enacted Public Law 89-199 'Education of the Handicapped Amendments of 1983', Part C, Section 622 (amended PL 91-230, Dec. 1983); and rehabilitation services for deaf–blind youth and adults as authorised by the Vocational Rehabilitation Act Amendments of 1983.

It is OSER's responsibility to establish national priorities, goals and objectives in co-operation with State and local education and rehabilitation agencies which will ensure the full range of educational, rehabilitative and lifelong services needed for all deaf–blind persons. There is much information available on the deaf–blind population, but the critical challenge seems to be on how to use it effectively to plan and develop alternative educational and rehabilitative services needed for this population on a short- and long-term basis. In 1981, the Special Education Programs (SEP) and the Rehabilitation Services Administration (RSA) in the Office of Special Education and Rehabilitation Services of the Department of Education jointly funded a one-year study to assess the service needs of deaf–blind individuals. The study examined educational and rehabilitative services available to deaf–blind persons throughout the United States and identified gains made in the services being provided for this group as well as significant areas in which needs were unmet or inadequately met.

The study, entitled the 'Needs Assessment of Services to Deaf–Blind Individuals', makes the following suggestions to SEP and RSA to assist them in planning future policies to improve educational and rehabilitative services for deaf–blind persons.

The federal government should assume the responsibility for annually determining the size and characteristics of the deaf–blind population.

A continued federal presence is desirable in the education of deaf–blind children and youth.

Encourage States to co-ordinate deaf–blind services at a decision-making level within their hierarchy of social services.

Programs for deaf–blind children's parents should be established to provide them with education and respite care, two areas now seriously lacking.

Every State needs to establish and maintain vision and hearing conservation programs, especially for persons who already have sensory impairments.

A federal program of job development and job placement is urgently needed to supplement the efforts of State Vocational Rehabilitation agencies and Commissions for the Blind.

Increased attention should be given to developing independent-living and alternate-living programs for deaf–blind adults.

Research efforts must be funded to identify, invent, and evaluate new methods for overcoming the disadvantages of deaf–blindness.

Federal support to recreational programs and services for deaf–blind persons should be increased.

The nature of the deaf–blind population demands that a concerted effort be made to provide elder care.

The assistance of deaf–blind consumers should be sought in planning all programs specifically directed at serving them.

Extend educational support for deaf–blind students from the present upper-age limit of 21 years up to 25 years of age (pp. ii-iii).

Now is the time for us to do what must be done at all levels of society and government to assure a better future on behalf of deaf–blind people throughout this nation.

Further Reading

A Cognitive Approach to Prevocational and Daily Living Skills Training (1975) Mountain Plains Regional Center for Services to Deaf–Blind Children

Carr, C., Zemalis C. and Evans, W. *Pre-Career Curriculum Guide for Deaf–Blind — Parts I and II* Southwestern Regional Center for Deaf–Blind

Community Residence Training Program Curriculum (1975) Perkins School for the Blind, Watertown, Massachusetts

Curricula for the Deaf–Blind. An Annotated Bibliography of Curriculum Development Materials Relevant to the Education of Deaf–Blind Children (1973) Mid-Atlantic North and Caribbean Regional Center for Services to Deaf–Blind Children, New York Institute for the Education of the Blind

Dantona, R. (1974a) 'Deaf–Blind Population: Implications for Rehabilitation', *Journal of Rehabilitation of the Deaf, 8* (1), 65–8

—— (1974b) 'Demographic Data, and Status of Services for Deaf-Blind Children in the United States' in Carl Sherrick (ed.), *1980 is now*, A conference on the future of deaf–blind children, John Tracy Clinic, pp. 25–33

—— (1980), Demographic Data For Planning Of Services For Deaf–Blind Persons: Implications For Special Education And Rehabilitation' in E.G. Wolf (ed.), *Proceedings The 1980's Partnership in Planning for Progress, Delivery of Services to Deaf–Blind Persons.* New York Institute for the Education of the Blind, pp. 8–17

—— and Salmon, Peter J. (1972) 'The Current Status of Services for Deaf–Blind Persons', *The New Outlook, 66* (3)

Lockett, T. and Rudolph, J. (1980) 'Deaf–blind children with maternal rubella: Implications for adult services', *American Annals of the Deaf, 125* (8) 968–76

Stuckless, R. (ed.) (1980) *Deafness and Rubella: Infants in the Sixties; Adults in the Eighties*, Report of a National Conference, Rochester, New York. National Technical Institute for the Deaf

Walsh, Sara R. and Holzberg, Robert (eds.) (1981) *Understanding and Educating the Deaf–Blind/Severely and Profoundly Handicapped. An International Perspective*, Charles C. Thomas, Springfield, Ill

Wolf, Enid G., Delk, Marcus T. Jr. and Schein, Jerome D. (1982). *Needs Assessment of Services to Deaf–Blind Individuals.* Redex, Inc. Rehabilitation and Education Experts, Inc., 1110 Fidler Lane, Suite 821, Silver Spring, Maryland 20910. Project funded under Contract No. 300-81-0426, jointly funded by Rehabilitation Services Administration and Special Education Programs, US Department of Education.

APPENDIX TO PART ONE: MENTAL HANDICAP REGISTERS: DATA ON COMMUNITY-BASED CLIENTS WHO HAVE SENSORY IMPAIRMENTS

David Ellis

Introduction

In recent years a number of reports have been published indicating the relatively raised prevalence of sensory impairments found in mental handicap populations (see Chapters 1 and 2). The two national British surveys by Ellis (1982) and by Kropka and Williams (1982) produced clear evidence of the raised prevalence but only for institutional populations. These data leave open the possibility that the raised prevalences within institutions might be due to a greater tendency to 'dump' sensorily handicapped retardates into institutions. The evidence from the community-based survey carried out by Mittler and Preddy (1981), however, suggested that community-based prevalences of sensory handicaps are similar to those in institutional populations.

It is always valuable to replicate population surveys, in order to validate earlier results. Yet community-based surveys are costly procedures. Moreover, a third component to be explored in this area, the prevalence of combined visual and hearing handicaps, was not available from the Mittler and Preddy survey.

The Case Register Study

The recent development in the United Kingdom of a larger number of mental handicap case registers, many of which have made good use of micro-computer technology, has provided a rich source of data on local mental handicap populations. This study sought the opportunity to approximate a community-based survey by asking for relevant data from several registers and pooling these. A list of case registers was compiled from various sources, and those registers reported to be still under development were excluded. Eventually 14 registers were contacted by letter during October and November 1983. The letter described the purpose of the enquiry, as summarized above, and asked register organizers to provide raw data summaries of the total case list, subcategorized in terms of age and dependency level (i.e. mild, moderate, severe or profound mental handicap). Separate summaries of all residents living *outside* National Health Service provision were also requested for each set of categories. Respondents were asked to show the co-occurrence of visual impairments and hearing impairments in a 2 × 2 table. Explicit definitions of sensory impairments were not imposed, in order to help limit the risk of incompatibility with the categories used by the registers. Instead, a simple two-part classification was suggested (e.g. 'blind' or 'partial sight'). The combined results obtained have the status of a 'straw poll', subject to the operational limitations experienced by each register, rather than a statistically rigorous population survey.

Results

Of the 14 registers approached, 6 usable responses were received. The resulting data are displayed in Tables A to C.

Discussion

While it is inappropriate to draw firm conclusions from the data provided, some broad trends can be observed. In Table A no children with sensory impairments under five years are reported. The reason for this is not clear and is contrary to what might be expected. More blind clients are reported in the younger age groups, and less in the older age groups than among the 'total' client populations. The opposite trend is found among deaf clients, most notably the larger proportion of older deaf people.

The interaction between visual and hearing impairments is also shown in Table A. In spite of the small numbers of clients involved, it is interesting that between one-quarter and one-third of clients with hearing handicaps also have visual handicaps. This range is broadly consistent with that noted in Chapter 3, although the wide variation between registers gives some cause for concern.

Table B carries data on level of dependency (in terms of degree of mental handicap or, in the case of the Sheffield Register, in terms of an aggregate of particular dependency characteristics). There is wide variation between registers in terms of the number of clients for whom no rating was available. Even so there is some evidence that blind clients are likely to be rated as more dependent than the 'total' client population, while deaf clients seem less likely to be rated as dependent. Reasons for these variations remain to be identified.

Finally some comparisons between community-based and hospital-based clients are available from three registers, as shown in Table C. The NHS populations have prevalences of visual and hearing handicaps broadly similar to those found in the two national surveys described in Chapters 1 and 2. By comparison the percentages for deafness and blindness in the community are relatively less, although still substantially larger than the prevalences found for these impairments in the normal population. The figures for partial loss of function, however, are much higher, and this must prompt the question, to what extent are 'partial' cases likely to be more seriously impaired than they appear to be? The 'community' data are certainly inconsistent with those found by Mittler and Preddy (1981) for

Table A: Mental Handicap Registers: Age Distributions and Co-occurrence of Sensory Impairments in Community-based Clients

Register		Age 0-4 No.	%	5-16 No.	%	17-29 No.	%	30-59 No.	%	60+ No.	%	Vision X Hearing	All No.	(D + Ph) %
	Total	23	3	157	24	213	32	223	33	53	8	D + B	—	
	B	—		2	25	4	50	2	25	—		D + Ps	—	
Salford	Ps	—		8	17	20	42	18	38	2	4	Ph + B	—	26.5
	D	—		1	17	2	33	2	33	1	17	Ph + Ps	9	
	Ph	—		12	43	9	32	5	18	2	7	All	9	
	Total	12	3	95	23	164	39	135	32	13	3	D + B	1	
	B	—		4	50	2	25	2	25	—		D + Ps	1	
Trafford	Ps	—		3	50	2	33	1	17	—		Ph + B	—	
	D	—		3	50	2	33	1	17	—		Ph + Ps	2	30.8
	Ph	—		3	43	2	29	2	29	—		All	4	
	Total	10	2	119	22	216	40	160	30	31	6	D + B	4	
Kensington,	B	—		6	46	5	39	2	15	—		D + Ps	4	
Chelsea and	Ps	—		29	32	33	36	21	23	9	10	Ph + B	1	42.6
Westminster	D	—		3	19	4	25	6	38	3	19	Ph + Ps	14	
	Ph	—		10	26	10	26	12	32	6	16	All	23	
	Total	9	3	88	31	96	34	74	26	14	5	Ph + Ps	1	
Islington	Ps	—		5	36	7	50	2	14	—	—			33.3
	Ph	—		—	—	2	67	1	33	—	—	All	1	
	Total	8	1	204	23	323	37	278	32	70	8	D + B	—	
South	B	—		4	20	6	30	8	40	2	10	D + Ps	—	
Glamorgan	Ps	—		5	6	18	22	33	40	27	33	Ph + Ps	—	5.6
	D	—		—	—	2	20	4	40	4	40	Ph + Ps	3	
	Ph	—		2	5	12	27	12	27	18	41	All	3	
	Total	62	2	663	24	1012	36	870	31	181	7	D + B	5	
Sum of	B	—		16	33	17	35	14	29	2	4	D + Ps	5	
Five	Ps	—		50	21	80	33	75	31	38	16	Ph + B	1	25.3
Registers	D	—		7	18	10	26	13	34	8	21	Ph + Ps	29	
	Ph	—		27	23	35	29	32	27	26	22	All	40	

Register		0-4 No.	%	5-15 No.	%	16-24 No.	%	25-44 No.	%	45-64 No.	%	65+ No.	%	Vision X Hearing	All No.	(D + Ph) %
	Total	80	3	895	28	1041	33	660	21	334	11	157	5	D + B	—	
	B	2	14	8	57	1	7	2	14	1	7	—	—	D + Ps	3	
Sheffield	Ps	4	4	24	27	22	25	24	27	10	11	5	6	Ph + B	1	16.9
	D	—		5	33	2	13	2	13	4	27	2	13	Ph + Ps	6	
	Ph	—		6	14	9	21	12	27	8	18	9	21	All	10	

Notes: Total = All clients on Register
B = Blind
Ps = Partial sight
D = Deaf
Ph = Partial hearing
All = All clients with *two* sensory impairments

Table B: Mental Handicap Registers: Distribution of Dependency in Community-based Clients with Sensory Impairments

Register		Dependency								Total
		Mild		Moderate		Severe and Profound		Not known		
		No.	%*	No.	%*	No.	%*	No.	(%)	No.
	Total	21	3	133	22	456	75	59	(9)	669
	B	—	—	—		7	100	1	(13)	8
Salford	Ps	—	—	11	24	34	76	3	(6)	48
	D	—	—	2	40	3	60	1	(17)	6
	Ph	—	—	3	13	20	87	5	(18)	28
	Total	198	45	69	16	171	39	98	(18)	536
Kensington,	B	3	25	1	8	8	67	1	(8)	13
Chelsea and	Ps	27	33	16	20	38	47	11	(12)	92
Westminster	D	8	53	1	7	6	40	1	(6)	16
	Ph	13	34	5	13	20	53	—	—	38
	Total	8	24	12	35	14	41	247	(88)	281
Islington	Ps	—	—	4	40	6	60	4	(29)	14
	Ph	—	—	1	50	1	50	1	(33)	3
	Total	42	31	2	2	93	68	746	(85)	883
South	B	—	—	—	—	9	100	11	(55)	20
Glamorgan	Ps	5	25	—	—	15	75	63	(76)	83
	D	1	33	—	—	2	67	7	(70)	10
	Ph	2	29	—	—	5	71	37	(84)	44
	Total	269	22	216	18	734	60	1150	(49)	2369
Sum of Four	B	3	11	1	4	24	86	13	(32)	41
Registers	Ps	32	21	31	20	93	60	81	(34)	237
	D	9	39	3	13	11	48	9	(28)	32
	Ph	15	21	9	13	46	66	43	(38)	113

Sheffield		'WESSEX' SPI Ratings								
		I/II		III		IV		Not known		
		No.	%	No.	%	No.	%	No.	%	
	Total	758	57	243	18	339	25	1827	(58)	3167
	B	1	7	1	7	12	86			14
	Ps	20	23	33	37	36	40			89
	D	4	27	3	20	8	53			15
	Ph	25	57	11	25	8	18			44

Notes: Total = All clients on Register
  B   = Blind
  Ps = Partial sight
  D   = Deaf
  Ph = Partial hearing
  %* = percentage calculated excludes 'Not known'
  (%) = percentage of TOTAL column

Table C: Mental Handicap Registers: Comparison between Community-based and Hospital-based Clients with Sensory Impairments

Register		Community clients		NHS clients	
		No.	%	No.	%
	Total	669		255	
	B	8	1.2	14	5.5
Salford	Ps	48	7.2	14	5.5
	D	6	0.9	10	3.9
	Ph	28	4.2	13	5.1
	Total	419			
	B	8	1.9		
Trafford	Ps	6	1.4		
	D	6	1.4		
	Ph	7	1.7		
	Total	536		393	
Kensington,	B	13	2.4	26	6.6
Chelsea and	Ps	92	17.2	49	12.5
Westminster	D	16	3.0	16	4.1
	Ph	38	7.1	44	11.2
	Total	281			
Islington	Ps	14	5.0		
	Ph	3	1.1		
	Total	883			
South	B	20	2.3		
Glamorgan	Ps	83	9.4		
	D	10	1.1		
	Ph	44	5.0		
	Total	2788			
Sum of Five	B	49	1.8		
Registers	Ps	243	8.7		
	D	33	1.4		
	Ph	120	4.3		
	Total	3167		600	
	B	14	0.4	32	5.3
Sheffield	Ps	89	2.8	36	6.0
	D	15	0.5	15	2.5
	Ph	44	1.4	19	3.2

Notes: Total = All clients on Register
B = Blind
Ps = Partial sight
D = Deaf
Ph = Partial hearing

children and young adults in a community-based survey. One reason for the lower prevalence rates may be the types of ascertainment procedures used by registers to identify clients and then to collect information about them. This seems likely to be a more difficult task in the community than in hospital settings, and may require a fairly complex organization to ensure a good response.

Acknowledgements

The compilation of these data was made possible by the kindness and goodwill of the organizers of registers who contributed material for the Appendix. I am most grateful to them for their help. Listed below are the Registers which contributed material, plus explanatory commentaries and annotations which accompanied each set of data.

Salford Case Register

Maureen Douglas
Salford Area Health Authority
Pendleton House, Broughton Road, Salford

Data reported as at December 1983. These data cover clients who were included in the 31 December 1983 census as having been in contact with the mental handicap services. Assessment of clients was carried out using a schedule devised by Dr Lorna Wing. Not all clients have been assessed yet and younger clients were given a lower priority for assessment. Most data concentrates on those in hospital or other residential care.

Dependency categories are defined as follows:	Mild	= IQ 70–90
	Moderate	= IQ 50–70, ESN(M)
	Severe/Profound	= IQ under 50, ESN(S)

Sensory impairments were identified by ratings of primary care personnel (nurses, teachers, parents, etc.). Vision was rated with spectacles on, and hearing rated with hearing aid, if these were usually worn. No detailed medical examinations were used, so 'partial' impairments, in particular, may be underestimated.

Trafford Mental Handicap Register

Dr. R. Lightup
Borough of Trafford Social Services Department
Warbrick House, Washway Road, Sale M33 1DJ

There are 565 people on the Register, but so far detailed assessments have been carried out on only a small percentage of them. The handicaps identified are those diagnosed by the community mental handicap team.

Kensington Chelsea and Westminster Mental Handicap Register

Mrs Jennifer Rohde, Register Organizer
Westminster Medical School
Department of Community Medicine, 17 Horseferry Road, London SW1P 2AR

Data reported as at 7 November 1983. Catchment area is two central London boroughs. The population is characterized by some unusual patterns of migration; young married couples who leave for the suburbs are replaced by younger singletons looking for, e.g., work or training.

There are many bedsitters, a low fertility rate and high abortion rate. Incomes range from extreme wealth to considerable poverty. Data on under-fives is held provisionally with no assessment completed, so they do not appear, other than in the classification by age. The Register uses the ICD classification of mental handicap, but many raters may still work on the older forms of classification, so there may be some confusion between the 'Moderate' and 'Severe' categories. Guidance notes for raters ask that vision be assessed with spectacles on, if prescribed. This may have been overlooked in some cases and 'partial sight' may include some visual defects which are corrected by spectacles.

Islington Register

Carol Jones, Community & Long Stay Unit
Islington Health Authority
Insurance House, Insurance Street, London WC1X CJB

Register is still under development and consequently only a minority of clients currently on record are living at home or in non-NHS establishments.

South Glamorgan Mental Handicap Register

Sally Pearson, Centre Administrator
Information Co-ordinating Centre
Whitchurch Hospital, Whitchurch, Cardiff CF4 7XB

Most data stored concern admission and assessment of in-patients at Ely Hospital. Clients in contact with Adult Training Centres and ESN schools are also recorded and registration is made only when such client contact is initiated. While the Register uses the ICD coding of mental handicap, a large proportion of data came from past assessments of former in-patients using the following categories: Not Subnormal; Mildly Subnormal, Severely Subnormal. Deaths are reported to the Register only if the client dies while in contact with one of the mental handicap services.

Sheffield Case Register

Trevor Parsons, Head of Register
The Ryegate Centre, Tapton Crescent Road, Sheffield S10 5DD

Data reported as at 30 September 1983.
Dependency categories are based on Kushlick's Social and Physical Incapacity (SPI) ratings. These ratings were made at the client's place of residence, where possible. The Kushlick ratings are defined as follows:

I/II (SPI = 9)	— No significant incontinence, ambulance or behaviour problems;
III (SPI = 5-8)	— Mild incontinence, ambulance or behaviour problems;
IV (SPI = 1-4)	— Severe incontinence, ambulance or behaviour problems.

'Poor Hearing' and 'Poor Vision' were rated with aids on, if supplied.

References

Ellis, D. (1982) 'Visually and mentally handicapped people in institutions. Part 1: Their numbers and needs', *Mental Handicap, 10* (4), 135–7

Kropka, B. and Williams, C. (1982) 'The deaf and partially hearing in mental handicap hospitals in England and Wales: preliminary results of the questionnaire survey. BIMH South Western Division' (unpublished), Royal Western Counties Hospital, Starcross, Devon

Mittler, P. and Preddy, D. (1981) 'Mentally handicapped pupils and school-leavers: a survey in North West England' in B. Cooper (ed.), *Assessing the Handicaps and Needs of Mentally Retarded Children*, Academic Press, London, pp. 33-51

PART TWO

AETIOLOGY AND MEDICAL ASPECTS

5 MEDICAL AND OPHTHALMOLOGICAL ASPECTS OF VISUAL IMPAIRMENT IN MENTALLY HANDICAPPED PEOPLE

Mette Warburg

Introduction

Mentally retarded people rely heavily on their eyesight for understanding their surroundings, and instruction is usually given by showing the mentally retarded clients how things are done and how the components of the world hang together. It is, therefore, important to know whether vision is normal in mentally retarded clients or pupils.

In this chapter, I shall discuss visual impairment in mentally retarded individuals. I shall begin with a survey of what is known about their numbers, and fortunately this has been extensively studied in the Netherlands, Sweden and Denmark.

Thereafter, I shall describe how visual acuity is measured in people who have difficulties talking or who do not talk at all.

It will be noted that the commonest cause of low vision is lack of spectacles and, since the majority of mentally retarded persons can use glasses, the prescription of spectacles is one of the cheapest ways of treating a handicapping condition among multi-handicapped people.

The discussion of the causes of visual impairment among mentally retarded persons is concerned only with the commonest disorders. Among mentally retarded patients there are as many different causes of low vision as in the non-retarded population, but mentally retarded individuals also have a number of rare diseases of the eye, not seen in the general population. These uncommon causes of visual impairment will not be considered here, but are described in the papers listed among the references at the end of this chapter.

Prevalence Studies

Legal blindness (i.e. visual acuity below 6/60 or 20/200 in the best eye) is more than two hundred times more frequent among mentally retarded children than among other children (Warburg, Frederiksen and Rattleff 1979). This was shown in a Danish screening of 7,700 mentally retarded children below 20 years of age. Five per cent of the mentally retarded children had severe visual impairment while this was present in 0.2 per 1,000 of children without mental retardation.

In Sweden 1,000 severely visually impaired mentally retarded persons of all ages were found among a total of 35,000 mentally retarded individuals. This is a mean prevalence of 2.9 per cent (Socialstyrelsen, Sweden 1973). In the general population the highest prevalence is 2 per cent, and this is only observed among old people. There is an exceptional distribution of the ages of the blind mentally retarded because only 49 per cent were over 21 years of age whereas in the general population 90 per cent of all legally blind people are over 20 years old (Goldstein 1974). Both the Swedish and the Danish study indicated that blind mentally retarded children and adolescents probably have an increased mortality.

This presumed high mortality is in good agreement with the high mortality among profoundly mentally retarded patients because one-third of these individuals are legally blind (Iivanainen 1974).

Assessment of Vision

It is astonishing to most nursing, hostel and other staff members to learn about the high frequency of severe visual impairment in their clients, who are often thought to be functioning as well as one could expect, their retardation taken into account. It is rarely appreciated that persons with a visual acuity below 6/60 or 20/200 can find their way about in well-known environments, find their food on the plates, and that children with such low vision can find and play with dolls, teddy bears and large building blocks. Small toys are not given to moderately retarded children because their motor development is retarded, and if speech is absent or deficient it may be difficult to observe that small or distant objects are not seen by the child.

There are several methods by which vision can be assessed even in pre- or non-verbal children. The examiner can point to a picture chart and ask the child to indicate a similar picture on a sheet in front of him (see Figure 5.1) (Hyvärinen, Näsänen and Laurinen 1980). Forced choice preferential looking techniques have also been used with mentally retarded persons (van Hof-van Duin, Mohn and Batenburg 1982; Lennerstrand, Axelson and Andersson 1983; see also Chapter 10, this volume). In this method, the child is placed in front of a sheet with two holes; behind the sheet a striped object is presented in one of the holes, while a neutral object, the colour of the sheet, is placed behind the other hole. An observer who is not told where the striped object is placed must then decide to which side the child is looking. The stripes are moved from one hole to the other and, when the child has seen them, smaller stripes are presented until eventually the child does not look at the stripes more frequently than at the neutral objects. Electrophysiological methods have also been applied to measure the vision, but they demand co-operation; moreover, expensive instruments are usually not available for routine testing of mentally retarded.

The bead test has been widely used (Frenkel and Evans 1980, Richman and Garzia 1983). In this test the patient is invited to eat small sugarbeads

Figure 5.1: Testing visual acuity in a non-verbal child. The child points to a picture similar to that shown by the examiner.

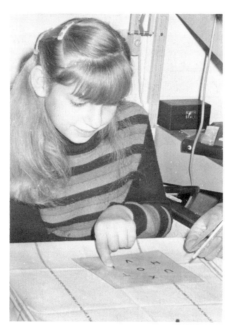

with a diameter ranging from 1 cm to 1 mm. The distance between the sugarbead and the patient is measured (see Figure 5.2).

Errors of Refraction

People whose vision is normal when they wear glasses are excluded from the definition of blindness or severe visual impairment. Mentally retarded persons have difficulties learning to wear glasses, and errors of refraction are frequent among the retarded. This has been shown in a great number of studies of patients from which it appeared that 25 to 40 per cent of mentally retarded patients needed glasses for distant vision. In the general population comparable errors of refractions are only found in 15 per cent. A comparison between the distribution of refraction among mentally retarded persons and other people is shown in Figure 5.3, which demonstrates that large errors of refraction are more common among mentally retarded and that mentally retarded persons are more apt to be hypermetropic than are members of the general population.

Errors of refraction can be measured objectively even in pre- or nonverbal persons, and it has been shown that a majority of those mentally retarded persons who need spectacles are also able to wear them although this may take time to learn (see Table 5.1; Figure 5.4; also Chapter 1 this

Figure 5.2: The bead test. A child with microcephaly reaches out for small sugar beads. The size of the beads and the distance between the table and the eyes of the child are noted.

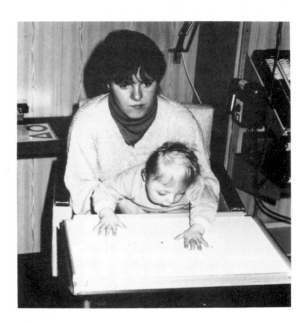

volume). A determination of the need of glasses is, therefore, an important part of the medical checklist in mentally retarded persons, but, unfortunately, very rarely done as a routine.

Old Age

Most people reaching old age need glasses for near-work, whether this means reading, sewing, playing cards or ludo or working in a sheltered workshop, but young persons caring for old mentally retarded patients are often unaware of this need. Glasses for near-work can be prescribed even for patients who co-operate poorly, and it has been shown that they utilize the spectacles well (see Table 5.1).

CAUSES OF SEVERE VISUAL IMPAIRMENT

Severe visual impairment is a visual acuity of no more than 20/200 (6/60) in the best eye *with the best correction with glasses.* In mentally retarded children the most frequent causes of severe visual impairment are: (1) cerebral visual dysfunction; (2) optic atrophy; (3) retinal disorders; (4) cataract, and (5) malformations of the eyes (see Table 5.2). Except for cerebral visual dysfunction, these groups of disorders are also the most prevalent among visually impaired children in the general population, but

Figure 5.3: Distribution of the refractive power of the eye. The refractive power, in diopters, is plotted along the abscissa and the number of patients, in per cent, along the ordinate. People with a refraction between minus 0.9 and plus 1.9 often need no glasses for distance, and such is the case for most people in the ordinary population. High myopia (near sightedness, minus powers) and high hypermetropia (far-sightedness, plus powers) are much more frequent among retarded than among ordinary people.

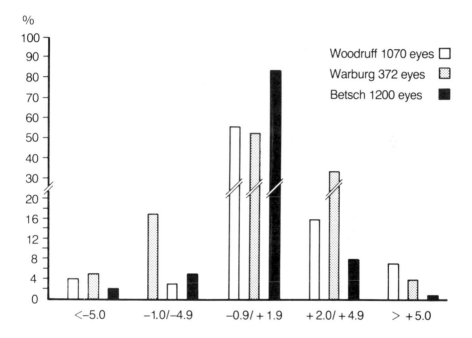

Table 5.1: Continued Use of Spectacles in Mentally Retarded Patients

Degree of MR	Ametropia (no.)	Prescription (no.)	Glasses used 2 years later (no.)
Glasses for distance			
Moderately retarded	27	27	18
Severely retarded	58	54	31
Profoundly retarded	7	4	2
Total	92	85	51
Glasses for near-work			
Moderately retarded	61	50	33
Severely retarded	116	58	40
Profoundly retarded	38	7	2
Total	215	115	75

Source: Warburg (1967).

Figure 5.4: Bifocal glasses worn by a patient with Down's syndrome. It is very common for patients with Down's syndrome and other causes of mental retardation to need glasses. The majority of these individuals can learn to wear not only ordinary spectacles, but also bifocals. This means that the elderly do not have to rely on staff to have their near-vision correction (glasses for near-work) brought to them when necessary.

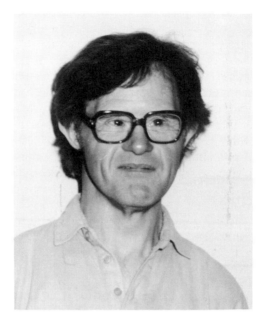

Table 5.2: Main Causes of Visual Impairment in Childhood

	Br. Columbia	New Zealand	The Netherlands		Denmark	
			MR[a]	MN[b]	MR	MN
	%	%	%	%	%	%
Cerebral visual dysfunction					20	
Optic atrophy[c]	19	8.5	27	13	39	19
Retinal disorders[d]	36	12	36	37	15	42
Cataract	17	22.5	16	8	7	9
Malformations	5	11.5	14	24	6	15
Others	23	45.5	7	18	13	15
Total	100	100	100	100	100	100

Nctes: a. MR = mentally retarded.
b. MN = mentally normal.
c. Optic atrophy and cerebral visual dysfunction are lumped together except in the Danish MR series.
d. Retinal disorders include retinopathy of prematurity, all types of tapeto-retinal degenerations and acquired chorio-retinal lesions.
Source: Adapted from Jan, Freeman and Scott (1979) (British Colombia); Sturman (1975) (New Zealand; Schapper-Kimmijser (1975) (The Netherlands); Warburg, Frederiksen and Rattleff (1979) (Denmark).

there are many causes of the conditions, and the causes are not the same in the mentally retarded and the ordinary group of visually impaired children.

Cerebral Visual Dysfunction

Twenty per cent of severely visually impaired mentally retarded children show no visual perception of light or react visually to only very large objects although the eyes appear normal on examination. There are several explanations and causes of this condition. Some educational psychologists hypothesize that these non-verbal children have become discouraged from communicating their visual sensations to the adults because their reactions were ignored. To other observers the explanation is a semantic problem; i.e. the majority of the patients show a developmental age no better than a neonate or even a premature infant and therefore cannot be expected to have a visual performance better than those. Whatever the explanation may be, further development of the children may in some cases lead to an increased performance of the eyesight.

In some cases there is clinical and pathological evidence of localized cerebral damage which explains the visual defect, and there are reports describing acquired, but transient visual cerebral dysfunction (Miller 1982).

Table 5.3 gives a survey of 52 patients with cerebral visual dysfunction. It is evident that the cerebral damage was widespread in all cases. In 12 of the cases, it was so severe that the patients died in childhood. Over the years, some patients showed mild improvement in their visual performance, such as a change from no perception to perception of light, or from perception of light to following 5 cm objects in front of their faces. In other cases, however, the faint visual performance declined over the observation period. It is important to know whether a child who does not see and shows no abnormalities of the eyes has a normal functioning retina. This can be examined by electroretinography (ERG). If ERG shows retinal impairment, improvement of vision cannot be expected.

There is no medical treatment for cerebral visual dysfunction. Teachers for the blind and retarded children direct their activities to areas in which their pupils are able to perform. They play with the children, giving them a chance to produce sounds at their will, invite them to move about and find interesting objects, first using the legs and arms then the feet and hands. The objects used have different smells thereby inviting the curiosity of the children, and play therapy often takes place on a sounding board which enhances the sounds produced by the children and the objects.

Although this does not improve sight, the interest in the physical world may be improved so much that the children begin using what eyesight they have when they handle and examine their toys.

Table 5.3: Mental Retardation and Cerebral Visual Disturbance: Aetiology of Mental Retardation and Change of Visual Performance

Aetiology	No.	Followed up	Visual performance Improvement	Decrease
Malformations of the brain	7	6	2	—
Cardiac arrest (surgery, submersion)	5	5	1	—
Meningitis, encephalitis	6	4	1	1
Perinatal cerebral haemorrhage	5	2	1	—
Postnatal cerebral haemorrhage	2	2	—	1
Accidental poisoning	1	1	—	—
Twin births	5	5	2	1
Low birthweight	1	1	—	—
Hyppsarrhythmia, unknown aetiology	8	8	4	1
Epilepsia, unknown aetiology	8	5	2	1
Other unknown aetiologies	4	3	2	—
Total	52	42	15	5

Source: Warburg (1983).

Optic Atrophy

The prevalence of optic atrophy (OA) is twice as high among mentally retarded as among other blind children (Table 5.4). It is diagnosed ophthalmoscopically when the optic nerve-head is pale, with very few capillaries visible. OA is usually due to lesions behind the eye, located either in the nerve, the chiasm or the central nervous system (CNS), but intraocular lesions may also result in OA. Visual evoked responses (VEP), an electrophysiological examination, may confirm the diagnosis in cases where ophthalmoscopy is equivocal.

Pre- and perinatal lesions.   Among institutionalized mentally retarded patients 16 per cent (Opitz, Kaveggia, Durkim-Stamm and Pendleton 1978) had lesions of the CNS which had occurred pre- or perinatally. Such lesions are often complicated by OA (see Table 5.5). The patients may have small brains (microcephaly), have too much fluid in the ventricles of the brain (hydrocephaly) or other developmental or acquired lesions (trigonocephaly, holoprosencephaly, porencephaly, etc.). Some of these lesions are part of syndromes wherein elements other than the lesions of the CNS are characteristic. Thus patients with defective closure of the skull or vertebral canal can have hydrocephaly as a complication of the hernia-

Table 5.4: Optic Atrophy: The Prevalence of Mental Retardation among Severely Visually Impaired Children (Acuity < 6/60)

	Br. Columbia		The Netherlands		Denmark	
	No.	%	No.	%	No.	%
Mentally retarded	64	54	89	64	118	67
Mentally normal	55	46	57	36	59	33
Total	119		146		177	

Source: The data are derived from Jan, Freeman and Scott (1977) (British Columbia); Schappert-Kimmijser (1975) (The Netherlands); Warburg, Frederiksen and Rattleff (1979) (Denmark).

Table 5.5: Optic Atrophy in Mentally Retarded Children

Aetiology	No.
Pre- and perinatal aetiology	29
Genetic aetiology established or presumed	10
Postnatal aetiology	12
Total	51

Note: Among 353 visually impaired mentally retarded children studied by Bleeker-Wagemakers (1981) 51 had optic atrophy. The table presents a classification of the causes.

tions of the cranial or spinal contents (encephalocele, meningo-myelocele). In other cases the pedigree of the family and clinical studies of the patient and his relatives may indicate other specific hereditary syndromes.

Birth lesions are suspected if there is information about twinning, perinatal respiratory distress or seizures, but infants with prenatal defects — inflammatory, genetic or toxic — may have a lower tolerance of an uncomplicated birth than normal children, and may therefore present respiratory distress or seizures in the first days of life.

Postnatal Lesions. Infections, such as meningitis and encephalitis, can lead to OA, but postnatal injuries, whether non-accidental or due to traffic or other accidents, are also observed as decisive events in children with mental retardation and OA.

Patients with OA are also found among mentally retarded children with seizures, cerebral palsy or hypotonia. Some of these patients have rare metabolic or other genetic syndromes, but in many cases the exact cause of the condition is unknown. Metabolic disorders present as if they were postnatal, because the intra-uterine environment has compensated for the metabolic error or because the deficient enzyme is not normally turned on until after birth. Only few inborn errors of metabolism can be treated today, but the diagnosis is important because a number of these diseases can be diagnosed prenatally, so that the family may have genetic counselling.

Tumours.   Tumours of the brain are very rare in infancy or early child-hood. Mental retardation is, therefore, not commonly caused by intra-cranial tumours, although these may give rise to acquired dementia. The only common type of tumour associated with mental retardation is tuber-ous sclerosis; here the children present with seizures, and the aetiology is often only revealed when small neurofibromata appear around the base of the nose in teenagers. All nervous tissue can become involved, thus also the optic nerve, but OA can also present as a consequence of other intra-cranial localizations of tuberous sclerosis.

Retinal Disorders

There are two important groups of retinal disorders giving rise to visual impairment among mentally retarded individuals, namely the various tapeto-retinal degenerations and retinopathy of prematurity.

Tapeto-retinal Degenerations

Tapeto-retinal degenerations are lesions of the retinal rods, cones and pigment epithelium (see Figure 5.5). There is a substantial number of different genetic and environmental disorders involving these structures. The main group of diseases is called retinitis pigmentosa (RP), itself comprising numerous different diseases and syndromes in which the natural history of visual impairment follows a common pathway.

In RP the patients are night-blind and have restricted visual fields (tunnel vision). A loss of central vision occurs in childhood or later, depending upon the clinical and genetic type of RP. Loss of central vision is accompanied by colour vision anomalies. Bone spicules, i.e. abnormal pigmentations, are seen in the mid-periphery of the retina by ophthal-moscopy, but they may occasionally be absent, in which case attenuation of the retinal vessels and a pale optic nerve may arouse the suspicion.

In some types of tapeto-retinal degenerations, the central part of the retina (the macula) is involved before the mid-periphery. Then night-blind-ness and tunnel vision are initially absent, and impairment of the visual acuity and colour vision anomalies are the first signs. These cases can be recognized by ophthalmoscopic observation of abnormalities in the macula.

The clinical diagnosis can be confirmed by electroretinography (ERG), a method in which the electrical signals produced by the retina are picked up by a contact lens placed on the cornea. It is possible to differentiate macular from peripheral disorders by recording the ERG when the eye is stimulated by light of different wavelengths.

The observed frequency of tapeto-retinal degenerations is almost the same among blind mentally retarded children and blind children from the general population (see Table 5.6), but very few partially sighted mentally retarded children with tapeto-retinal degenerations have been notified as

Figure 5.5: Cross-section of the eye. Most cases of visual impairment are due to lesions of the optic nerve or the retina. Malformations may involve all layers of the eye, and cataracts are located to the lens. The refractive power of the eye depends upon the curvature of the cornea, the size of the lens and the length of the eye, measured from the centre of the cornea to the fovea centralis.

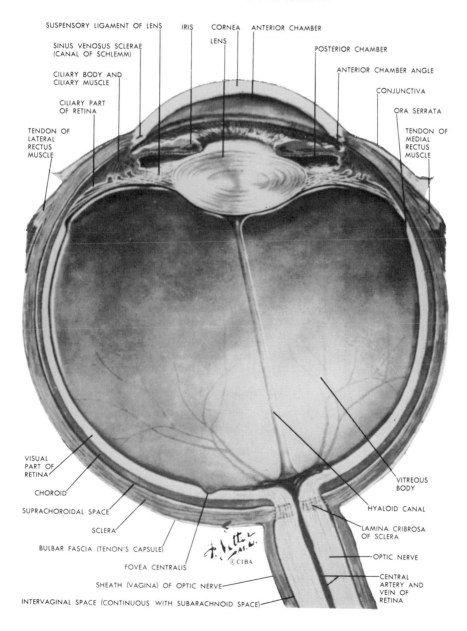

Source: Illustration by Frank H. Netter. From *Clinical Symposia.* Copyright CIBA-GEIGY. Reproduced with permission.

Table 5.6: Tapeto-retinal Degenerations: Prevalence of Mental Retardation Among Severely Visually Impaired Children

	Mentally retarded	Normal	Total
Tapeto-retinal degenerations	78	112	190
All blind children	363	449	812

Source: Adapted from Schappert-Kimmijser (1975).

opposed to the substantial number of partially sighted children without mental handicap who have tapeto-retinal degenerations.

This means that it is quite difficult for the staff to detect incipient RP and other retinal disorders in mentally retarded children. Night-blindness is not observed because the patients are indoors in the evening. Tunnel vision results in a tendency of the children to overturn objects on the table or stumble over things on the floor, but poor motor co-ordination may provide an easy explanation for this behaviour.

Colour vision anomalies can be explained away as a child's lack of understanding colour matching or colour naming. Thus visual impairment is only apparent when it becomes severe, and surveys of visual impairment among mentally retarded persons tend to under-estimate the number of cases with tapeto-retinal degenerations. However, patients with RP will all eventually have severe visual impairment, if they live long enough. The age at which they become blind depends upon the type of RP present.

The main causes of tapeto-retinal degenerations among mentally retarded children are Leber's congenital amaurosis, Batten's disease, and the Bardet-Biedl syndrome (see Table 5.7). These diseases are hereditary, and a diagnosis thus leads to the opportunity for genetic counselling.

Leber's Congenital Amaurosis.　In this disease, all affected children are blind or severely visually impaired from birth. All cases are assumed to be hereditary, but there are many different genetic types of Leber's amaurosis. Non-retarded young adults with Leber's amaurosis frequently have keratoconus (coned-shaped cornea), but otherwise they are healthy. In mentally retarded persons with Leber's amaurosis, nephronophthisis, polycystic kidneys and hearing loss may be observed.

Ophthalmoscopy reveals either a normal retina, or disseminated salt-and-pepper pigmentations, a pallor to the optic nerve-head and attenuated retinal arteries. The ERG is extinguished.

Batten's Disease.　Batten's disease and Leber's amaurosis are equally frequent among mentally retarded blind children (see Table 5.7). The development of Batten's disease is shown in Figure 5.6. The patients are healthy in infancy, but night-blindness and visual impairment begin at three to six years of age, mental retardation and seizures present between six and twelve years, then speech becomes slurred and eventually spoken language

Table 5.7: Tapeto-retinal Degenerations Among Mentally Retarded Children

	1975		1981	
	No.	%	No.	%
Leber's congenital amaurosis	26	31	22	41
Batten's disease	24	29	16	30
Bardet-Biedl syndrome	12	14	8	15
Other types of TRD	22	26	8	15

Note: There are several types of tapeto-retinal degenerations among mentally retarded children. The commonest are tabulated, and it appears that a national study (Schappert-Kimmijser 1975), and a study of patients from an institutions for blind retarded children (Bleeker-Wagemakers 1981) show the same distribution of the disorders in question.

disappears. In late stages the patients loose perception of light and become bedridden and tetraplegic.

The retinal pigmentations are initially observed in the macula, but within the first ten years of life they spread to the entire posterior pole of the eye, and ERG becomes extinguished.

There are abnormal storage products in neuronal and lymphocytic preparations observed in light- or ultramicroscopy, which distinguish Batten's disease from other types of RP. Batten's disease is undoubtedly an inborn error of metabolism, but the defect has not yet been identified.

Bardet–Biedl syndrome. In this hereditary disease, the patients present obesity, hypogenitalism, polydactyly, mild mental retardation and retinal pigmentations (see Figure 5.7). Renal failure and liver dysfunction have been described in some cases, but are rare. The mental retardation is borderline or mild, and these co-operative patients are often educated with visually impaired children and adolescents without intellectual problems. Residual vision is often present until the fourth decade of life or later.

Treatment of Tapeto-retinal Degenerations. Although medical treatment has been claimed to improve tapeto-retinal degeneration, follow-up of the patients has failed to show any effect. Visually impaired mentally retarded children have been mainstreamed in special schools before mainstreaming was introduced for educationally normal blind children, but teachers of sighted mentally retarded children have difficulties assessing mentally retarded children with retinal degenerations when visual acuity is good even though dark adaptation and peripheral vision are impaired. The signs and prognosis of the disorders must, therefore, be explained to staff and parents.

Hearing loss is a complication of some disorders with retinal degeneration, and even mild hearing impairment of 30-40dB is educationally very disadvantageous. The adults must remember to speak directly in front of the children, having their own faces well illuminated. It is important having an audiological examination performed on all visually impaired persons, and especially in mentally retarded persons with retinal degenerations.

Figure 5.6: The natural history of Batten's disease. The figure shows the ages at which the clinical signs have been first observed. The first signs are visual impairment leading to blindness. Seizures may appear at any age, and speech and gait disturbances appear almost simultaneously with mental deficiency.

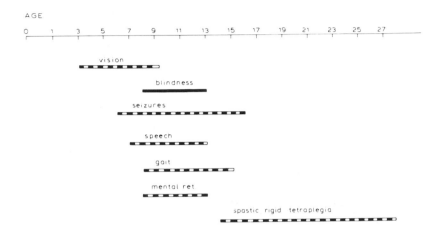

Figure 5.7: Young boy with the Bardet–Biedl syndrome. Ten-year-old boy with obesity and hypogenitalism typical of the Bardet– Biedl syndrome. Most patients have an extra finger or toe, and all have retinitis pigmentosa, i.e. abnormal pigmentations seen in the retina. These are associated with tunnel vision, loss of visual acuity, night-blindness and disturbed colour vision.

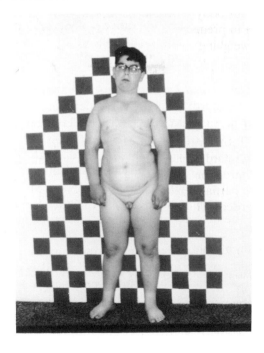

Retinopathy of Prematurity

Retinopathy of prematurity (ROP) was previously termed retrolental fibroplasia because the first cases described had a fibrous plate behind the lens. After it was understood that oxygen treatment of premature infants was one of the most important causative agents, oxygen tension has been kept as low as possible in the incubators where the prematures are supervised. Recent cases have therefore presented a less serious damage with a wrinkling or folding of the retina, but visual impairment becomes severe if the macula is involved or the retina becomes detached.

The prevalence of ROP has not declined over the years, presumably because premature infants with increasingly low birthweights have been carried through; the smallest neonates have the highest risk of ROP.

In 1975 ROP was seen among 10 per cent of 812 blind non-retarded children studied in the Netherlands (Schappert-Kimmijser 1975). Among the blind mentally retarded children the prevalence was almost the same, i.e. 12 per cent, and a study performed six years later (Bleeker-Wagemakers 1981) showed that 9 per cent of 353 blind mentally retarded children had ROP (see Table 5.8). Among blind mentally retarded children with ROP, spastic palsy is common; the patients are often disturbed, and rocking, handflapping and eye manipulations are frequently seen (see Figure 5.8).

Treatment. In most cases treatment is not possible, but some centres are studying the benefit of removal of vitreous strands by vitrectomy, i.e operations on the vitreous body. Prevention of ROP through careful monitoring of oxygen tension in premature babies has reduced the incidence considerably in neonates weighing over 1,000 g at birth.

Cataract

Cataract is found in 14-22 per cent of all legally blind children. In the Netherlands (see Table 5.9) cataract appeared in 20 per cent of all visually impaired mentally retarded children and in 15 per cent of visually impaired without mental retardation. While 67 per cent of the non-retarded children with cataract were partially sighted, this was the case in only 31 per cent of the mentally retarded. This shows that assessment of mentally retarded

Table 5.8: Retinopathy of Prematurity

	Mentally retarded	Normal	Total
ROP	43	36	79
All blind	363	449	812

Source: Adapted from Schappert-Kimmijser (1975).

Figure 5.8: Eye poking in a boy with complete blindness caused by retinopathy of prematurity. The orbits are sunken due to the eye pressing and to atrophy of the globes.

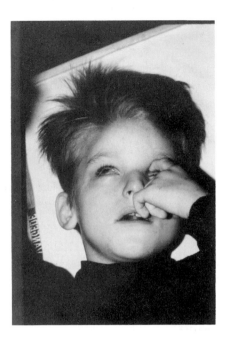

children with mild visual impairment from cataract has been problematic. The Netherlands is the country in which the most comprehensive assessment of visual impairment in the mentally retarded has been performed; in other countries failure of assessment and notification of visual impairment in mentally retarded children is much more pronounced, and the number of mentally retarded children with incipient cataract needs to be studied.

There are many causes of congenital and acquired cataract in mentally retarded children; the main causes are listed in Table 5.10.

Maternal Rubella.   Maternal Rubella in pregnancy has been the single most common cause of congenital cataract, but immunization of girls against Rubella has now been introduced in many countries, and congenital Rubella will hopefully disappear in the future. The Rubella cataract is often associated with hearing loss, congenital heart defect and apparently serious mental retardation and is thus a very handicapping disorder. It occurs in epidemics, and the deaf and blind children resulting from these are now being given special education. Previously these children were regarded as mentally retarded, but it is possible that many of them suffered from lack of stimulation rather than lack of intellectual capacity.

Chromosomal Aetiology.   Most mentally retarded patients with chromosomal aberrations have Down's syndrome, and in some of these cases

Table 5.9: Prevalence of Childhood Cataract

Cataract	Mentally retarded	Normal	Total
Blind	55	34	89
Partially sighted	30	82	112
Unknown acuity	10	6	16
Total with cataract	95	122	217
All blind	363	449	812
All partially sighted	117	371	488
Total visually impaired	480	820	1300

Source: Adapted from Schappert-Kimmijser (1975).

Table 5.10: Aetiology of Childhood Cataract among Mentally Retarded People

	No.	%
Genetic	3	4
Chromosomal	9	13
Rubella	22	32
Toxoplasmosis	6	9
Pre- or perinatal	29	42
Other causes	1	1
Total	69	100

Source: Bleeker-Wagemakers (1981).

cataract may develop in young or middle-aged adults. There has been a tendency to refrain from operating on patients with Down's syndrome, but the operations are well tolerated and quite safe if the patients can be kept quiet for a few days after the operation. Spectacles are needed afterwards to get the full benefit of the extraction, but even without glasses the resulting visual acuity is better post-operatively than before. In recent years artificial lenses are implanted after the cataract has been removed, thereby reducing the need of glasses for those with near-vision.

Vision deteriorates if the cataract is left unoperated and then the patients become anxious, sometimes hallucinated and usually very uncooperative.

Pre- and Perinatal Cataract. These are the cases in which the aetiology is not fully understood. A premature birth, especially when associated with low blood sugar values, is a common history in mentally retarded blind persons with congenital cataracts. Sometimes there is a simple causal relation, but in other cases the patient has one of the many less well understood syndromes with cataract that are being studied intensively these days. A definitive diagnosis requires a clinical, metabolic and genetic examination of the patient and his relatives (Merin 1974).

Injuries.   Injuries to the eyes may also result in cataract, whether the trauma involves blunt or penetrating lesions. In mentally retarded persons injuries are sometimes self-inflicted; frequent banging of the head with fists is dangerous and may lead to the development of a cataract. In such patients cataract extraction has a poor prognosis.

Senile Cataract.   Like other elderly people, mentally retarded persons may develop a senile cataract, and the incidence is increasing because more survive to old age than before.

Many elderly mentally retarded persons now live in hostels or sheltered homes where they are not having regular medical checks, and the number of patients with senile cataract is not known. These patients not only lose their sight if unoperated but some will have serious complications of the eyes. Cataract extraction with implantation of an artificial lens can restore their eyesight and contact lenses or glasses can be prescribed post-operatively to patients without artificial lenses. The staff in sheltered homes need to be informed about cataracts and should be encouraged to send their clients to ophthalmological examinations if there is a suspicion of loss of sight.

Malformations

Between 12 and 18 per cent of blind children have malformations of the eye. Although almost half of all legally blind children are mentally retarded, only about one-third of those blind from malformations of the eyes are mentally retarded (see Table 5.11). In the statistics, malformations mean eyes of abnormal size (microphthalmos, anophthalmos), eyes with visible growth defects (colobomata of the iris, the choroid or the optic nerve or aniridia) or multiple malformations (see Figure 5.9). The causes of malformations of the eye in mentally retarded persons are varied. Some cases are due to prenatal infections, chromosomal abnormalities are found in others, but the majority are due to rare syndromes (see Table 5.12). If malformations of the eye are present together with other malformations, a precise diagnosis can be established, and then it is often possible to calculate the risk of recurrence of the syndrome in siblings. If a woman has an increased risk of having children with microphthalmos, it is now feasible to follow the growth of the eye of the foetus by ultrasonography so that there is an option of abortion if microphthalmos or anophthalmos is present.

TREATMENT OF VISUAL IMPAIRMENT

Treatment of visual impairment in mentally retarded persons has been mentioned in the previous paragraphs. It will be noted that the most preva-

Table 5.11: Malformations of the Eye: Prevalence of Mental Retardation among Legally Blind Children

	Mentally retarded	Mentally normal	Total
Malformations	47	105	150
All legally blind children	363	449	812

Source: Adapted from Schappert-Kimmijser (1975).

Table 5.12: The Causes of Malformations Among Mentally Retarded Patients

Aetiology	No.	%
Prenatal infections	16	19
Chromosomal	6	7
Identified syndromes	17	19
Provisionally identified syndrome	36	42
Unidentified syndromes	11	13
Total	86	100

Source: Warburg (1981).

Figure 5.9: Complicated malformations. Mentally retarded girl with microphthalmos and coloboma of the iris in the right eye and coloboma of the choroid in the left. She has a congenital heart defect, cleft palate and dwarfism due to congenital dysfunction of the hypophysis and the thyroid.

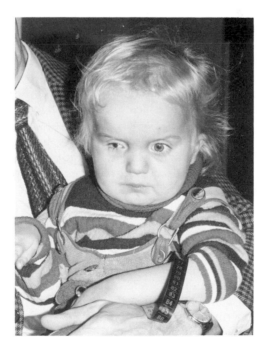

lent causes of low vision are uncorrected errors of refraction; it has also been shown that many mentally retarded persons can use glasses, and optical correction should always be tried even if it takes a long time for some of the mentally retarded patients to get used to spectacles.

Contact lenses are common in the ordinary population; their usefulness among mentally retarded persons has not been studied, and in my experience they are rarely tolerated.

Old mentally retarded persons like all other elderly people need glasses for near-vision. It needs a well-informed staff to see that they are used correctly. I have, therefore, prescribed bifocals to many of my mentally retarded patients, and this has worked well.

Reading aids, telescopes and loupes are commonly prescribed to ordinary visually impaired people, but utilization is difficult and mentally retarded patients do not profit from such aids.

Congenital cataract is found in about 20 per cent of visually impaired children and senile cataract is becoming more prevalent now, because more mentally retarded persons get old. Cataracts should be operated in mentally retarded patients when vision becomes reduced; if possible, artificial lenses should be implanted, and the patients without lenses should be fitted with glasses for near and distant use. If contact lenses are prescribed, the patients must be seen regularly because inflammation of the outer eye is common among the mentally retarded and may give rise to corneal scarring unless the contact lenses are removed.

Even in cases where neither intra-ocular lenses nor glasses can be used, removal of dense cataracts will improve vision, and there is thus only a need to hesitate operating on mentally retarded patients who are prone to automutilation.

There are many causes of visual impairment for which there is no medical or surgical treatment, namely retinal degenerations, optic atrophy or malformations. Patients with such disorders need special education by teachers knowledgeable in the education of mentally retarded persons. Mobility training teachers teach the visually impaired individuals to use other sensory information than sight to understand their environment. The mobility teacher and other teachers for the blind retarded also teach the staff to stimulate the clients to move about or handle objects and they provide objects that the blind and partially sighted will enjoy handling.

CONCLUSIONS

Legal blindness is more than two hundred times more frequent among mentally retarded children than among other children. The main causes of severe visual impairment or legal blindness among the mentally retarded are cerebral visual dysfunction, tapeto-retinal degenerations, retinopathy of prematurity, cataract and ocular malformations. These conditions comprise

90 per cent of all cases. Little is known about the prevalence or causes of moderate visual impairment among mentally retarded children, and almost nothing about the frequency of visual impairment among adult mentally retarded people although screening procedures have shown that it is much larger than in the general population (see Chapter 1, this volume).

Some causes of visual impairment in mentally retarded persons are correctable either by glasses, by operations or by medical treatment; the establishment of an aetiological diagnosis may indicate the risk of recurrence of the disorder in the family.

Syndromes or diseases which are rare in the general population are seen more frequently among mentally retarded persons, and understanding their causes will improve the opportunity to prevent the eye disorder or the associated retardation.

It is distressing to know that many mentally retarded persons, children and adults alike, have visual defects that are unidentified, that some of the patients could have their eyesight restored and that those whose disability has not been noticed are at a risk of being considered more retarded than they really are.

References

Bleeker-Wagemakers, E.M. (1981) *On the Causes of Blindness in the Mentally Retarded,* Bartiméus-The Netherland, Doorn

Frenkel, M. and Evans, L. (1980) 'The Nonpareil test of visual acuity in the young and retarded', *Ann. Ophthalm, 12* (7), 811

Goldstein, H. (1974) 'Incidence, Prevalence and Causes of Blindness', *Public Health Review, 3* (1)

Hyvärinen, L. Näsänen, R. and Laurinen, P. (1980) 'New visual acuity test for pre-school children', *Acta Ophthalmologica* (Kbh), *58,* 507-11

Iivanainen, M. (1974) *A Study on the Origins of Mental Retardation.* Clinics in Developmental Medicine No. 51, Spastics International Medical Publishers, with Heinemann Medical Books Ltd., London

Jan, J.E., Robinson, G.C., Kinnis, C. and MacLeod, P.J.M. (1977) 'Blindness due to optic-nerve atrophy and hypoplasia in children: an epidemiological study', *Developmental Medicine and Child Neurology,* 19, 353-63

—— Freeman, R.D. and Scott, E.P. (1977) *Visual Impairment in Children and Adolescents,* Grune and Stratton, New York

Lennerstrand, G., Axelson, A., Andersson, G. (1983) 'Visual acuity testing with preferential looking in mental retardation', *Acta Ophthalmologica* (Kbh), *61,* 624-33

Merin, S. (1974) 'Congenital cataracts' M.F. Goldberg (ed.) *Genetic and Metabolic Eye Disease,* Little, Brown and Co., Boston, pp. 337-55

Miller, N.R. (1982) in Walsh and Hoyt (eds.), *Clinical Neuro-ophthalmology,* 4th edn., Williams and Wilkins, Baltimore, London, pp. 142-4.

Opitz, J.M., Kaveggia, E.G., Durkin-Stamm, M.V and Pendleton, E. (1978) 'Diagnostic genetic studies in severe mental retardation', *Birth Defects: Orig. Art. Ser.,* 14/6B, pp. 1-38

Richman, J.E. and Garzia, R.P. (1983) 'The bead test: A critical appraisal', *Am. J. Optometry Physiological Optics,* 60, 199-203

Schappert-Kimmijser, J. (1975) *in* J. Schappert-Kimmijser (ed.), 'Causes of severe visual impairment in children and their prevention' *Documenta Ophthalmologica, 39,* 224-8

Socialstyrelsen redovisar (1973) *Utvecklingsstörda med ytterligare handicapp.* Allmänna Förlagets Distribution, Vällingby

Sturman, D. (1975) 'Blindness in childhood in New Zealand', *Transactions of the Ophthalmological Society NZ, 27,* 45-52

van Hof-van Duin, J. Mohn, G. and Batenburg, A.M. (1982) 'Simple tests of visual function in multiply handicapped children', *International J. Rehabilitation Research, 5,* 239-40

Warburg, M. (1967) 'Brillebehandling', *Psykisk utvecklinshämning, 69,* 31-8

—— (1981) 'Diagnostic precision in microphthalmos and coloboma of heterogeneous origin', *Ophthalmic Paediatr. Genet., 1,* 37-42

—— (1982) 'The natural history of Jansky-Bielchowsky's and Batten's diseases' in D. Armstrong, N. Koppang and J.A. Rider (eds.), *Ceroid-lipofuscinosis* Elsevier Amsterdam, New York, Oxford, pp. 35-44

—— (1983a) 'Congenital blindness' in A.E. Emery and D.L. Rimoin (eds.), *Principles and Practice of Medical Genetics,* pp. 471-81

—— (1983b) unpubl.

—— Frederiksen, P. and Rattleff, J. (1979) 'Blindness among 7700 mentally retarded children' in V. Smith and J. Keen (eds.), *Visual handicap in children,* Clinics in Developmental Medicine No. 73 Spastics International Medical Published with Heinemann Medical Books Ltd. London, Philadelphia, pp. 56-69

6 MEDICAL AND OTOLOGICAL ASPECTS OF HEARING IMPAIRMENT IN MENTALLY HANDICAPPED PEOPLE

Sybil Yeates

Introduction

Recent attempts at identifying the numbers of mentally handicapped people who also have some degree of hearing loss have shown that this figure is considerable (Wigram 1983; see also Chapter 2, this volume). It is, therefore, surprising and discreditable that, as late as the 1960s, many children examined in special schools and training centres did not have their hearing tested in any way. They were said to be 'untestable' and unhappily this situation was accepted without much comment or questioning. It is not entirely excused by the recent improvement and availability of objective tests of hearing, as in many cases simple clinical tests would have been appropriate. Therefore diagnosis was generally left to observation by parents and staff, which could not be considered as satisfactory. In addition, when diagnosis was made, the attitude towards treatment was very ambivalent. Often comments were made to the effect that it was useless to amplify the sounds of speech which the patient would not understand, even if heard. Other excuses included the assumption that many patients could not learn to use or would not tolerate a hearing aid. Also some patients with severe loss were categorized as being 'too deaf' to benefit from the use of amplification. (Such is, in fact, rarely the case.)

If such a state existed in schools and junior training centres it was hardly surprising to find it, in more marked form, amongst centres and hospitals for the adult mentally handicapped. Neither can we be complacent and allege that diagnosis, treatment and, most importantly, attitudes have suddenly changed. Perhaps they are changing slowly, but a great deal remains to be altered. Further education for otologists, medical audiologists, paediatricians, psychiatrists and general practitioners has to be achieved. If this training promotes diagnosis there is then the need for training those concerned with the ongoing treatment, i.e. parents, teachers, carers and nursing staff, etc. Only then shall we prevent a situation where hearing aids, once issued, are put to rest in drawers and cupboards, or where several unmarked, different aids are put away together and nobody can match the aid to the patient until the next clinic visit.

AETIOLOGY OF HEARING LOSS

The causes of hearing loss may be divided into four main groups:

1. Genetic causes, i.e. occurring before or at conception, including recessive genetic causes, dominant genetic causes, X-linked genetic causes, and primary chromosomal abnormalities.
2. Causes occurring during pregnancy, including infections.
3. Perinatal causes, i.e. occurring at or around birth, including the problems of prematurity and low birth weight, anoxia due to multiple causes and hyperbilirubinaemia in the neonatal period.
4. Postnatal causes, i.e. occurring after birth.

Whereas the causes outlined above give rise to sensori-neural or nerve deafness, postnatal causes include both sensori-neural and conductive types of hearing loss.

In sensori-neural hearing loss the pathological condition affects the inner ear, the cochlear nucleus or higher auditory pathways, but the outer ear and middle ear are undamaged. However, in conductive hearing loss the problem lies in the outer or middle ear, while the inner ear remains intact. In such cases an auditory stimulus placed on the mastoid bone bypasses the damaged area, and is heard normally, e.g. a tuning fork is heard better when placed on the bone that when held very near the external auditory meatus. Similarly, pure tones are heard better when an oscillator is placed on the mastoid process than when they are played through headphones into the external auditory meatus to pass to the tympanic membrane. In other words, bone conduction remains normal while air conduction of sound is diminished. When it is possible to do an audiogram the typical difference between air and bone conduction can be seen; the 'air-bone gap'.

There are many conditions in which both middle and inner ears are damaged. There is then a mixed loss, i.e. a conductive loss together with a sensori-neural loss.

Infections such as meningitis, encephalitis, measles and mumps, give rise to sensori-neural loss, as do damage from noise and the very important hearing loss of old age (presbyacusis). On the other hand there are congenital abnormalities, infections and other conditions of the middle ear which give rise to varying degrees of conductive hearing loss which are extremely important.

It will be apparent that such a group of causes bears a strong similarity to any table which could be drawn up to demonstrate the aetiology of mental subnormality. Thus it is not surprising to find a very significant number of individuals who unhappily suffer from a whole spectrum of problems including both mental subnormality and hearing loss.

Genetic Causes

Recessive Genetic Causes

This can be divided into two groups. The first, and the commonest cause of

Figure 6.1: Audiogram Showing a Conductive-type Hearing Loss.

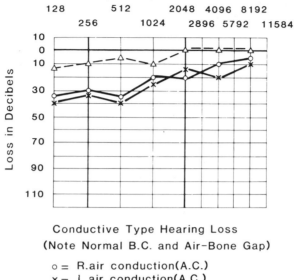

Conductive Type Hearing Loss
(Note Normal B.C. and Air–Bone Gap)

o = R.air conduction(A.C.)
x = L.air conduction(A.C.)
△ = Unmasked bone conduction(B.C.)

profound hearing loss, is clinically undifferentiated autosomal recessive deafness. Fraser's (1976) study of 2,355 deaf children of school age in the British Isles found an incidence of 25 per cent. The second group consists of the syndromes that are inherited recessively and contain specific groups of symptoms and signs, including deafness.

Clinically Undifferentiated Autosomal Recessive Deafness. The prevalence of hearing loss of the type found in recessive deafness is 1 in 1,000 of the population. The prevalence of severe mental subnormality approaches 4 per 1,000 of the population (Wing 1984). Thus it seems likely that there will be some individuals who suffer from both conditions but in whom the causes are not linked, and when Fraser (1976) studied 72 adult mentally handicapped females, he found 14 with clinically undifferentiated autosomal recessive loss.

Recessive Syndromes. There are three main syndromes, including hearing loss, which are inherited in a recessive manner: Pendred's syndrome (deafness with goitre), Usher's syndrome (deafness associated with retinitis pigmentosa) and Abnormal ECG syndrome or Jervell and Lange–Nielsen syndrome (deafness associated with prolongation of the Q–T interval in an ECG). None of these is usually associated with mental subnormality, but it may be useful to mention certain other conditions at this point which bear some resemblance to the above.

Foetal hypothyroidism due to a biochemical defect in thyroxine synthesis, which is very similar to the defect found in Pendred's syndrome, may be inherited in a similar way. This gives rise to hypothyroidism, some degree of mental retardation and hearing loss, sometimes associated with motor problems such as diplegia. Pendred's syndrome is distinguished by means of the Perchlorate Test, which is recognized as being conclusive evidence of the condition (see Table 6.1). Infants are now screened routinely after birth for hypothyroidism so cases of hearing loss with some degree of mental subnormality from this cause will be minimized although damage from the intra-uterine period may well remain. However, in the adult population of the mentally subnormal, where treatment was delayed, more cases will undoubtedly be found.

When retinitis pigmentosa is found together with pituitary dystrophy and polydactyly it constitutes the Laurence–Moon–Bardet–Biedl syndrome (also known as the Bardet–Biedl syndrome, see Chapter 5, this volume). In some cases of this syndrome there is some degree of mental handicap and also in some cases there is a very definite hearing loss. It is, therefore, worthy of mention here. There is some tendency for the hearing loss to appear several years after the initial diagnosis; this should be remembered and careful observation of the patient's hearing should be maintained. The inheritance of the syndrome is rather complex, but is often labelled as recessive (see Chapter 7 this volume).

Pathological Changes In The Ear Found in Recessive Conditions.   In clinically undifferentiated autosomal recessive deafness, the degeneration has usually been limited to the cochlea and the saccule, with haemorrhages and thromboses in the important very small vessels that supply the 8th nerve endings. More extensive damage has been found in the syndromes, affecting the vestibular apparatus.

Table 6.1: Principle of Perchlorate Test: Diagnostic of Pendred's Syndrome

1.	Perchlorate ions (ClO_4^-) are capable of discharging inorganic iodide from thyroid gland.
2.	In the normal thyroid gland, the inorganic iodide is quickly transformed to the organic form and *very little* inorganic form is left in the gland.

The test

1.	Give the patient a dose of radioactive inorganic iodide; take a Geiger count.
2.	Give the patient a dose of potassium perchlorate ($KClO_4$).
3.	The normal gland will have *used* the radioactive iodide and converted it to an organic form; but the iodine remains *in* the gland, simply in another form.
4.	In Pendred's disease the gland cannot use the inorganic iodide, therefore the perchlorate discharges it *away* from the gland.
5.	Take another Geiger count, over the gland; in the normal gland the *count remains the same*, as the radioiodine remains *in* the gland, simply in another form.

In Pendred's disease the radioactive iodide has been 'discharged from the gland' as it has stayed in *inorganic* form. Therefore the Geiger count *over the gland* falls as the radioactive iodide has been sent off to other parts of the body by the potassium perchlorate.

However, knowledge about the pathological changes remains limited and the most important gap in our knowledge is associated with the time when the changes occur. Evidence from animals suggests that in many hereditary forms of hearing loss the condition is not present at birth but occurs very quickly afterwards. There is an obvious analogy here with phenylketonuria and the necessity for further research is obvious. Similarly the reason for the association of deafness with so many disparate conditions is still unknown.

Dominant Genetic Causes

As with the recessive type, dominant genetic hearing loss can be divided into two main groups, i.e. clinically undifferentiated autosomal dominant loss and hearing loss forming part of a syndrome which is inherited in a dominant form.

Clinically undifferentiated autosomal dominant loss. This is not as common as the recessive type. Again using Fraser's (1976) study of school-children he found that the dominant type of loss accounted for 11.6 per cent of the deaf children in the study, i.e. less than half as many as were caused by recessive loss. There is an even more striking comparison when we look at his study of 72 adult mentally handicapped females. While he found 14 cases of autosomal recessive loss, he found no cases of autosomal dominant loss. However, this is a more difficult figure to ascertain accurately, as will be mentioned below when discussing the clinical differences between recessive and dominant hearing loss.

Dominant Syndromes. The main syndromes inherited in a dominant manner are the auditory–pigmentary syndromes, of which Waardenburg's syndrome is the most important. Besides hearing loss this has three main features. These are a white forelock, heterochromia and lateral dystopia. Of these features lateral dystopia, or an increase in the distance between the medial canthi, is the one thought to be truly diagnostic of the syndrome. Of the various signs listed above, any number or combination may be present, and they may also be modified in many and various ways. However, although there are reports of mental subnormality existing with this condition (Amini-Elihou 1970), including a case seen regularly by the writer, the two conditions are thought to coexist fortuitously.

Apart from the auditory–pigmentary syndromes, there is an important group of conditions in which multiple congenital deformities are associated with deafness and sometimes with mental subnormality. These are often the result of malformation of the branchial arches occurring in utero. Probably the best known is mandibulo-facial dysostosis or Treacher–Collins syndrome, and mental handicap undoubtedly occurs in some of these patients. There are abnormalities of the outer and middle ears, and sometimes also of the inner ears. (Tomograms are necessary to try and ascertain the extent of the damage.) The eyes tend to show an anti-mongoloid slant, with coloboma of the lower eyelids. As implied by the name, there is marked hypoplasia of both the malar bone and the mandible. There may also be macrostomia, with a high palate and malformed teeth, and blind fistulae occurring in the area between the angles of the mouth and the ears. The number of signs and symptoms found in any one case vary across a wide range. In most cases the hearing loss will be conductive in type, but when the inner ear is deformed there will be a mixed sensori-neural and conductive deafness. Because of the abnormalities of the outer ears, with deformed or absent pinnae and blind or absent external auditory canals, the amplification has to be by bone conduction. This adds to the problems of treating those patients who also show intellectual deficit.

Cranio-facial dysostosis (Crouzon's disease) is another member of the multiple congenital deformities group, in which the head is pointed and high. It is sometimes associated with both mental subnormality and hearing loss. Acrocephalosyndactyly (Apert's syndrome) is associated with cranio-stenosis of the coronal suture, facial dysostosis, hypoplasia of the maxilla and also with syndactyly of the fingers and toes. This is often accompanied by more severe mental handicap and sometimes with deafness. In both these conditions, with their accompanying cranial malformations, hearing loss is likely to be conductive, although occasionally there is also a sensori-neural element.

Other conditions which merit mention are the 'deafness–earpits' syndrome, in which abnormalities of the outer ears are associated with earpits and possibly sinuses between the ear and the mouth or in the neck, and the Pierre–Robin syndrome in which cleft palate is associated with micrognathia and sometimes with deafness. Mild mental subnormality may sometimes be seen in the latter syndrome, but slowness of development may only be due to repeated attacks of conductive hearing loss due to the recurrent chronic secretory Otitis Media which are so often seen in this condition. The last two conditions to be noted are otopalatal–digital syndrome and oculo-auriculovertebral dysplasia. In both cases abnormalities of the outer and middle ears may lead to conductive deafness and there may also be mild mental subnormality.

In all the syndromes mentioned in this group, although inheritance may be labelled as 'dominant', in many cases there appear to be mutant genes and differences in penetrance.

When skeletal abnormalities are combined with conductive hearing loss it may be only too easy to diagnose 'mental subnormality' which is not borne out as treatment progresses and the child becomes older. This is particularly well illustrated in Pierre–Robin syndrome where the mandibular development improves as the child gets older and development is speeded up as the frequency of middle ear problems decreases.

Other dominantly inherited types of hearing loss such as Alport's syndrome (nephritis associated with sensori-neural loss) and Otosclerosis may, of course, coexist fortuitously with mental subnormality.

Pathological Changes In the Ear Found in Dominant Conditions. In dominant-type sensori-neural hearing loss the whole of the inner ear is much more commonly involved than in the recessive type, but in the cases discussed above where mental subnormality is a distinct feature of the condition the importance of conductive hearing loss should be noted.

X-Linked Genetic Causes

There is a clinically undifferentiated type of X-linked hearing loss but this is so uncommon that we need not discuss it further.

There is, on the other hand, a syndrome inherited in this manner in which both mental handicap and hearing loss are quite commonly found. This is Hunter's syndrome, one of the group of mucopolysaccharidoses. In this syndrome the typical dwarfism and the coarsening of the facial features, sometimes referred to as 'gargoylism', are found, together with the biochemical changes due to abnormal metabolism of the high molecular carbohydrates. The degree of mental retardation is very variable between cases.

Figure 6.2: Pierre–Robin Syndrome, Lateral View

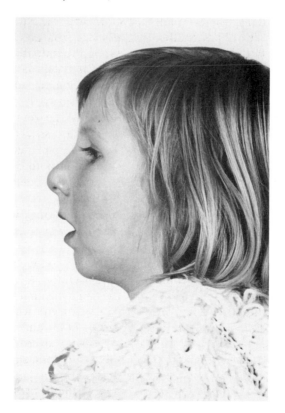

Figure 6.3: Hunter's Syndrome

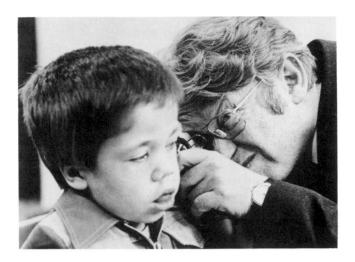

The other mucopolysaccharidoses are inherited in recessive fashion and mental handicap is severe in some, e.g. Hurler's syndrome and Sanfilippo syndrome, and very uncommon in others, e.g. Morquio's syndrome and Maroteaux–Lamy syndrome. While hearing loss is typical of the X-linked syndrome, it can also be seen in some of the recessive syndromes. There seems to be evidence that abnormal metabolites can be laid down in the middle ear, and many other areas of the body, and a conductive-type hearing loss is not uncommon in any of these conditions.

Characteristics of Genetic Hearing Loss

If a mentally handicapped person is suspected of having a hearing loss which was genetically determined, it is important to attempt to classify this. Although the patient may be unlikely to have children, there are important implications for the rest of the family.

Although sections have been divided into firm groups, it must be stressed that, often, distinctions become very blurred, and the advice of a clinical geneticist should always be sought by the family. There are some guide-lines which are helpful. In recessive hearing loss both parents may be expected to have normal hearing while more than one sibling may be deaf. If the parents are related, then there is a greater chance of recessive loss occurring. If the patient is capable of doing an audiogram (see Conditioning Tests), then this is likely to show a severe loss, worse in the high frequencies. It is often referred to as 'a left-hand corner' audiogram, for reasons which can be seen in Figure 6.5.

On the other hand, in dominant-type loss one parent is often affected and a very obvious family history of deafness in grandparents, aunts, uncles, cousins, etc. may be seen. The hearing loss itself is much less severe,

Figure 6.4: Audiogram of Girl with Autosomal Recessive Hearing Loss. No Bone Conduction Recorded; ○ Right Ear, × Left Ear.

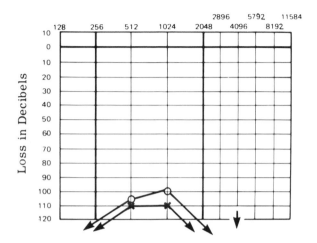

Figure 6.5: Typical Audiogram of Clinically Undifferentiated Autosomal Recessive Hearing Loss; ○ Right Ear, × Left Ear

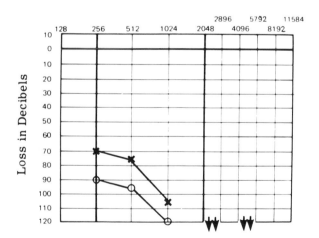

and is flat in type, tending to be of equal severity across all the frequencies. A very important factor here is that a dominant loss may be so small that it is missed. This is particularly true in older patients who did not have the benefit of routine hearing tests in childhood. Or the loss may be unilateral and may have passed without much comment. This means that occasionally a dominant-type loss may appear to have 'missed' a generation, but careful audiological examination of the family may bring one of the above to light. This difficulty may possibly have contributed to the fact that Fraser found no cases of dominant-type loss in his study of 72 adult mentally handicapped females. A commonly found form of audiogram in dominant-type loss is shown in Figure 6.6.

X-linked hearing loss is, as has been said, much rarer than the other types, but tends to give an audiogram similar to the dominant variety, when it is possible for the patient to co-operate in audiometric exam.

Primary Chromosomal Abnormalities

Hearing loss and mental subnormality are found together in a variety of chromosomal abnormalities. The commonest is Down's syndrome, and this merits a very special mention. Children with Down's syndrome are widely known to have recurrent upper respiratory tract infections. They are mouth-breathers and they show Eustachian malfunction. This leads to repeated attacks of chronic secretory Otitis Media, with the attendant conductive-type hearing loss, generally worse in the low frequencies but often extending across the whole frequency range. In high-grade Down's children who are developing speech, this recurrent hearing loss will slow down progress. It is important to treat this condition in all cases of Down's syndrome where the condition can be shown to exist. Because the secretory Otitis Media is likely to recur, it is probably sensible to start with conservative treatment, but if this is unsuccessful there is no reason to deny these children the surgical intervention (i.e. myringotomies with insertion of grommets or Good's tubes) that is indicated. Where there is a real contra-indication to surgery, e.g. in cases of congenital heart disease, amplification should be used. With proper programmes and teaching, most patients with Down's syndrome can learn to use a hearing aid and the popular myths that a small hearing loss does not matter or that these patients cannot deal with amplification must be sternly refuted. There are some cases of Down's

Figure 6.6: Typical Audiogram of Clinically Undifferentiated Autosomal Dominant Hearing Loss; ○ Right Ear, × Left Ear

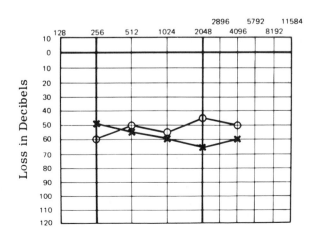

syndrome in which sensori-neural loss can be diagnosed and, very import-antly, there is a real need to treat the presbyacusis occurring in older patients with Down's syndrome. The quality of life for such patients can be very significantly improved by the use of suitable aids.

Other much rarer chromosomal abnormalities are associated with both mental subnormality and deafness. These include Patau's syndrome where there is an extra chromosome in pairs 13-15. There are gross congenital malformations including the skull, eyes, nose and palate. The fingers and hands are often abnormal, with many cases showing polydactyly. The genitalia are often abnormal, especially in males. There is also usually a congenital heart defect. There are feeding difficulties due to hare lip and cleft palate, which is often severe. Obviously many of these infants do not survive.

Edward's syndrome (Trisomy of 17-18) is another rare syndrome which must be mentioned in the same group. Here there is an abnormally shaped skull, with low-set ears which are also often abnormally shaped. The sternum is noticeably short, giving a typical appearance to the chest. There are usually flexion deformities of the fingers and the feet may be rocker-bottom in type. Limited hip abduction is common and the genitalia are often ambiguous. Again there are feeding difficulties, in this case associated with extreme micrognathia. Also there is often congenital heart disease.

In 'Cri-du-chat' syndrome, there is deletion of the short arm of chromo-some 4-5. The presenting symptom is represented in the name of the syndrome, i.e. a high-pitched, mewing cry. Some of these infants are microcephalic and they have micrognathia with low-set ears. Some have congenital heart lesions. In clinical practice these infants are more often seen and hearing loss may be encountered, although not a common feature.

Again, in practice various other deletions or partial deletions have been seen, where both mental subnormality and very definite sensori-neural hearing loss have existed together with other features (see Figures 6.7 and 6.8).

The last condition to be mentioned in this group is Turner's syndrome (XO), but mental subnormality is not a particular feature of the condition, although hearing loss may occur.

The importance of mentioning this rare group of disorders is to stress that, when chromosomal abnormalities have been diagnosed, hearing should be thoroughly investigated.

Causes Occurring During Pregnancy

Having discussed a rare group of disorders we now turn to some commoner reasons for finding the combination of mental abnormality and hearing loss.

Figure 6.7: Boy with Translocation of Chromosome 17

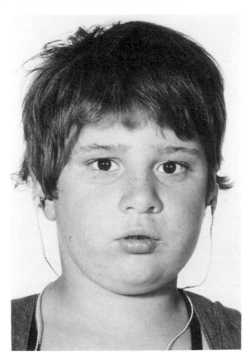

Infections During Pregnancy

Rubella.   The commonest infection occurring in pregnancy which can give rise to a whole spectrum of symptoms and signs, including mental subnormality and hearing loss, is Rubella. This is still very often seen in the adult mentally handicapped population and, unfortunately, in spite of the Rubella vaccination programme, cases still appear. Hopefully, with a recent increase in the uptake of vaccination, the condition will become rarer. However at the moment, when enquiry is made of any collection of young adult females, there are still large numbers who have not been protected. Some improvement can be expected by the practice of offering the vaccine to newly-delivered mothers, but obviously this has highlighted the number of unprotected pregnancies that still take place. All medical and paramedical personnel have a duty to promote Rubella vaccination at every opportunity. A great deal more is necessary in terms of education and informative propaganda.

The full Rubella syndrome is associated with visual defects, hearing defects, congenital heart lesions, microcephaly associated with mental subnormality and cerebral palsy. At birth there is marked hepatosplenomegaly and often a purpuric rash. The sufferer is infectious and serological tests are diagnostic.

Figure 6.8: He is severely handicapped, and has a very severe sensori-neural loss. Photographed at age 8 years.

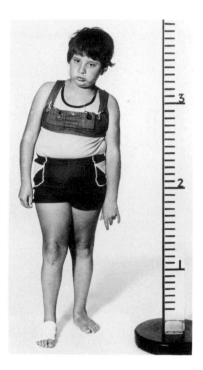

The damage is caused by infection during the first trimester of pregnancy and the earlier the infection the more widespread is the damage. Occasionally the maternal attack is sub-clinical with a minimal rash, so the patient is unaware of the infection and is not offered the opportunity of termination of pregnancy.

Cytomegalovirus (CMV).   This virus can cause widespread damage to a developing foetus, while having little effect on the mother. An infant can show retarded development and a hearing loss, often with visual problems in addition.

Unfortunately this infection cannot be detected in pregnancy, as many adults are already serologically positive, but virological studies in the infant are diagnostic. Since routine tests for CMV have become more widespread, the diagnosis has been seen more frequently in cases where previously no obvious cause would have been found.

Toxoplasmosis.   Toxoplasmosis is a protozoal infection. Like CMV, it causes little problem to an adult or an older child but it invades growing tissues and in the early months of pregnancy can cause widespread damage to the growing foetus. It can result in mental subnormality and often in

Figure 6.9: Infant with severe hearing loss, following maternal Rubella in pregnancy. Diagnosed at age of 7 months. No other symptoms of Rubella syndrome. The infection occurred at 16 weeks of pregnancy.

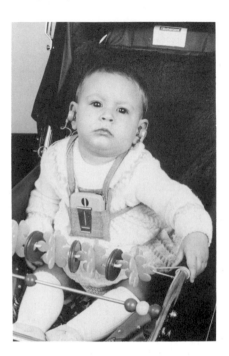

ocular lesions, but also occasionally damages the developing ear.

Again, diagnosis is in the infant after birth, and not in the pregnant woman. As with CMV, a high percentage of the population shows positive results for both infections and a positive result in a pregnant woman is, therefore, not significant.

Syphilis.   Fortunately advances in treatment have cut down the incidence of congenital syphilis to the point where it is now rarely seen. However in adult populations of the mentally handicapped it is likely that the results of this infection will be seen including hearing loss.

Drugs in Pregnancy

This subject has received so much publicity that problems arising now are very rare. The chief culprits of former years were drugs of the streptomycin group, particularly Dihydrostreptomycin. Adults deafened by the use of this drug are not particularly liable to be found in any groups of the mentally handicapped. However, when it is remembered how widely it was used at one time in the treatment of tuberculosis, there is no doubt that sporadic cases will be found amongst the adult mentally handicapped population, especially any who recovered from tuberculous meningitis.

In recent years Gentamicin and allied drugs present the main problems in causing hearing loss, but their use during pregnancy is limited to life-saving situations and blood levels are monitored very carefully. (See also Meningitis.)

Congenital Abnormalities of the Middle Ear

This is another cause of conductive hearing loss. The types of abnormality that are found are many and various, and they cannot be attributed to any simple or single cause. There are complex interactions of genetic and environmental factors occurring during embryogenesis. The conditions range from almost complete absence of the middle ear, as occasionally seen in Treacher–Collins syndrome, to minor abnormalities of the inter-ossicular joints and ligaments. In some cases the abnormality is unilateral and there is a completely normal second ear with only unilateral deafness. Often abnormalities of the middle ear, in mentally handicapped patients with well-defined syndromes, are associated with general abnormalities of the skull.

In those cases where gross abnormalities are seen, tomograms are necessary before any surgical intervention is considered. In some cases where the pinnae and external auditory canals are missing, tomograms may reveal one or both middle and inner ears to appear normal. In such cases, an otologist may consider the construction of a passage into the middle ear. However, this is not without problems as the newly formed initial canal shows a very marked tendency to close itself up again, and operations are always carried out in several stages. When successful there is the considerable bonus of allowing a patient to use a normal hearing aid, with an ear mould, rather than a bulky and obvious bone conduction aid.

More minor abnormalities may be suspected in children showing a conductive hearing loss, diminution of compliance of the middle ear and abnormal appearance of the tympanic membrane on otoscopic examination, but in whom no glue or very little abnormal secretion is found at operation. It is also common for glue ear and minor abnormalities of the middle ear to coexist. In these cases insertion of the grommet does not give the expected improvement. The surgeon may then perform a tympanotomy, in which a flap of the tympanic membrane is turned back so the contents of the middle ear can be directly viewed. He may then be able to reposition misplaced ossicles, e.g. replace the stapes over the oval window, refashion unsatisfactory ossicular chains, mobilize ossicular chains which have become rigid because of abnormal intra-ossicular ligaments, etc. There are many variations which may be amenable to intervention by a skilled otological surgeon. However, parents should always be involved in the discussion before any decision is made to operate, as the results of intervention are very variable even in the best hands. Parents should be fully aware of this before giving consent to any of the more complex operations on the middle ear.

Perinatal Causes

Prematurity

Infants born prematurely are particularly prone to both hearing loss and intellectual deficit. In the case of the ear the fragile, underdeveloped blood vessels of the inner ear are very prone to haemorrhage, thus decreasing the blood supply of the Organ of Corti. In addition, blood extravasated into this area appears to have a toxic and irreversible effect on the cells of the area (Dollinger 1927; Kelemen 1963). Of course, if obstetric manipulations are needed, the risk of damage becomes greater.

Similar problems seem to occur in 'dysmature' or low-birthweight infants and in these cases the problem may also be exacerbated by anoxia resulting from poor placental function. Careful monitoring in utero is intended to minimize these dangers.

Anoxia

Again, careful monitoring by obstetricians and neonatal paediatricians is all directed towards prevention of anoxia before, during and after birth. Anoxia at any of these times can damage the infant and the results include both cerebral damage and damage to the ear.

A large number of problems can give rise to anoxia and these include very severe toxaemia with infarction of the placenta, long labours with difficult presentations and difficult forceps deliveries, emergency situations such as placenta praevia or prolapsed cord, situations occurring in the newborn period such as respiratory distress syndrome (Hyaline Membrane disease), etc. When one thinks of the possible outcome to the infant of any of the very large numbers of situations which may be responsible for anoxia it is hardly surprising that foetal monitoring has become much more widespread and the incidence of delivery by Caesarean section increased.

In the case of the ear, not only is haemorrhage in the inner ear more likely but there may be damage to the cochlear nuclei in the brain.

Damage by anoxia is very commonly the cause of cerebral palsied individuals who also show mental handicap of varying degree and high frequency hearing loss. (See also Differential Diagnosis.)

Hyperbilirubinaemia

The commonest cause of increased serum bilirubin levels in the neonatal period is probably Rh incompatibility, although this is now less frequent as susceptible mothers are given anti-D-immunoglobulin after the first pregnancy, in the immediate post-partum period. However AB–O incompatibility must also be remembered and physiological jaundice in a small premature baby can also be dangerous.

For years now serum bilirubin levels have been carefully watched in susceptible infants or, indeed, in any jaundiced infant. Exchange transfusions have been given whenever danger levels have approached.

However, there are still adults who managed to survive but in whom toxic damage occurred by the product of red cell breakdown, i.e. unconjugated bilirubin, especially in the basal ganglia as well as in the cochlear nuclei and the central auditory pathways. Such patients commonly show athetoid cerebral palsy and high-frequency hearing loss. They may, or may not, show some degree of mental handicap. (See Differential Diagnosis.)

Lastly, on a subjective basis, it would seem a wise precaution for hearing levels to be watched carefully in any infants where there has been concern about jaundice in the new-born period, e.g. when phototherapy was used, irrespective of any particular level of serum bilirubin measurement (Fenwick 1975).

Postnatal causes

Meningitis

This is one of the most dangerous and commonest causes of hearing loss in childhood. A survey of world literature showed that possibly 5 per cent of children with meningitis are left with hearing loss. Mental handicap is a possible sequel of the disease. As far as hearing loss is concerned, the type of causal organism does not seem to be important. In addition, the severity of the disease does not seem to correlate with the legacy of hearing loss, and neither does the length of time between onset of symptoms and onset of treatment. (In one of my cases, a three-year-old boy complained of hearing loss before the diagnosis was made.) Hearing loss resulting from meningitis is usually very severe or profound. If the patient has already acquired speech then enormous efforts must be made to preserve it or the parents will simply watch while the patient's speech deteriorates rapidly and progressively (see Figure 6.10).

Figure 6.10: Audiogram of a Post-meningitic Patient

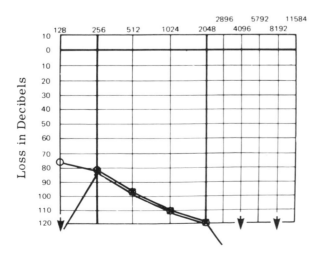

The usual treatment of meningitis is by the drugs Chloramphenicol, Penicillin and Sulphonamide. Occasionally the organism is not susceptible to this combination and it may be found that Gentamicin is required as a life-saving drug. In these cases, the drug may have to be used in doses which may border the ototoxic level, but blood levels are monitored and the patient observed with scrupulous care.

Another drug which was once accused of ototoxicity when used in the treatment of meningitis was Ampicillin (Gamstorp and Hanson 1974). However, subsequent work proved that this was only the case when given in doses exceeding 250 mg/Kg per day (Jones and Hanson 1977).

The reason why meningitis is associated with both mental handicap and hearing loss becomes apparent when the anatomy of the ear is considered. The cochlea has a minute bony canal (the aqueduct of the cochlea), which allows the perilymph (fluid between the membranous and bony parts of the inner ear) to drain into the subarachnoid space. Thus there is a direct pathway for organisms to travel between the subarachnoid space and the organs of the inner ear. Exudate has been found around the auditory nerve, resulting in fibrosis. Vascular thrombosis also occurs in the internal auditory vessels. In addition, the rise of intracranial pressure may be an important factor in causing mental defect and hearing loss. Encephalitis can cause similar problems to those described as typical of meningitis.

The number of patients having suffered from meningitis who also suffer from residual neurological problems varies from 5 to 20 per cent, as shown in various studies. The incidence of sequelae is high in infants and highest in the neonatal group (Dodge and Swartz 1965). In a series of 129 children with mental retardation resulting from postnatal disease, 14 were identified as post-meningitic. It is obviously extremely important to monitor the progress of meningitic patients from the earliest stages of the illness, to minimize the effects of sequelae as far as this is possible.

Other Infections Causing Hearing Loss

Measles and mumps can also cause profound unilateral sensori-neural hearing loss. They are probably the commonest cause of severe unilateral deafness. In addition, both diseases can also cause encephalitis with resulting profound mental retardation.

In some cases, both conditions may coexist but difficulty in diagnosing unilateral deafness in severely mentally handicapped patients is obvious and, almost certainly, depends upon electro-diagnostic tests.

Noise-induced Loss

Hearing loss produced by constant, or even intermittent, exposure to very high sound intensities has been recognized for a very long time. (Metalsmiths were probably the first individuals who realized that exposure to a very high intensity noise, even for a brief period, produced a loss of hearing which gradually recovered if the noise was not repeated.) However, for more than a century the subject has been studied in detail and with the noisy machinery introduced since the Industrial Revolution, and the need to protect workers, the results have become very significant and often the cause of litigation. While some employers may have been negligent in not providing protection, employees have also often been negligent in not using it. Even more recently loud disco music has provided another hazard and, perhaps worst of all, the use of personalized stereo headphones to listen to music has now to be taken into account. The person using such apparatus may fail to appreciate the intensity of the sound source so close to the hearing apparatus. What is more, the temporary auditory fatigue produced by a short session may cause the same person to increase the intensity as it is used for longer periods.

The critical sound pressure level, which has been calculated from two-hour exposures to octave-band noise, is around 70-75db SPL(A) for noises above 1,000 Hz (Jerger 1973). It may be greater than this with low-frequency sounds. The changes are greater as the length of exposure is increased and also if the frequency of the sound is increased. Thus, a sound of 75dB SPL will produce very little change in hearing, no matter for how long it is heard. However, 90dB SPL will produce a significant change in hearing threshold two minutes after the cessation of the stimulus and an intensity of 105db SPL will produce about twice as much change for the same length of exposure. From this it will be seen that many individuals risk damage to their hearing by loud sounds. People with moderate mental handicap who are able to do simple repetitive tasks in noisy environments need special care and protection. While their more able colleagues may even consider litigation against neglectful employers, these workers need helpful supervision and explanation. It is necessary for workers in charge of their welfare, e.g. social workers, factory welfare officers and managers in charge of factory or hostel, to be aware of the dangers. The same precautions apply when people of lesser ability use personal stereos for long periods or where special clubs are continually using disco music of unacceptable intensities.

Noise-induced deafness is sometimes preceded by or accompanied by tinnitus, a symptom of extreme discomfort, not easy to treat, and particularly difficult for the mentally handicapped patient to understand.

Presbyacusis

The hearing loss of old age, which often appears in the fifties, may be common to all individuals, whatever their mental capacity. It is extremely irritating to active, able-bodied persons in middle life, perhaps carrying out very responsible jobs, but they can recognize the problem and seek help. In their less fortunate brethren, the hearing loss may easily be missed and the ensuing problems attributed to worsening mental defect. This is particularly the case because the hearing loss is generally worse in the high frequencies, especially in the early stages. This means that low-frequency sounds are heard and normal responses are given to them. However, in speech, where frequencies vary from 64Hz to 8,129Hz, some words may be heard correctly, others not at all and yet others are partially heard and therefore misinterpreted. It is easy to understand why an older person with this form of hearing loss often reacts inappropriately in conversation. This is very easily misinterpreted as a behavioural problem. The phrase, so often used to wicked effect, is: 'They hear when they want to.'

The hearing levels of the adult mentally handicapped population should be kept under regular observation. In this case, many misunderstandings and frustrations might be prevented.

In addition, efforts should be made to help ageing people to use a hearing aid. If it is remembered that some of their 'difficult' behaviour is in fact caused by a hearing loss, then the motivation to give consistent help with amplification must surely be increased. If speech is limited by reason of mental handicap, then further isolation is caused by the onset of hearing deficit. Again, every effort should be made to keep as many links as possible between the patient and his environment and thus minimize the problems which invariably increase as isolation increases.

Unfortunately presbyacusis increases as the patient gets older and conductive hearing loss also occurs (i.e. the conduction of sound by bone). Obviously if the patient learns to use an aid when the loss is at an early stage, it will be much easier for him and his carer. Aids can easily be changed as required, once use has been established.

Chronic Secretory Otitis Media

It is now necessary to think about the commonest cause of minor hearing loss in childhood and its particular relevance to those children who also show general retardation of development. Around one in five of children entering a nursery class at the age of four years has suffered from a small recurrent conductive hearing loss which, although much less than most sensori-neural losses, has nevertheless been sufficient to interfere with the normal acquisition of language (Hamilton and Owrid 1974; Nietupska and Harding 1982). If not diagnosed and treated, such a loss interferes with early education. The cause of this type of conductive hearing loss is almost invariably Chronic Secretory Otitis Media, commonly known as 'glue ear'. This is seen in children who are prone to recurrent upper respiratory tract infections, who are often mouth-breathers and who often snore. They may, or may not, complain of earache. They often have enlarged adenoids. In such children the Eustachian tube becomes blocked, leading to poor aeration of the middle ear. A healthy middle ear cavity is air-filled and, when aeration is interfered with, the mucous membrane lining the cavity secretes fluid into it. This fluid cannot escape when the Eustachian tube is blocked and, therefore, accumulates and thickens. Finally this thick secretion, known as 'glue' for obvious reasons, interferes with the compliance and movement of the tympanic membrane and the ossicles. This causes conductive deafness, which is generally worse in the low frequencies (see Figure 6.1).

Some children who are mentally retarded are particularly prone to the predisposing factors mentioned above. The commonest example, and the children most often seen in practice, are those with Down's syndrome. The importance of treating these children has already been stressed. However, the principle applies to any retarded child who presents with hearing loss due to glue ear. If speech is developing slowly, it is extremely important to remove any factor which hinders this. If there is no speech, then there may be a better chance of some development if the child's hearing is optimal. If it seems that there may be very little likelihood of speech developing, then one wishes to keep the child in touch with all the everyday sounds as much as possible, so that situational understanding can develop to its fullest extent. Also it is worthwhile remembering that glue ear can cause recurrent earache, with considerable discomfort. A normal child will be able to convey this message whereas the child with less ability may not be able to localize the cause of his suffering to those who are looking after him. Examination of the ears by otoscopy and acoustic impedance is very important in such a child who is obviously ill and in discomfort.

The treatment of chronic secretory Otitis Media may either be conservative or by surgery. Conservative treatment consists of the use of decongestants and antihistamines, or antibiotics. Co-trimoxazole used regularly for one month appeared, in a double-blind controlled trial, to give some improvement in around 60 per cent of cases. This does not mean that the condition will not recur. Recurrence is very typical of the condition and many cases end up with surgical treatment. This consists of myringotomy followed by removal of the glue by suction, and insertion of a small drainage tube. This tube is not inserted to allow further secretion to get out of the middle ear, but to allow air to get in. A middle ear cavity filled with air is generally healthy. There are two types of tube in use, the commonest of which is the grommet. A larger, broader tube, which allows greater aeration and tends to stay *in situ* longer than the grommet, is known as Good's tube. This is probably useful for children with mental handicap who are known to be particularly prone to factors leading to chronic secretory Otitis Media. There is a considerable risk that children who have grommets inserted on one occasion may need them again. (Their stay *in situ* is very variable, between two months and two years.) As it is particularly desirable to minimize the risk of further operations in children with mental handicap, there is probably a firm case for the use of the more expensive Good's tubes in all such children who have myringotomies.

Otosclerosis

This condition, inherited in a dominant fashion, generally causes a conductive hearing loss, although it may also affect the cochlea, giving rise to sensori-neural loss. Onset is usually in adolescence or later in life and any mentally handicapped boy or girl from a family where other members had a late onset of deafness should be carefully watched.

Although the name suggests hardening of the bone in the ear, in fact the normal bone is replaced by spongy bone of immature type, usually commencing in the region of the promontory on the medial wall of the middle ear (Ballantyne 1978). The oval window, which is the main connection between middle and inner ears, lies above the posterior end of the promontory. The spongy bone is gradually laid down around the rim of the oval window. It then affects the footplate of the stapes, which sits snugly in the oval window and is responsible for conducting sound from the air of the middle ear to the perilymph of the inner ear. The footplate of the stapes gradually becomes more fixed and symptoms become more marked.

Unless the otosclerosis involves the cochlea, the audiogram shows a typical conductive loss, i.e. air-conduction loss, worse in the low frequencies. The bone conduction is normal except for a small diagnostic feature. This is a 'notch' in the bone conduction at around 2 KHz known as Carhart's notch.

Surgical treatment by stapedectomy is very effective and treatment should be available to mentally handicapped persons. There is no place for pretending that treatment is less important in a patient unfortunate enough to have another handicapping condition. For patients where surgery is contra-indicated, every effort should be made to introduce amplification.

DIAGNOSIS OF HEARING LOSS

Tests

Diagnosis of hearing loss employs four main methods, i.e. (1) distraction tests; (2) co-operative tests involving speech; (3) tests involving a conditioning technique, and (4) objective tests which require very little or no co-operation from the patient. The idea that *all* retarded individuals require objective tests is untrue. Many can be tested by the other methods and those without speech can understand the conditioning technique if their mental age exceeds 2½ years. For all subjective tests, a suitably quiet environment is essential. A sound-proofed room is optimal but is not usually available. Ambient noise of more than 30dB SPL interferes significantly with the tests.

Distraction Tests (7 months–2 years in children with no other problems)

These are routinely done when infants reach the age of 7–9 months. To obtain accurate results it is necessary for the infant to have satisfactory head control. If this is still incomplete, then the tests may be attempted with the infant lying supine. However, it is convenient in these cases if the result can be checked by a non-invasive objective test.

If head control is complete, the retarded infant may fail to respond because of central reasons, i.e. lack of interest or understanding of the stimuli, rather than lack of hearing. In such cases results are often ambiguous and impossible to interpret with accuracy, and an objective test has to be carried out.

It is very important that distraction tests are carried out accurately and with the correct apparatus. The methods used are as follows:

1. The rim of a china cup is stroked gently with the bowl of a teaspoon. The cup should never be tapped with the spoon, as it is essential to keep the intensity of the sound at 35-40dB SPL(A). This test is not frequency-specific but the sound is interesting to babies and young children, and it forms a useful introductory test.
2. A high-frequency rattle, e.g. the Manchester rattle or the Nuffield rattle, should be used. Both are specific for testing high-frequency hearing at around 8kHz. The manchester rattle should be gently rolled and not shaken. The Nuffield rattle should be used as if the tester is stirring a cup of coffee.
3. Voice sounds should always be used. The high-frequency sound 'ss-ss-ss' (a repeated pure sibilant) is useful for testing hearing at around 4kHz. The sound should be very quietly made and it is optimal if the tester has the use of a sound level meter to ensure that intensity does not exceed 35-40dB SPL. The sounds 'oo-oo-oo', or 'ba-ba-ba', can be used to test low-frequency hearing. A few conversational sentences should also be used, including the child's name, in a very soft voice but not a whisper. The latter cuts out low-frequency sounds.

All these tests, with the exception of the Nuffield rattle, should be used at 3 feet, on a level with the meatus of the ear, and ensuring that the tester is *not* within the child's visual range. It is crucial that all sounds are kept at the screening level of 35-40dB SPL, and that *no* other apparatus is used. Unhappily it is only too common for retarded children to be tested with loud bells or the rattling of keys, etc. These non-specific tests are not only useless but dangerous, and hearing loss often remains undiagnosed.

For further details of all tests, see Yeates (1980) and Chapter 11, this volume.

In retarded children, distraction tests can often be used in older age groups when they would not be useful in more able children. As the child increases in awareness and knowledge of his surroundings, he may not bother to turn and identify the simple sounds described.

Co-operative Tests Involving Speech (2 years onwards, in children with no other problems)

There are many of these, but all depend upon a child's comprehension of simple words. Some use toys and others pictures. In all cases the method is similar, i.e. the tester names the objects and then, using a loud conversational voice, asks the child to identify each object in turn. If the child is successful then the tester can cover his mouth, to prevent lip-reading, and gradually lower his voice to the screening level of 35-40dB SPL. If the child can still identify the objects correctly, he obviously has enough hearing for speech development to continue optimally.

Although commonly used with children there is no reason why such tests cannot be used with mentally handicapped adults who have some speech and who often enjoy them. The McCormick Test is particularly useful, as it employs 14 toys but a smaller number can be used if the patient is of limited ability (McCormick 1977). The toys are paired, so their names contain similar vowels, but different consonants, e.g. shoe spoon, plane and plate. This helps to identify people with high-frequency loss who hear the vowels but do not hear the consonants accurately and, therefore, give muddled results. (See also Presbyacusis.)

Conditioning Tests (Performance Tests)

These depend upon teaching patients to carry out a simple motor task, e.g. putting a brick in a box, every time they hear an auditory stimulus. A patient having a mental age of $2^{1}/_{2}$ years is generally considered capable of understanding the concept. Once understood, the process is generally enjoyed and the ensuing sense of achievement and the praise given by the examiner is much appreciated. The auditory stimulus can be either a drum or the voice. The drum, with its vibro-tactile element, is usually suitable for patients with a hearing loss, to ensure that they are really conditioned to the noise. It is easy for inexperienced testers to give the patient many other clues and the more able patient may be conditioned to movements of the tester's head, eyes, etc. which he makes unconsciously when producing the auditory stimulus. When voice is used, the word 'Go', which is a useful low-frequency sound, can be used initially, with a very loud voice. When the process starts, visual and auditory stimuli are given together, i.e the patient can see the drum being banged or the tester's lips moving as he says 'Go'. When this stage is understood, the tester removes the visual stimulus, usually by gradually moving behind the patient. After this is established, the intensity of the auditory stimulus is lowered until a threshold is reached. If voice is used, a high-frequency sound can also be used, such as the sibilant 'ss-ss'. The stages are the same. The availability of a sound level meter to measure the hearing threshold obviously improves the test.

Once the whole process is understood, the patient can be introduced to pure tones, either using a free-field audiometer or, finally, an audiometer in which headphones are used. In this way each ear can be tested separately and thresholds at 125Hz, 250Hz, 500Hz, 1000Hz (1kHz), 2kHz, 4kHz and 8kHz can be established. The production of a reliable audiogram depends entirely upon the ability of the patient to understand the concept and the patience of the examiner in working through all the preliminary stages carefully and thoroughly. (A fuller description of pure-tone audiometry is found in Chapter 11, this volume.)

Objective Tests

There are a large number of patients of very limited ability where the examiner remains puzzled by the results or where there are no results at all. This is where we can use one or more of the range of objective tests. These are fully described in Chapter 11, so need not be discussed here.

Differential Diagnosis

It should first be pointed out that at an early stage children are often presented to doctors because of poor speech development. The commonest causes of this are mental handicap or hearing loss. Sometimes the mental handicap is almost immediately obvious, but, in other cases, a proper developmental exam is necessary to show that the child is retarded not only in speech but also in other parameters of development. A useful clue is the presence or otherwise of 'inner language' or the child's ability to use toys appropriately in symbolic play.

The deaf child of normal ability shows normal symbolic play, while the

Figure 6.11: This profoundly deaf child with a meningitic hearing loss is shown at the age of 16 months. Note his appropriate play continues. In fact he went on to pour a cup of tea which was handed to his mother.

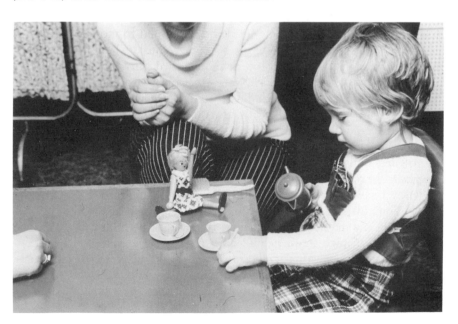

Figure 6.12: A child aged three years, with delayed speech due to a mild hearing loss. (The family show an unusual syndrome: multiple epiphyseal dysplasia tarda with osteochondromatosis and sensori-neural hearing loss. It is inherited in a dominant fashion and the symptoms increase with age. It is not uncommon for the initial presentation to be because of so-called 'osteo-arthritis' in a big joint, in a young adult.) In spite of delayed speech this child shows completely normal 'inner language'. The toys are handed in a random fashion without comment, so the child may produce her own arrangement.

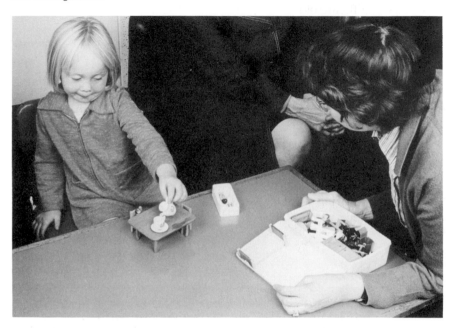

mentally handicapped child often piles the toys in a characteristic and meaningless way. However, it should be remembered that the retarded child may also be deaf. Autistic children often appear totally unreactive to sound, but I have had two typically autistic children who also had severe hearing loss in addition to their characteristic behaviour patterns. The first remained undiagnosed for several years, his reactions being thought to be part of his autistic behaviour. The second was the subject of much argument in his early years, being transferred from one school to another, but when I saw him he was able to do an audiogram and there was no doubt about his organic hearing loss. Both children subsequently used hearing aids, but neither developed any speech, nor was this expected.

The pitfalls of high-frequency hearing loss have been mentioned several times. Diagnosis is often difficult and parents and teachers will deny hearing loss, quoting examples of many reactions to sound. However, a high-frequency loss can add to the behavioural problems of a mentally handicapped person very considerably, and great efforts should be made to exclude the diagnosis beyond doubt. (Note that when high-frequency hearing loss is combined with athetoid cerebral palsy, then the patient may *wrongly* be labelled as mentally handicapped.Great experience is needed to separate the problems.)

A conductive hearing loss in Down's syndrome can similarly cause difficulties in social and intellectual progress. The use of a hearing aid when necessary may alleviate such problems or surgical treatment may be appropriate. The 'difficult old person' may be difficult, or more difficult, by reason of presbyacusis.

It is clear that it is of the greatest importance to be capable of diagnosing hearing loss at any stage of the life of a mentally handicapped person. It would be optimal if regular, routine tests could be established for these members of the community, and these tests should be very carefully and accurately carried out. It must be stressed that careless, random, non-specific tests are not only useless but dangerously inadequate.

TREATMENT OF HEARING LOSS

Treatment of hearing loss in general can be divided into several parts, which are all necessary, and which together help the patient in an optimal way.

Hearing Aids

The most obvious way of helping someone who cannot hear sound normally is to amplify it. Remember, however, that amplified sound is distorted to some degree and the greater the amplification the greater the distortion. Having said that, it remains absolutely essential to diagnose the quantity of the loss at the various frequencies, as accurately as possible. This is much more difficult in the mentally handicapped person, particularly when reliance is on objective tests where results are only given for the high frequencies. Having used all the results available, to get as accurate a picture as possible, a careful choice of suitable hearing aid must be made. The question whether the patient will tolerate body-worn aids or post-aural aids best should be discussed with those who know him well. If body-worn aids are to be used, remember that the patient can easily move the controls and switches; while this may be desirable for the more able patients, it may be a distinct disadvantage for the more seriously handicapped. The cords attaching the ear pieces or moulds to the aids may annoy handicapped patients who will pull at them, thus pulling out the moulds and they may well destroy the cords or the moulds or both. Conversely, the patient may find it irresistible to pull the aids from behind his ears, bringing out the attached moulds. Being small, the whole piece of apparatus may be conveniently lost, thrown or even eaten. In such cases body-worn aids securely fixed in a harness, with the cords mainly hidden under dungarees or a T-shirt, may be more practicable. It may be necessary to experiment with an individual to decide which type of aid is most adequate. Both body-worn and post-aural aids are now available to suit all types of hearing loss. When appropriate, miniature post-aural aids are available for some types of loss.

When the external auditory meatus is absent or malformed it is not possible to fit an earpiece and a bone conductor hearing aid may be used. An oscillator attached to the headband is worn over the mastoid process. It is attached to a body-worn aid, which supplies the required amplification. This is a cumbersome piece of apparatus, but nevertheless I have seen mentally handicapped patients who learned to use it.

Hearing aids are expensive, especially where it is necessary to prescribe a commercial aid and not use one of the NHS aids which are bought in bulk in the UK, on contract from certain manufacturers. Because of this

Figure 6.13: Different types of body-worn and post-aural aids. Although the top left body-worn aid (OL 56) has not now been issued for some time, elderly patients still ask for it as it is very simple to operate. Many of these aids will still be found in hospitals or hostels for the mentally handicapped. They give moderate amplification, often suitable for presbyacusis. The other body-worn aid, the Oticon P 15 P, gives powerful amplification, and has the benefit of two microphones incorporated in one aid. One of the post-aural aids (bottom, centre) is specific for high-frequency loss.

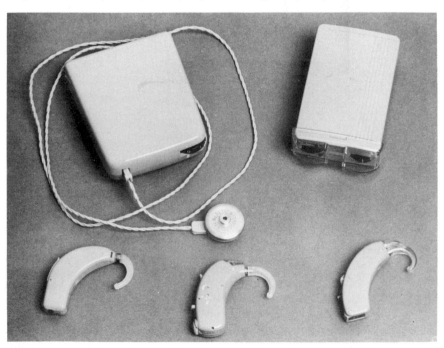

Figure 6.14: Illustrations showing the making of a 'mould' or earpiece. Plastic silicone material is used by the technician to make an impression of the patient's ear (first picture on left). This is then trimmed (second picture) and sent off to the factory where the mould is manufactured from a cast. The mould may be 'hard' or 'soft' or may have a 'soft tip'. It may be made in a special non-allergic material for patients liable to otitis externa. Tubing is incorporated in the mould and this can then be joined to the tubing of the post-aural aid. With a body-worn aid the mould clips on to the receiver head which can be seen in Figure 6.13 (top left). It is essential that moulds fit well and that the ear is free from wax before impressions are taken. Poorly made and poorly fitting moulds mean that aids cannot be used because of the noisy feedback that occurs. The importance of good moulds cannot be stressed too much.

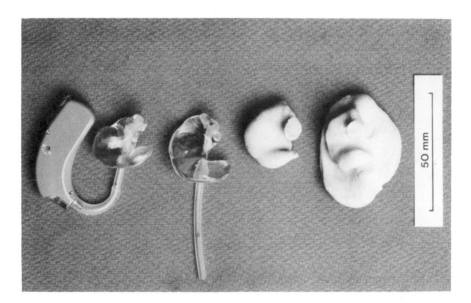

some prescribers use a cheaper aid, even if it is not optimal for the patient's hearing loss. Remarks are often made that the aid will be misused anyway or that it will *not* be used or that it does not matter if a subnormal patient does not hear optimally because of his intellectual deficit. Aids should only be dispensed as part of a total programme of rehabilitation. It is always essential to involve those caring for the patient, a teacher of the deaf whenever available or a speech therapist with special interest in mental handicap, and most importantly a psychologist who can work out a programme based on behavioural modification in liaison with the people already mentioned (see Chapter 17, this volume). Using such a programme, involving very small steps towards the use of the mould and the aid, can result in the most unlikely candidates accepting and benefiting from amplification. This work requires faith, dedication and the utmost patience but the rewards are eventually very great. This is written from experience, having

Figure 6.15: Abnormality of the pinna, with absent external auditory canal. If both ears show similar abnormalities a bone conductor hearing aid must be used.

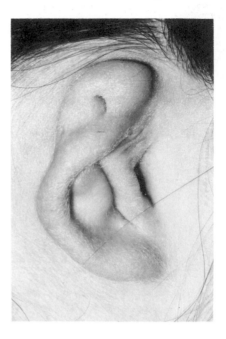

watched the work of enthusiastic teams, undaunted by problems which others have forsaken. When such a team is involved and when results are obtained, it becomes possible to replace an initial aid, issued for a trial period, by the expensive commercial aid which may be required by the patient for the best audiological results.

Education and Training

Parents or carers must be involved in all education and training. If a patient learns to use an aid and begins to learn some simple signs, the whole long process can be destroyed if he returns home to an environment where 'it doesn't matter' or 'it takes too long'. Similarly teachers in schools for the mentally handicapped must be aware of the programme and its importance. They must ensure that aids are brought to school and should have simple instruction in their use. If they are removed, they should be capable of replacing them. They should be able to turn to a teacher of the deaf for help and guidance, and perhaps these teachers should be more adequately trained in helping multi-handicapped children. The same remarks apply to the workers in centres for the adult mentally handicapped and they should have access to speech therapists who, again, must be involved in setting up programmes for individuals.

Figure 6.16: Post-aural Aid *In Situ* — When Covered by Hair It Is Very Inconspicuous

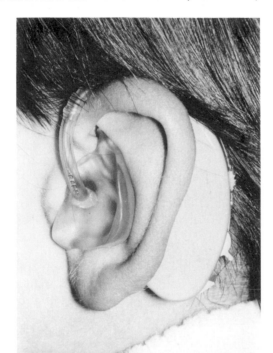

The more able patients may be capable of benefiting from lip-reading, an area where teachers of the deaf and speech therapists should be able to help. Both should also have access to speech trainers, with use for suitable patients. These give amplification to the patient by means of earphones and can be adjusted to the patient's requirements. The interest of patients of very limited ability may be aroused by the use of a speech trainer with music, especially music involving a vibro-tactile element. On the other hand, in the more able patients, limited speech can be increased and improved by its use.

Sign Language

There are many different types of sign language now in use. For severely deaf patients without other handicaps, Signed English is probably now the method of choice. But in mentally handicapped patients the simpler Makaton system is now widely used (see also Chapter 19, this volume).

Even with patients of very limited ability the system of Total Communication must be recommended (Morris 1978). This consists of a combination of amplification, oral language, lip-reading and a suitable signing system. This offers the best to patients who need and deserve the best that we can give them. It gives them the opportunity to benefit where they are able to do so and provides the maximum opportunity for keeping them in touch with their environment, their day-to-day life and those around them. The aim for each patient should be defined, should be realistic and should then patiently be kept in mind, with enthusiastic recognition of each very small achievement.

CONCLUSIONS

Much more education is needed to enhance the treatment of those people who are both mentally handicapped and deaf. While lip-service may be paid to this, far too little effort has been put into providing the highly specialized teams who are able to diagnose and train this very handicapped section of the community. Far too often it has been easier to regard the task as impossible or unnecessary and great pools of ignorance still exist amongst the professionals responsible, who do not know what can be achieved by these teams. However, in some regions multi-professional units are being set up, not only to diagnose and treat but also to pass on their skills to district workers. We hope they may flourish.

Audiological Apparatus in Common Use

Clinicians who routinely test mentally handicapped people will need suitable audiological material and apparatus. The following list is not comprehensive, but to be used for guidance when, for example, specialist teams are being assembled.

Material for Distraction Tests
1. The STYCAR hearing box (Sheridan Tests for Young Children and Retardates) includes the Nuffield rattle. Available from the NFER Publishing Company Ltd., Darville House, 2 Oxford Road East, Windsor, Berks., SL4 1DF.
2. The Manchester rattle is available from the Department of Audiology and Education of the Deaf, University of Manchester, Manchester, UK.

Material for Co-operative Tests Involving Speech
1. The STYCAR hearing box contains material for the Sheridan 6 Toy Test and 7 Toy Test; also the cards for the Sheridan 6 and 12 High Frequency Picture Tests.
2. The McCormick test box; enquiries to Dr B. McCormick, c/o Department of Audiology, University of Nottingham, Nottingham, UK.

3. The Michael Reed Picture Tests: use the same principles as the McCormick and Sheridan Tests; available from Royal National Institute for the Deaf, 105 Gower Street, London WC1E 6AH, UK.
4. The Manchester Picture Test, as described in Chapter 11, available from Department of Audiology and Education of the Deaf, University of Manchester, Manchester, UK.

Audiometers

1. Free Field Audiometer, measuring hearing at 250Hz, 500Hz, 1kHz, 2kHz and 4kHz and producing tones up to 80dB, in steps of 5dB. Also useful for distraction tests. Available from Peters of Sheffield.
2. A portable Pure Tone Audiometer, capable of measuring air and bone conduction and with masking noise facility. Headphones preferably fitted with ear muffs.
3. Acoustic Impedance Bridge for tympanometry, with ability to measure Stapedial Reflex. Preferably a fully automated model, with hand-held probe.

Play Material

1. Selection of miniature doll's house furniture and figures, suitable for assessment of symbolic play.
2. Play bricks: 1 inch cubes.
3. Peg-men in boat (8 small figures fitting into circular holes in the boat). Useful in all tests requiring the conditioning technique.
4. A drum (can be used with very deaf patients when teaching the conditioning process, and for distraction tests).

Sound Level Meter

This is essential equipment. Various models are available from Dawe Instrument Limited., Concord Road, Western Avenue, London W3 OSD, UK.

Acknowledgement

I would like to thank MTP Press, Lancaster, for permission to use illustrations from Yeates (1980).

References

Amini-Elihou, S. (1970) *J. Genet. Hum.*, *18*, 307
Ballantyne, J. (1977) *Deafness*, Churchill Livingstone, Edinburgh
Dodge, P.R. and Swartz, M.N. (1965) *New England Journal of Medicine*, *272* (19)
Dollinger, A. (1927) *Ergebn, Inn. Med. Kinderheilkeit*, *31*, 373
Fenwick, J.D. (1975) *Otolaryngology and Otology*, *89*, 925

Frazer, G.R. (1976) *The Causes of Profound Deafness in Childhood,* Balliere Tindall, London

Gamstorp, I. and Hanson, D.R. (1974) *Developmental Medicine and Child Neurology, 16,* 678-9

Hamilton, P. and Owrid, H.L. (1974) *British Journal of Audiology, 8*

Jerger, J. (1973) *Modern Developments in Audiology* (2nd edn.) Academic Press, New York

Jones, F.E. and Hanson, D.R. (1977) *Developmental Medicine and Child Neurology, 19,* 593-7

Kelemen, G. (1963) *Archives of Otolaryngology, 77,* 365

McCormick, B. (1977) *Public Health,* London *91,* 67-9

Morris, T. (1978) Paper from the Rycroft Centre, Royal Schools for the Deaf, Manchester

Nietupska, O. and Harding, N. (1982) *British Medical Journal*

Wigram, R. (1983) Personal communication

Wing, L. (1984) Personal communication

Yeates, S. (1980) *The Development of Hearing; its Progress and Problems,* MTP Press, Lancaster

7 GENETIC ASPECTS OF VISUAL AND AUDITORY IMPAIRMENT IN MENTALLY HANDICAPPED PEOPLE

Anthony Holland

Introduction

Severe mental handicap is a common lifelong disability with an estimated prevalance of 3 to 4 per 1,000 of the population (Akesson 1961; Wing 1971) with ten times that number having lesser degrees of handicap. In certain causes of mental handicap the association with auditory or visual impairment is well recognized, but in many others sensory deficits may develop insidiously and remain undiagnosed and untreated. In population studies of children it has been estimated that a genetic defect is responsible for over one-third of all causes of severe mental handicap, up to one-half of the causes of blindness (Bryars and Archer 1977) and one-third of the causes of deafness (Fraser 1964). In a proportion of these disorders there is a single genetic abnormality responsible for both the mental handicap and the sensory impairment. In other genetic disorders, sensory loss is not invariable but is more likely to occur because of structural abnormalities to the eyes or ears or because of a predisposition to infections or other disorders.

This chapter is concerned with the genetic causes of mental handicap associated with auditory and visual impairment. It is not a detailed glossary of all such disorders but it attempts to explain the mechanisms behind these conditions and to enable those involved to recognize when a genetic cause is likely and its implications.

The recognition of mental handicap is often not easy, but it may be suspected after birth because of the presence of characteristic features known to be associated with causes of mental handicap or because the baby fails to make normal progress. Later, the triad of major diagnostic features includes: developmental delay; the failure or delay in gaining basic living skills, and intellectual impairment, assessed using standardized tests. The term 'mental handicap' does not in itself suggest a cause. A reason for the handicap should always be sought so that sound advice regarding specific treatments, the likely extent of the handicap and possible recurrence risks can be given.

What Is Meant By Genetic?

Each cell in the human body has 23 pairs of chromosomes (except in the ova and spermatozoa where there is only one of each pair). Twenty-two pairs of chromosomes, called autosomes, are similar in both sexes. The pair of 'sex chromosomes' differ, females having 2 X chromosomes and males one X and a smaller Y chromosome. A set of 23 chromosomes is therefore inherited from each parent (carried in the ova and spermatozoa), making up the total of 46 chromosomes (23 pairs) in the fertilized ovum. The fertilized ovum and subsequent cells divide by a process called mitosis and differentiate forming the different organs of the developing foetus, each new cell receiving copies of the 23 pairs of chromosomes (see Figure 7.1).

The chromosomes contain the basic genetic material, deoxyribose nucleic acid (DNA), which codes for all proteins (e.g. enzymes, hormones and structural proteins). A section of DNA coding for a particular substance is referred to as a 'gene'. It has been estimated that there is enough DNA for up to 3 million genes in the total human 'genome', but there are probably approximately only 60,000 functioning genes, the rest of the DNA having regulating or, as yet, unrecognized functions. Each chromosome of a pair (homologous chromosomes) contains similar genes, the gene for one protein being at the same site (locus) on each of the pair. These genes, however, are not necessarily identical and it is the specific relationship between functionally similar but not necessarily identical genes

Figure 7.1: Photograph of a normal human male karyotype (46 XY). The 23 pairs of chromosomes have been arranged according to size and position of the centromere. The chromosomes were stained using a Giemsa banding method. Courtesy of J. Martin, Institute of Psychiatry.

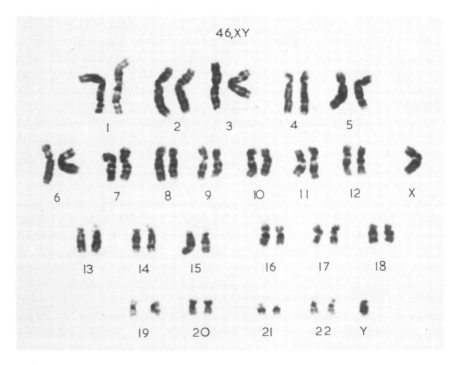

at a given 'locus' that is one factor in determining the varying expression of disease states as well as normal variation between individuals. When the genes at a particular locus on a pair of chromosomes are identical the individual is said to be 'homozygous', and if they differ 'heterozygous', for that locus.

A particular cause of mental handicap can be said to be 'genetic' if it is known to be due to a structural rearrangement of the chromosomes, an abnormality of the number of chromosomes, or a defect of the basic unit of inheritance, the gene.

GENETIC CAUSES

Genetic causes can be divided into three broad groups. The first is chromosome disorders and as many as 1 in 200 new-born babies may have such an abnormality. Individuals with these disorders, for example Down's syndrome, may have a characteristic appearance. The chromosomes can then be examined by culturing and staining white blood cells and the diagnosis confirmed. The second is a group of disorders due to abnormalities of the genes themselves. These disorders are frequently difficult to diagnose but may give rise to a characteristic change in the levels of certain amino acids (the basic units that make up proteins) which can be detected by examination of the urine or blood (e.g. phenylketonuria). These disorders are frequently inherited in a characteristic manner, the mode of inheritance being referred to as autosomal dominant, autosomal recessive or X-linked. The third group of genetic disorders are considered to be 'multifactorial' in that no specific chromosome or gene defect has been identified but family studies or recurrence rates suggest an inherited component. One such condition is spina bifida, which in its severe form may lead to mental handicap.

The Relationship Between Genetic Abnormalities and Mental and Sensory Handicap

Although each cell in the body contains the same genetic material, it is clearly expressed in different ways. The cells of different organs produce specific proteins relevant for their function. In general, if chromosome or gene abnormalities are present at the time of conception, then they will be passed on to all cells. If, for example, that particular gene or chromosome abnormality prevents the cells of the brain producing a protein essential for its normal development, or if it allows the accumulation of substances that in excess are toxic to the nerve cells, then mental handicap may result. Similarly the developing visual and auditory systems can be affected.

Within the group of genetic disorders there is considerable variation on the degree of mental and sensory handicap. At one extreme, severe developmental delay occurs after a period of normal development but leads rapidly to deafness, blindness and death within two to three years. An example of this is Tay-Sachs disease, an autosomal recessive disorder affecting lipid storage (Volk and Schneck 1975). At the other extreme there may be mild, or no, mental handicap, and the development of sensory loss later in life. An example of this is Refsum's syndrome (Refsum 1952). The degree to which mental, visual or auditory handicap occurs is dependent on the specific chromosomal and/or biochemical defect and its significance for the developing nervous and sensory systems. Given the numbers of genes and the complexity of genetic and biochemical inter-actions, there is the potential for a large number of disorders with varying degrees of handicap. The detection of sensory loss in any given condition may largely depend upon the initial realization that, given a particular cause for a disorder, additional handicaps are known to develop.

Chromosome Disorders Associated with Mental and Sensory Handicaps

Chromosomal disorders are due to changes in the chromosome number, or the losses and additions of parts of chromosomes. The loss of whole or sections of chromosomes may result in the loss of several thousand genes and is frequently incompatible with life or gives rise to a foetus that has been unable to grow or develop properly. The addition of chromosomes has a similar devastating effect and the majority result in miscarriage. The reason for the deleterious effect of extra genetic material is unknown.

The cause for many chromosomal abnormalities is not known. Increased maternal age at conception increases the likelihood of Down's syndrome and other disorders in which extra chromosomes are inherited (Penrose 1967). Exposure of the ovaries or testes to X-rays or specific chemicals may also be important. Many of the chromosome abnormalities are sporadic and due, for example, to a defect in the separation of the chromo-somes during the formation of an ovum or spermatozoon (this is referred to as 'non-dysjunction'). The risk of recurrence is related to such factors as maternal age. There are, however, a minority of cases where a chromosome abnormality is carried by one or other parent. The parent is said to carry the chromosomes in a 'balanced state' and is normal but carries a high risk of passing on the abnormally arranged chromosomes to his or her children who may then be affected if their chromosomes are 'unbalanced'. These and other chromosomal rearrangements can be detected by examining the parents' or the child's chromosomes.

The recognition of a chromosome disorder depends on a variety of factors including the presence of characteristic abnormalities known to occur in particular chromosome disorders, multiple structural anomalies suggesting the embryo was abnormal from a very early stage, advanced maternal age and a family history of a similar disorder or of multiple miscarriages. In the majority of cases of severe mental handicap, chromosome analysis is appropriate. The finding of such abnormality provides a diagnosis, may help in genetic counselling and may help in determining the prognosis and the occurrence of any associated handicaps.

Down's Syndrome (Trisomy 21). This chromosomal disorder affects approximately 1 in every 600 births. Langdon Down (1866) first described the characteristic appearance of the syndrome now named after him in 1866 and it was finally established by Lejeune in 1959 that an extra 21 chromosome (Trisomy 21) was the underlying abnormality. This type of chromosome abnormality accounts for over 95 per cent of all individuals with Down's syndrome. The extra 21 chromosome is due to 'non-dysjunction' of the chromosomes at the time of ovum or spermatozoon formation. Polani in 1960 described an individual with the features of Down's syndrome, not associated with increased maternal age, but due to a different chromosome abnormality in which there was a 'translocation' of the 21 chromosome on to chromosome 15, where it remained attached. Under these circumstances the mother was a carrier of the abnormality but unaffected, having a normal complement but abnormally arranged chromosome 21 pair in each cell. The child had the features of Down's syndrome, having inherited a normal and an extra piece of chromosome 21 from mother and a normal 21 chromosome from father. The 'translocation' Down's syndrome is much rarer (approximately 5 per cent of all those with Down's syndrome) and has a high risk of recurrence in those families that carry the abnormality. A third classification of individuals with Down's syndrome, accounting for less than 1 per cent, has been described and is termed 'mosaicism'. In this group the chromosomal abnormality develops shortly after the division of the fertilized ovum has begun and not all the cells carry the extra 21 chromosome and therefore the individual may be less severely affected.

The effect of this extra genetic material can be observed in many of the body's structures, in measureable biochemical abnormalities and in susceptibility to disease states. The eye is abnormal and abnormalities of the cornea (keratoconus), cataracts, squints (strabismus) and Brushfield spots (not of pathological significance) occur. In one study, 5 per cent of individuals with Down's syndrome were found to be blind due to cataracts or secondary to keratoconus (Cullen 1963). Falls (1970) suggested that cataracts could be found in all those with Down's syndrome if the eyes were examined with a slit lamp. The recognition of this risk allows appropriate and cost-effective screening programmes among those with Down's syndrome.

Abnormalities of the outer, middle and inner ear have been described and deafness may be an important factor in the well-recognized speech delay of Down's syndrome. Structural and functional abnormalities contribute to hearing loss and up to 60 per cent of individuals with Down's syndrome may have some hearing loss in childhood (Downs and Balkany

1977). The risk of middle ear infection is higher and if untreated, may contribute to later hearing loss (Brooks, Wooley and Kanjilal 1972).

There has been little systematic research comparing the development of sensory loss between these three types of Down's syndrome. Further research is needed to examine the possibility of preventing the development of these abnormalities or at least reducing their impact by early treatment.

Edward's Syndrome (Trisomy 18).   This disorder occurs in 1 in 3,500 live births and is associated with severe mental handicap. Few survive into childhood. Cataracts and small eyes (microphthalmos) have been reported (Taylor 1968) and deafness is common. The skull has an unusual shape with a protruding occipital region, the eyes are widely spaced and the chin small. Heart abnormalities among others are frequently found. These findings usually suggest the possible diagnosis of this syndrome and the finding of an extra chromosome 18 would confirm the diagnosis. As with Down's syndrome, the incidence increases with increasing maternal age.

Patau's Syndrome (Trisomy 13).   This occurs in 1 in 7,600 live births and is associated with severe handicap, multiple abnormalities and a very short life expectancy. Both eye defects and deafness are reported. Only 5 per cent survive beyond three years (Magenis, Hecht and Milham 1968). An extra chromosome 13 is found on chromosome analysis and rarely it may be due to a balanced 'translocation' of this chromosome in one or other parents and a recurrence in future pregnancies is likely. Counselling with the offer of amniocentesis in future pregnancies would be appropriate.

Other Trisomy Syndromes.   The addition of a whole or part of other chromosomes has been described, including chromosomes 4, 8, 9, 10 and 20. They usually cause severe defects and may have associated sensory impairments. They can be identified by appropriate chromosome analysis and, if present, suggest the possibility that a parent is a 'balanced' carrier of the chromosome abnormality.

Aniridia–Wilm's Tumour Association.   The previously recognized association between aniridia (failure of the iris of the eye to develop) and Wilm's tumour of the kidney occurring in childhood has now been shown to be related to a specific absence (deletion) of part of chromosome 11 (Riccardi, Sujansky, Smith and Francke, 1978). The extent of other abnormalities, including mental handicap, may be related to the extent of the chromosome loss. Parents may carry this abnormality in a form that does not affect them but can be passed on to subsequent children. Genetic counselling and the offer of amniocentesis in future pregnancies is therefore important. Wilms tumour has been reported to occur in about 1 in 70 cases of aniridia.

Other 'Deletion' Syndromes. The absence of parts of other chromosomes are also associated with severe defects. These include chromosomes 4, 5 ('Cri-du-chat' syndrome), 9, 13 and 18. If these are suspected, then chromosomal analysis is appropriate and will identify the abnormality.

Sex Chromosome Disorders. Losses and additions of sex chromosomes have less severe effects than such changes in autosomes.

There are two major sex chromosome abnormalities: Klinefelter's syndrome, affecting 1 in 500 males, in which the males have an extra X chromosomes (XXY) and Turner's syndrome, affecting 1 in 5,000 females, in which females have only one X chromosome (XO). The former may be associated with mild mental handicap and other abnormalities, but the latter usually with normal intelligence although over 50 per cent may have some perceptive hearing impairment.

In the last few years an abnormality on the X chromosome has been found to be associated with mental handicap in males. The association of mental handicap and this particular chromosome abnormality has been called the 'Fragile-X syndrome' because the chromosome abnormality has the appearance of a narrowing near the tip of the long arm of the X chromosome. It is not thought to be associated with additional sensory handicaps but the potential for prenatal diagnosis and the possible high prevalence of this syndrome has made it the centre of much research (De Arche and Kearns 1984).

Single-Gene Disorders Associated with Mental and Sensory Handicaps

The common feature of these disorders is that there is an absence or deficiency of an enzyme needed to convert one substance to another in a particular metabolic pathway or to control the storage of such substances (e.g. lipids and glycogen) in the tissues. This is shown schematically in Figure 7.2.

A deficiency of enzyme 'a' will give rise to an increase in substance 'A' as this cannot be metabolized to 'B', and, unless there is an alternative metabolic pathway, to a deficiency of 'B', 'C' and 'D'. Deficiencies of enzymes 'b' and 'c' may have a similar result, the symptoms depending upon the effect of the excess of some and deficiency of other metabolites. Similarly, deficiencies of enzymes in 'storage' pathways lead to the damaging abnormal accumulation of material within tissues. There are many different cells in the nervous, visual and auditory systems each with special metabolic requirements. Although the genetic abnormalities are very different between diseases, their end effect may be similar, for example retinal pigmentation and degeneration and thus visual impairment may be the feature of several disorders. In one group of disorders, the gangliosidoses, the absence of a gene coding for an enzyme involved in lipid

Figure 7.2: Schematic Representation of a Metabolic Pathway

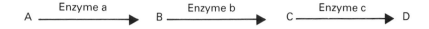

storage gives rise to the accumulation of lipids in a variety of tissue including the nervous and visual systems. Genetic disorders affecting the production of enzymes in other parts of this particular metabolic pathway will have similar effects. It seems likely that some of these disorders will be due to genetic abnormalities of the genes responsible for controlling the 'expression' of the genes coding for the enzyme, rather than the gene coding for the enzyme itself (regulator genes).

Each enzyme is coded for by the genes at the same locus on a particular pair of chromosomes. The effect of an abnormality of the genes coding for a particular enzyme depends on a variety of factors including whether both genes coding for that enzyme are abnormal, the mode of inheritance and the biochemical significance of such a loss. These disorders are inherited in different ways according to whether the responsible gene is carried on an autosome (as opposed to one of the sex chromosomes) and are then inherited in an 'autosomal recessive' or 'autosomal dominant' manner or whether they are carried on the X chromosome and are then said to be inherited in an 'X-linked' manner.

There are many single gene disorders that can cause visual and auditory impairment. The disorders included in this chapter are associated with mental handicap and sensory impairment and have been divided according to their pattern of inheritance: autosomal recessive, autosomal dominant and X-linked.

Autosomal Recessive Disorders

For a child to develop such a disorder both parents must be 'carriers' of the same abnormal gene and both the abnormal genes must be inherited by the child. Each parent will have a normal gene as well as the abnormal gene at that locus and, therefore, have a 50 per cent chance of passing on the normal or the abnormal gene. There is, therefore, with each child, a 25 per cent ($\frac{1}{2} \times \frac{1}{2}$) chance that they will inherit both normal genes (homozygous normal) or both abnormal genes (homozygous affected) and a 50 per cent chance that they will inherit only one abnormal gene (and therefore be clinically unaffected like their parents) and be a carrier (heterozygote). Most of us are carriers of some abnormal genes, but the chance of two people carrying the same abnormal gene marrying and having children is rare. This may not be the case for all genes in certain populations where marriages tend to be within the same ethnic or religious group and the chance of carriers for the same genetic disorder marrying is increased. In the majority of cases the fact that both members of a couple are carriers of the same abnormal recessive gene may only become apparent after they have had an affected child.

Galactosaemia.   This is a rare disorder occurring in 1 in 30,000 live births (Lee 1972) and, if untreated, leads to rapid deterioration in infancy and death. There are two related variants of the disorder, the classical form being an inability to break down galactose-1-phosphate due to an enzyme deficiency. There is 'failure to thrive' in the early weeks of life, a suscepti-bility to overwhelming infections and cataract development. The liver and spleen enlarge and jaundice develops. The diagnosis can be confirmed by specific blood and urine tests and the early removal of dietary galactose may arrest the deterioration and prevent further mental retardation and cataract formation. Lee (1972) followed up 60 affected individuals and found 16 per cent with residual visual impairment due to cataracts and evidence of mental retardation.

Mucopolysaccharidoses.   This is a group of disorders that have rather similar clinical pictures, although varying in severity, in which there is early mental deterioration resulting from an inability to breakdown mucopoly-saccharides which accumulate in certain tissues. Early development may be normal, but coarse facial features and mental retardation soon develop. There are a variety of subtypes (e.g. Hurler's syndrome and Sanfilippo's syndrome) that are inherited in an autosomal recessive manner. One form, Hunter's syndrome, is X-linked, affecting males only. There is the patho-logical deposition of lipid material with the cells of the brain and the visual and auditory systems and in Hurler's syndrome there is corneal clouding, retinal degeneration and deafness as well as severe mental handicap. There is usually a deteriorating course and death by the age of ten years.

The diagnosis is based on the clinical picture and by the demonstration of abnormal mucopolysaccharide excretion in the urine and accumulation in tissues. Rare conditions (e.g. 'I' cell disease associated with corneal clouding) may mimic this type of disorder and therefore detailed bio-chemical analysis is necessary before genetic guidance and advice concern-ing prognosis can be given.

Gangliosidosis.   In this rare group of disorders there is an abnormality of lipid storage due to the absence of specific enzymes. This group includes Tay–Sachs disease (GM 2 gangliosidosis) and GM 1 gangliosidosis. In the former a period of normal development is followed by rapid deterioration, enlargement of the head, convulsions and progressive sensory impairment. There is a characteristic 'cherry red spot' in the central retinal area of the eyes which is indicative of retinal degeneration. The cause is a deficiency of the enzyme Hexosamidase A, which is reduced in carriers (heterozygotes) and very low or absent in affected individuals (homozygotes). This disorder is exceedingly rare in the general population, but among the Ashkenazi

Jewish population up to 1 in 30 may be carriers and preconceptual and prenatal diagnosis is possible by measurement of hexosamidase A in potential carriers and in the foetus.

Niemann−Pick Disease (Sphingomyelin Lipidosis).   There are at least four different types of this disorder that vary as to age of onset and the degree of mental handicap. The basic abnormality is the absence of the enzyme sphingomyelinase and in the most severe form there is abnormal lipid accumulation in cells, a rapid deterioration and death before two years of age. The age of onset is later in some forms and macular degeneration and blindness occurs. The forms can be distinguished by the nature of the clinical presentation and on specific enzyme assays. Prenatal diagnosis is possible.

Metachromatic Leukodystrophy.   In this lipid storage disease, development up to two years of age is usually normal. This is followed by a relatively slow decline of motor skills and intellectual functioning. The retina becomes discoloured by lipid deposition and a 'cherry red spot' similar to Tay−Sachs disease is observed on examination. The disorder is due to an absence of the enzyme arylsulphatase A or B. This can be shown to be low in heterozygote carriers of the disorder and prenatal diagnosis is also possible. A diet low in vitamin A has been tried with variable success. The life expectancy is usually five to six years.

Gaucher's Disease (Cerebroside Lipidosis).   There are several forms of this disorder, varying in severity. These are thought to be due to different abnormal genes that may be inherited at a particular locus. Following a period of normal development the child develops enlargement of the liver and spleen and in some forms neurological deterioration, sensory impairment and early death. The exact nature of the change depends on which form of the disease has been inherited. The enzyme defect can be detected and prenatal diagnosis is possible.

Homocystinuria.   The major features of this disorder are dislocation of the lenses in the eyes, mental retardation and a tendency to blood clot formation. These features are not invariably present and one-third or more of individuals having this disorder are usually mentally normal. The basic disorder is an absence of the enzyme cystathionine synthetase. A number of individuals have been shown to improve on vitamin B6 (pyridoxine). Some have a different biochemical abnormality and, if prenatal diagnosis is proposed, the exact biochemical defect must be established.

Laurence−Moon−Bardet−Biedl Syndrome (also known as the Bardet− Biedl syndrome, see Chapter 5, this volume). The frequency of this disorder is not known. It is associated with mild mental retardation, degeneration of the retinal cells (characterized by retinitis pigmentosa), the death of the cells of the optic nerve, cataracts, hormonal changes, extra fingers and toes (polydactyly) and obesity. A total of 273 individuals with this disorder were reviewed by Bell (1958). The life span appeared to be normal. The basic abnormality is unknown and there is no specific treatment. Alstrom's syndrome is similar but not associated with mental handicap and should be clearly distinguished from this disorder.

Usher's Syndrome. This is thought to be a recessive disorder characterized by possible mild mental handicap, retinitis pigmentosa and sensorineural deafness (Vernon 1979). There may be at least two variants of this disorder, one mild and the other severe. The genetic evidence is based on the observation that this disorder occurred in certain cases of first-cousin marriages (Lang 1959) and in certain populations. Davenport (1978) found that 90 per cent of reported cases had severe congenital deafness and the onset of retinitis pigmentosa occurring before puberty, whereas the rest had a less severe hearing loss and retinitis pigmentosa developing after puberty. The underlying abnormality of this disorder is unknown. The diagnosis is based on the triad of mild intellectual impairment and progressive visual and auditory loss. The early recognition of this condition is important as educational help, before sensory loss is profound, may help to minimize the overall social handicap.

Ichthyosis (Sjogren–Larsson Syndrome). This disorder is associated with a marked abnormality of the skin, severe mental retardation and increasing weakness of the limbs. Macular degeneration, leading to blindness, has been reported in 25 per cent of individuals.

Refsum's Syndrome. This disorder is included because of its association with progressive blindness (due to retinitis pigmentosa) and deafness. It is not associated with severe mental handicap but individuals are reported as having below average intelligence. The underlying abnormality is a disorder of lipid metabolism due to an absence of the enzyme phytanic acid oxidase with the resultant excess of phytanic acid in blood and other tissues. Dietary restriction and a treatment called 'plasmaphoresis', whereby the phytanic acid can be removed from the blood, has been shown to prevent deterioration (Gibbard, Page, Billimoria and Retsas 1979).

Cockayne Syndrome. This is a very rare disorder characterized by senile-like changes occurring in infancy. Growth and development are normal for the first two to four years of life, but this is followed by a fall off in growth, changes in the skin, mental handicap, moderate perceptive deafness, retinal degeneration, optic atrophy and corneal opacities. Other changes affect the skeletal system and the kidneys and the hair may become sparse and grey (Cockayne 1946; MacDonald, Fitch and Lewis 1960). The cause is unknown and the prognosis poor.

Autosomal Dominant Disorders

In these disorders the presence of one abnormal gene is sufficient to give rise to the disorder. The pattern of inheritance is characteristic in that, unlike in autosomal recessive disorders, there is usually one affected parent and often other affected family members. Children of an affected individual carry a 50 per cent chance of being similarly affected. The inheritance of these disorders is complicated by two factors. The first is that, although the abnormal gene is present, it may not be manifest. This is related to what is termed the degree of 'penetrance' of the disorder. The second is the high occurrence of new 'mutations' whereby the abnormal gene causing the disorder has occurred for the first time in that family. Therefore, a detailed examination of several members of the family is frequently necessary before advice can be given concerning recurrence risk.

Treacher–Collins Syndrome.   This disorder may vary considerably in severity. At its most severe the features are of mental handicap, an abnormal development of the facial bones, downward slanting eyes, colombomata of the eyes (abnormalities of the iris) and small ears resulting in deafness. The expression of the disorder varies within families and the severity cannot be predicted from the severity of others within the family. The deafness may be helped with aids, and plastic surgery may be of value with certain deformities. Most individuals with this disorder are, however, mentally normal even if they have some hearing impairment.

Dystrophia Myotonica.   This disorder varies considerably in severity. The onset may be delayed until adult life and is characterized by muscle weakness, stiffness and a difficulty in the relaxation of muscles, cataract formation and, in males, testicular atrophy. Lens opacities may be detected early in the disorder by slit lamp examination. Mild to moderate mental handicap may occur and may be the only feature in childhood. The underlying biochemical defect is not known, but 'linkage' to certain blood groups may be of value in prenatal diagnosis (Gibson and Ferguson-Smith 1980). This evidence suggests that the abnormal gene is carried on chromosome 19.

Neurofibromatosis (Von Recklinghausen's Disease).   This disorder may be found in 1 in 3,000 live births. The diagnosis may be suspected on the finding of several (at least six) 'café au lait' patches on the skin. These may increase in number and skin nodules also develop numbering several hundred. These benign tumours may occur elsewhere in the body including the eye socket or more commonly the auditory nerve, causing deafness. Occasionally the tumours become malignant. Up to one-third of affected individuals may become mentally handicapped. The underlying genetic abnormality is unknown.

Tuberous Sclerosis (Epiloia).   This disorder has been estimated to occur in 1 in 20,000 to 1 in 40,000 live births. The characteristic features are:

epilepsy, mental retardation and a rash on the face called 'adenoma sebaceum'. Although this disorder is inherited in an autosomal dominant manner, in nearly half the cases neither parent has the disease and up to 50 per cent of individuals may have the disorder as a result of a new mutation. The child is normal at birth but early in life develops characteristic skin patches on the trunk, adenoma sebaceum on the face and occasionally nodules in the retina and less frequently cataracts. Epilepsy may develop as a result of nodules developing in the brain tissue. These can be demonstrated using computer X-ray scans (CAT scans). The degree of mental handicap is variable and may relate to the number of abnormalities within the brain. Overall about one-third of affected individuals are of normal intelligence. The cause is unknown and genetic counselling is dependent on a detailed family history and examination of the parents of an affected child to assess whether one or other is affected and therefore has the abnormal gene or whether it was due to a new mutation (Zaremba 1968).

X-linked Disorders

Some disorders characteristically affect males only but have been inherited from the mother. In these disorders the abnormal gene is carried on the X chromosome and is said to be 'X-linked recessive'. If, of the two X chromosomes carried by the mother, the male inherits the one carrying the abnormal gene, he is affected by the disorder caused by that abnormal gene having only one X chromosome. A male child, therefore, has a 50 per cent chance of inheriting the disorder from a carrier mother and the female child a 50 per cent chance of being a carrier.

Some genetic disorders only affect females and are inherited in a 'X-linked dominant' manner. Affected females are heterozygotes, one X chromosome carrying the abnormal gene and the other the normal gene at that locus, but because of the 'dominant' nature of that gene the individual develops the disorder. If the one X chromosome in the normal chromosome complement of males carries the abnormal gene, the foetus is non-viable.

Hunter's Syndrome (Mucopolysaccharidosis Type II). This disorder is similar to the autosomal recessive forms of mucopolysaccharidosis but is inherited in an X-linked recessive manner, affecting males only. It differs from Hurler's Syndrome Type I in the manner of inheritance and in addition there are no corneal changes. The major characteristics are the facial appearance, dwarfism, enlargement of the liver and spleen and mental retardation. Deafness has occasionally been reported. There is an excess of chondroitin sulphate B and heparitin sulphate in the urine which may be diagnostically helpful. Specific sulphatase enzymes are deficient and prenatal diagnosis is possible by enzyme assay of foetal cells obtained by amniocentesis.

Incontinentia Pigmenti.   This disorder affects females only and is inherited in an X-linked dominant manner. The child is normal for the first few months of life and then develops 'bullous' lesions of the skin which change over time giving an atrophied appearance to the skin. The teeth and nails are poorly developed, the skull may be small, some develop cataracts and corneal opacities and up to one-third may be mentally handicapped.

Disorders of Possible Genetic Aetiology Associated with Mental and Sensory Handicap

Cornelia de Lange Syndrome.   The major characteristics of this disorder are small stature, abnormal facial features with excess facial hair, severe mental handicap and abnormalities of the hands, feet, eyes and ears. The degree of handicap and life expectancy is variable although the majority are severely affected. The aetiology is unknown, although chromosome abnormalities have been reported (Craig and Luzzatti 1965). An empirical recurrence risk of between 1 per cent and 3 per cent is usually given, but in certain cases chromosome analysis can be helpful in giving more specific guidance.

Pierre–Robin Syndrome.   The features of this disorder may be the result of a number of causes, some of which may be genetic. There is poor development of the mouth, in particular the mandible, and mental retardation of varying degree. One-third of individuals with this syndrome are also found to have eye abnormalities and glaucoma may be a complication.

Norrie's Disease.   This is one cause of congenital blindness (present at birth) and is thought to be genetic in cause. It may be associated with deafness. Warburg (1968) reported that 9 out of 35 individuals with this disorder were severely handicapped and another 11 mildly affected. It has to be differentiated from other causes of congenital blindness such as maternal Rubella.

Congenital Hypothyroidism.   An underactive thyroid gland is an important cause of potentially reversible mental handicap. The thyroid gland may fail to develop or rarely there may be a loss or absence of an enzyme necessary for the child's thyroid gland to produce thyroxine. The diagnosis should be established as soon as possible after birth as giving thyroxine will prevent handicap. Failure to thrive, unexplained jaundice and a large foetal umbilical hernia are some of the features that suggest this diagnosis. It may also be associated with deafness. In the UK the majority of children are screened for this at birth.

RESEARCH AND NEW ADVANCES

A large proportion of the causes of severe mental handicap are now recognized to be 'genetic'. The labelling of a condition in this way may be associated with two major concerns: firstly, does this mean other children will be affected and, secondly, because it is genetic does that mean we can do nothing about it? The answer to the former depends upon an accurate diagnosis of the condition and knowledge of its inheritance. The answer to the latter question is dependent on a prior knowledge of the disorder and in particular of any previous attempts at specific treatments or of any association with additional handicaps that could be ameliorated.

Carrier Detection and Prenatal Diagnosis

Genetic counselling has largely relied on empirical observations of recurrence risks and a knowledge of the laws of inheritance of autosomal recessive and dominant and X-linked disorders. There have been considerable advances which have enhanced the accuracy and predictability of such counselling for single-gene disorders.

Genetic counselling may be sought for several reasons. A couple may already have one affected child and wish to know the risk of subsequent children being affected, a particular disorder may be known to occur in the family or there may be concern because of factors such as advanced maternal age or a genetic disorder may be particularly prevalent in a given population. In all cases the approach to this must be based on sound diagnosis and on proper biochemical and/or chromosomal examination of affected individuals and possibly normal members of the family. With the greater understanding of the biochemical abnormalities of many of these disorders, carrier detection is possible. Many of these conditions are rare and population screening for carriers would be inappropriate, but, in specific populations where the disorder (and thus carriers) are common, screening and counselling may be appropriate. This is now offered, in the case of Tay–Sachs disease, to Ashkenazi Jewish couples because of the high carrier frequency in that population. In all autosomal recessive disorders, if only one parent is a carrier, then the children cannot be affected and under those circumstances the couple reassured. If they are both carriers, then prenatal diagnosis is possible and selective termination carried out if so wished. Similarly the identification of the carrier status of the mother in the case of X-linked inheritance and either parent in autosomal dominant disorders would be of considerable benefit. In these conditions there is frequently a family history and the fear of having an affected child is present even before a family is started. Recent advances in the ability to detect abnormal genes is now making this possible. In these cases advice before the child is conceived may be crucial because the exact biochemical nature of the disorder may have to be established and in some cases detailed study of different generations within the family is necessary. Accurate prenatal diagnosis is now possible for about 60 single-gene disorders, some of which cause mental handicap (Patrick 1984).

Amniocentesis and Chorionic Villus Biopsy

Prenatal diagnosis has been dependent on the procedure called 'amniocentesis'. This involves the removal of a small quantity of amniotic fluid that surrounds the foetus in the uterus and which will contain foetal cells. This is a relatively simple procedure that involves inserting a small needle, under local anaesthetic, through the abdominal wall into the uterus and drawing out a small amount of fluid through a syringe. This is done under guidance, using an ultrasound scanner so that the placenta can be avoided. It is a quick and relatively simple procedure but has a possible risk of miscarriage in about 1 per cent of cases. The major drawback is that it cannot be performed until the sixteenth week of pregnancy and the results may not be available until the eighteenth or twentieth week. Termination at this stage is a major procedure both psychologically and physically. A technique called 'chorionic villus biopsy' allows the examination of foetal tissue as early as the eighth week of pregnancy and early and safer termination can be offered. This technique, as yet still experimental, can be used for chromosome culture and for the collection and subsequent analysis of the DNA of the foetus. Over the next few years more disorders causing mental handicap may be detected by this method.

Treatment of Genetic Disorders

Advances in genetics have largely enabled prenatal diagnosis to be carried out with the offer of termination of pregnancy if the foetus is affected. The identification of the particular chromosome or gene defect will, however, lead to a more fundamental understanding of the disorder. The ultimate aim of such research must be to correct or replace the abnormal genetic material. DNA can be introduced into cells but this is a long way from being able to introduce a specific segment of DNA into the correct place in the correct chromosomes. Transplantation of tissue with cells not containing the genetic defect into the foetus or child may be one method of partially providing the missing or abnormal gene, which is the basis of many of these disorders, and thus at least providing a small amount of the gene product (e.g. missing enzyme). There are many other genes involved in the functioning of individual genes and the link from gene, to gene product, to the functioning system is far from understood.

There are other areas of research looking at whether the effects of the presence of abnormal chromosomes or genes can be modified by diet or specific treatments. Phenylketonuria and galactosaemia are examples whereby radical changes in the diet prevent the development of mental handicap. There are also claims, as yet not satisfactorily proven, that vitamin supplements may improve the functioning of individuals with Down's syndrome. Given the presence of a genetic disorder, there may still be interventions that can modify the severity of the disorder and further research is needed in this area.

The long-term goal of genetic research must be the identification of the specific genetic defect in these disorders and the correction of that defect or the modification of its effect. At present the correct recognition of a genetic disorder will enable sound genetic counselling to be given, guide in our assessment of degree and types of impairment, and may eventually enable more radical treatment of the basic genetic defect.

Acknowledgements

My thanks to Dr Lachlan Campbell and Dr Mary Honeyman for their helpful suggestions during the preparation of this chapter and for their patient and constructive criticisms of the various drafts.

References

Akesson, H. (1961) *Epidemiology and Genetics of Mental Deficiency in a Southern Swedish Population*, University of Uppsala, Sweden

Bell, J. (1958) 'The Laurence-Moon syndrome' in *The Treasure of human inheritance*, 5 (3), 51-69, Cambridge University Press

Bryars, J.H. and Archer, D.B. (1977) *Trans. Ophthalmol. Soc., U.K.*, 97, 26.

Brooks, D.N., Wooley, H. and Kanjilal, G.C. (1972) 'Hearing loss and middle ear disorders in patients with Down's syndrome (mongolism)', *J. Ment. Defic. Res.*, 16, 21-9

Cockayne, E.A. (1946) 'Dwarfism with retinal atrophy and deafness', *Arch. Dis. Child.*, 21, 52

Craig, A.P. and Luzzatti, L. (1965) 'Translocation in de Lange's syndrome', *Lancet II*, 445-6

Cullen, J.F. (1963) 'Blindness in mongolism (Down's syndrome)', *Brit. J. Ophthal.*, 43, 331

Davenport, S.L.H. (1978) 'The heterogeneity of Usher's syndrome', *Vth International Conf. on Birth Defects*. Montreal, Aug., 1977

De Arche, M.A. and Kearns, A. (1984) 'The fragile X syndrome: the patients and their chromosomes', *J. Med. Gen.*, 21, 84-91

Downs, M. and Balkany, T. (1977) 'Audiological and otological findings in Down's syndrome', *Amer. Speech and Hearing Convention*, Chicago

Falls, H.F. (1970) 'Ocular changes in mongolism', *Ann. N.Y. Acad. Sci. 171*, 625-36

Fraser, G.R. (1964) 'Review article: profound childhood deafness', *J. Med. Genet.*, 1, 118-51

Gibbard, F.B., Page, N.G.R., Billimoria, J.D. and Retsas, S. (1979) 'Heredopathia atactia polyneuritiformis (Refsum's disease) treated by diet and plasma-exchange', *Lancet I* 575-8

Gibson, S.L.M. and Ferguson-Smith, M.A. (1980), 'The use of genetic linkage in counselling families with dystrophia myotonica', *Clin. Genet.*, 17, 443-8

Lang, H. (1969) 'Retinal degeneration and nerve deafness', *Brit. Med. J.*, 2, 1096

Langdon Down, J. (1866) 'Observations on an ethnic classification of idiots', *Clin. Lectures and Reports, London Hospital, 3,* 259

Lee, D.H. (1972) 'Psychological aspects of galactosaemia', *J. Ment. Defic. Res., 16,* 173-91

Lejeune, J., Gautier, M. and Turpin, R. (1959) Études des chromosomes somatiques de neuf enfants mongoliens', *C.R. Acad. Sci. (Paris), 248,* 1721-2

MacDonald, W.B., Fitch, K.D. and Lewis, I.C. (1960) 'Cockayne's syndrome. An heredo-familial disorder of growth and development', *Pediatrics, 25,* 997

Magenis, R.E., Hecht, F. and Milham, S. (1968) 'Trisomy 13 (D1) syndrome: studies on parental age, sex ratio and survival', *J. Pediat., 73,* 222-8

Patrick, A.D. (1984) 'Prenatal diagnosis of inherited metabolic disease' in C.H. Rodeck and K.H. Nicolaides (eds.), *Prenatal diagnosis.* Proc. of the 11th study group of the Royal College of Obstetricians and Gynaecologists, London

Penrose, L.S. (1967) 'The effect of change in maternal age distribution upon the incidence of mongolism', *J. Ment. Defic. Res., 11,* 54-7

Polani, P.E., Briggs, J.H., Ford, C.E. Clarke, C.M. and Berg, J.M. (1960) 'A mongol girl with 46 chromosomes', *Lancet 1,* 121

Refsum, S. (1952) 'Heredopathia atactica polyneuritiformis', *J. Nerv. Ment. Dis., 116,* 1046-50

Riccardi, V.M., Sujansky, E., Smith, A.C. and Francke, U. (1978) 'Chromosomal imbalance in the aniridia-Wilm's tumour association: 11p interstitial deletion', *Pediatrics, 61,* 604

Taylor, A.I. (1968) 'Autosomal trisomy syndromes: a detailed study of 27 cases of Edwards' syndrome and 27 of Patau's syndrome', *J. Med. Genet., 5,* 227-52

Vernon, M., (1969) Usher's syndrome deafness and progressive blindness. Clinical cases, prevention, theory and literature survey. *J. Chronic dis., 22,* 133-51

Volk, B.W. and Schneck, L. (eds.), (1975) *The Gangliosidoses,* Plenum Press, London

Warburg, M. (1968) 'Norrie's disease', *J. Ment. Defic. Res., 12,* 247-51

Wing, L. (1971) 'Severely retarded children in a London area: prevalence and provision of services', *J. Psychol. Med., 1,* 405-15

Zaremba, J. (1968) 'Tuberous sclerosis: a clinical and genetic investigation', *J. Ment. Defic. Res., 12,* 63-80

General Reference Texts

Smith, D.W. (1982) *Recognizable Patterns of Human Malformation. Genetic, Embryologic and Clinical aspects* (Third edn.), W.B. Saunders Co., Philadelphia and London

Tredgold's mental retardation (1979) edited by M.J. Craft, Bailliere Tindall, London

PART THREE

FUNCTIONAL AND DEVELOPMENTAL ASPECTS

8 COGNITIVE DEFICIT AND MOTOR SKILL

Feriha Anwar

Introduction

Mentally handicapped people have consistently been found to be inferior to non-handicapped subjects on measures of physical development, gross-motor and fine-motor abilities (Annett 1957; Ellis 1963; Cratty and Martin 1969; Bruininks 1974; Gibson 1978; O'Connor and Hermelin 1978; Anwar 1981a; Hogg 1982). The motor behaviour of the retarded individuals is usually considered to be poor not because they are unable to perform the necessary movements, but rather because they are too slow or clumsy or show unco-ordinated movements. Furthermore, in cases in which more severe intellectual defect is present, motor function has been found to decrease correspondingly, a condition usually associated with extensive brain damage. Extensive research studies on motor movements have shown that even the simplest actions are planned in advance using prediction and inferences made on the basis of a certain number of cues (Mounoud 1982). These cues are interpreted by means of what can be called representations (as suggested by Mounoud 1982; Mounoud and Hauert 1982; Karmiloff-Smith 1984) or schemas (as proposed by Adams 1971 and Schmidt 1975) which are elaborated in the course of development. The inference, therefore, is that motor planning itself is an intellectual function, based in part on such mental representation, thus the person with congenital or acquired intellectual retardation will usually be clumsy even when a neurological physical examination reveals no evidence of cranial nerve, motor or sensory dysfunction.

According to Gubbay (1975), in terms of clinical neurological function it is often inappropriate to consider any part of the nervous system in isolation, for the central nervous system is regarded as a nerve network where activation in any one area has widespread implications regarding factors of input, output, facilitation and inhibition. From a psychological point, O'Connor and Hermelin (1978) also propose that perception and cognition are not two qualitatively different operations, but represent different aspects of the same processing activity by which one structure interacts with another. These authors regard the successive stages of this process as interactive and interdependent and in studies with sensorily and cognitively impaired children (O'Connor and Hermelin 1978) have shown that sensory deficits affect cognition and congenital impairment in turn influences perceptual organization. The following chapter by O'Connor and Hermelin presents their theoretical views on the effect of sensory handicap on cognitive defect in detail.

Severe sensory handicaps restrict all aspects of severely subnormal people's development from infancy to adulthood. There is no doubt that the presence of an additional sensory disability, as for example impaired vision, in a mentally retarded person would produce a corresponding effect which would be greater than that expected from the sum of the two disabilities. The present chapter will attempt to delineate the effect of mental handicap on the development and acquisition of motor skills and motor proficiency.

Motor Performance

The mentally deficient child exhibits increasing degrees of awkwardness for increasing complexities of intellectually challenging physical tasks. Where a series of movements presents no real challenge to motor planning for a child with intellectual retardation, there is no real difficulty or clumsiness. Thus automatic movements, such as walking or running, may be executed perfectly. However, it has also been noticed that in severe retardation even such automatic movements may be carried out with a certain degree of inefficiency. Specifically, experimental findings suggest that the breakdown of well-integrated movement, however simple, occurs when it has to be newly learned rather than repeated.

Definition

One of the major handicaps in interpreting the literature on the motor characteristics of the mentally retarded person is the difficulty presented by the plethora of overlapping terms used to describe motor proficiency and development. Terms like 'motor ability', 'motor skill', 'motor development' and 'motor proficiency' tend to be used interchangeably to denote either the same or a different meaning. For the present purpose the distinctions drawn by Fleishman (1964) will be used. According to Fleishman, *motor ability* describes a more general trait of an individual inferred from a consistent pattern of motor responses on measures related to a variety of performance tasks. In contrast, Fleishman suggests that *motor skill* be applied to performance of an individual on specific tasks or a limited group of tasks. The term *motor development* will be used to refer to changes in performance with increasing age, and *motor proficiency* will be used to refer to performance(s) on a wide variety of tasks requiring motor coordination and planning in a manner similar to that proposed by Bruininks (1974). Thus what one can presume from such a distinction is that, whereas training may change motor performance or skills on specific tasks, abilities contribute to a wide range of skilled performances and are less influenced by the effects of training and environment. The purpose of the present chapter will be to evaluate the potential of severely subnormal people to acquire simple motor skills in three- and two-dimensional space (Anwar 1981a) and to discuss the implication of isolated research findings and the relevance of such findings for an overall theoretical framework within which varied and disparate streams of work on motor skills in the mentally retarded could be integrated.

It appears that, as far as motor skill in the mentally retarded is concerned, the experimental evidence to date has been fragmented and concerned mostly with phases or levels of development in disparate domains. From such a perspective and the range of deficits observed in processes one can at best only infer that the representation of motor skills in the mentally retarded does not appear to follow a pattern characteristic of normal development.

Information Processing in Motor Skills

Mentally handicapped individuals appear to have a limited capacity for information processing. Ellis (1963) proposed that the generally low performance of retarded people on motor tasks is due to a limited capacity for information intake and a more rapid decay of that information over time. Motor skill requires the processing of sensory information at the initial stage, during the movement and at the completion of the movement in the form of knowledge of results (Anwar 1983a).

Research on human performance traditionally fragmented the problem with studies of sensory efficiency on the one hand and motor performance on the other. An appreciation of the importance of what takes place between the reception of signals by the sense organs and the initiation of responses by the muscle groups has emerged since the work of Craik (1947, 1948). Craik considered the human operator as a link in a communication channel — receiving, processing and transmitting information from display (input) to control (output).

Information-processing theory assumes that human behaviour can be analysed in terms of discrete stages in a process. In viewing a response as only the end product of a series of processes, it becomes possible to specify the correlates of observed performance deficits more accurately than could otherwise be done.

Even a simple perceptual-motor task requires the integration of sensory, perceptual information from various sensory modalities and such inter-modality integration of information is necessary at various stages in the processing chain. For example, in the first instance, some specific sensory input must determine for the subject the plan of the motor act itself, e.g. where to point, where to reach, what to draw and so on. During the movement itself, the information from the kinaesthetic sense regarding the position of the hand must be related to the visual frame of reference for accurate guidance. At the completion of the motor act the sensorily acquired knowledge of results or feedback must be stored and subsequent improvements in any motor task would be determined by the facility with which this information is acquired, organized, stored and made accessible. Thus, not only does a simple perceptual motor task make cognitive demands on the subject, but it would seem that a strong relationship exists between cognitive development and motor performance. This view has been well documented by Connolly (1970), Newell and Kennedy (1978), O'Connor and Hermelin (1978), Mounoud (1982) and Anwar (1983a).

A person must be able to utilize information from various sensory modalities in order to learn new motor skills. Two important sources of information are derived from vision and kinaesthesis. When learning a motor skill, a subject must encode information from these two sources and store it in a format suitable for subsequent movement planning, execution and evaluation. O'Connor and Hermelin (1978) proposed that inadequacies of coding at the input stage may account for some of the problems experienced by the mentally handicapped. Coding was defined by these authors as the translation of information from one repre-sentational system to another. O'Connor and Hermelin suggested that the classification of any particular input and its appropriate tagging for reference constituted the basic operation in perception, learning a recall.

As mentioned earlier, in most motor skills the utilization and integration of information must occur at the various stages: during the planning of the movement, during the actual motor sequence, and at the completion of the response when some sensory information may be used to appraise the accuracy of the response itself. It could be, for example, that in persons with cognitive deficit the comparison of two kinds of input, visual and kinaesthetic (intermodality integration) may be difficult — i.e. cognitive capacity may determine how much information from more than one sensory input would be processed. Experiments were conducted to evalu-ate further this hypothesis (Anwar 1981a, b, 1983a) and to determine if deficits in motor performance are related to accessibility of information from memory.

In a number of studies on motor skills, subjects with cognitive deficit were compared with those without any deficit, i.e. children of normal intelligence, and comparative studies were also made within the retarded group over different tasks. A group of mentally retarded people with specific aetiology, e.g. Down's syndrome, and another group of mentally handicapped subjects, were usually selected who were matched for mental and chronological age but did not suffer from other physical handicaps or autism. The mental age of Down's-syndrome and non-Down's-syndrome adolescents usually ranged between four and six years and the chronological age was 13-17 years. The IQ of mentally handicapped gener-ally ranged around 35 points. Where comparative data were obtained from normal children, they were matched for mental age to the persons with cognitive deficit.

Visual Motor Localizations

In experiments on three-dimensional space, subjects were required to point to a visual target located at arm's length in front of the subject (Anwar 1981b). The reference points defining the task were primarily visual. Two different experimental conditions were as follows: (1) *In the visually directed (VD) condition without knowledge of results* (KR), as the subject localized the target, he/she could not see the pointing hand and also received no knowledge of results. In such a task the mentally handicapped persons were as accurate as normal children of the same mental age. (2) *In the visually directed condition with visual knowledge of results*, the child could not see his/her hand until the visual target was localized, but could see both the extent and direction of his/her error at the completion of an incorrect response. Such use of visual error information was made differentially by those subjects with cognitive deficit and normal children. The mentally handicapped adolescents were unable to improve localization accuracy on such a task when given visual knowledge of results — on the contrary, these subjects were affected by such visual feedback. Normal children, of the same mental age, were found to improve significantly when given visual knowledge of results. In such a task visual information gave knowledge about the subjects' target localization accuracy, that is the extent and direction of error. In order to be used effectively, visual information would have had to be stored in short-term memory, coded and subsequently used to correct the motor movement on the next trial. The mentally handicapped could not use such visual error information accurately to improve localization accuracy to a visually presented target.

In comparison, on a similar *visually directed target localization, kinaesthetic information in the form of knowledge of results* was effectively used by mentally handicapped subjects. In such a condition the subject pointed to a visual target and, at the completion of the response, the subject was made to feel with his/her pointing hand, which was hidden from view, the extent and direction of the pointing error for that trial. Such error information was effectively used by the mentally handicapped adolescents and their response accuracy improved significantly over trials.

Statistical comparisons between groups on these two feedback conditions revealed that the mentally handicapped children were significantly more accurate when given kinaesthetic information than when given visual knowledge of results, whereas the reverse was the case for the normal controls. Thus, in visually directed pointing, mentally retarded subjects were able to improve accuracy by effective utilization of kinaesthetic but not of visual knowledge of results. The matched group of normal children on the other hand was able to improve accuracy considerably under both conditions but was better able to utilize visual than kinaesthetic error information.

What conclusions can be drawn from these experiments? Feedback enables the subject to compare information received from knowledge of results with knowledge of his/her own performance, and to modify his/her subsequent performance in the light of this information. Thus, in order that such appropriate modification can occur, the visual or kinaesthetic information acquired from knowledge of results had to be stored in and retrieved from memory. It seems possible that visual error information could not be used effectively by mentally handicapped children for the modification of subsequent kinaesthetic/proprioceptive positioning movements. This deficiency might indicate a failure of transfer of sensory information and its representation in an alternative modality for output. Alternatively, the results could suggest a relatively more rapid deterioration of visual as compared with kinaesthetic information.

Drawing Ability

The results reported above were from target localization experiments where it was found that perhaps one of the reasons why persons with cognitive deficit are unable to acquire this skill adequately is because of limitations in their storing, processing and integration of visual information with motor output. The experimental paradigm utilized imposed artificial demands on the subject. Other than the fact that the mentally handicapped are unusually clumsy, errors in visuo-motor calibration are usually either not noticed or corrected. However, one skill which has been extensively noticed to be difficult for those with cognitive deficit is drawing. The effect of variations in the modality of input on drawing skill has revealed interesting results (Anwar 1983a, b).

Following the perception of a stimulus, copying, drawing and reproducing requires that the visually derived information must be translated into a motor response. There is considerable evidence to indicate that brain-damaged or retarded children exhibit drawing difficulties both in copying and reproducing simple shapes (Hermelin and O'Connor 1961; Abercrombie 1970). Individuals must be able to use information from various sensory modalities in order to learn new motor skills. Two important sources of information are derived from vision and kinaesthesis and from memory based on these souces. For example, in copying a simple geometric figure, there must be a mechanism which analyses the visual stimulus and another which transforms this visual pattern into a kinaesthetic motor code. Such integration of perceptual information determines the coordinated patterns of movement sequence which is required in order to reproduce the movement. In an experimental condition where normal and mentally handicapped people (matched for mental age) were asked to copy simple shapes, no group differences were found. Thus no overall differences in performance were observed when no memory was involved (Anwar 1985, in press).

Visual Versus Kinaesthetic Input. The two sources of visual and kinaesthetic information were varied at the input stimulus stage (Anwar 1983a). In the kinaesthetic condition the mentally handicapped adolescent was unable to see the stimulus as his/her finger was traced along the shape by the experimenter. In the visual condition, the stimulus was shown for about the same time as it took to trace or outline the stimulus shape. The subjects were asked to reproduce the shapes from either visual or kinaesthetic memory, i.e. after either vision or touch. Overall the results clearly demonstrated the advantage that kinaesthetic tracing had on reproducing skills. Thus the kinaesthetic tracing condition was significantly better than the visual condition for Down's and non-Down's-syndrome adolescents. Furthermore, it was found that, in the visual input condition, the non-differentiated group of subnormal adolescents was significantly better than the group with Down's syndrome (Anwar 1983b). This result replicated the earlier finding by O'Connor and Hermelin (1961) where Down's-syndrome children were found to be significantly worse than other mentally handicapped children in reproducing a visual stimulus from memory. Overall, the kinaesthetic percept elicited a better approximation from both groups of subjects. There were also some qualitative advantages for the tracing condition; for example, the mentally handicapped adolescents were invariably quicker in reproducing the stimulus shapes after kinaesthetic than after visual input.

The intra-modality processing in the kinaesthetic tracing conditions probably enabled both groups of mentally handicapped persons to represent the shape better for either or both of the following reasons:

Firstly, in tracing, by forcing attention to each aspect of the shape, the method in a sense demonstrated to the subject how to begin and organize a series of steps for response. Kinaesthetic tracing may also have provided the mentally retarded adolescents with knowledge of specific stimulus features rather than with only a global impression. There is some evidence that normal children extract only the relevant salient features of a visual stimulus (Yarbus 1967; Olson 1970). If the mentally handicapped child has not learnt to do this spontaneously, then one would assume that stimulus information presented in a manner which favours discrete and successive processing may have led to improved internal representation.

Secondly, as kinaesthetic tracing was congruent in action within the subsequent act of drawing, it probably required little translation of perceptual information into a different representational code. Implicit in this explanation is the suggestion that, for the subnormal, the visual perceptual input may not be easily translated into a movement plan. Thus the severely subnormal adolescents were particularly handicapped when visually derived and stored information had to be translated into a set of motor movements as compared with visual information. Kinaesthetically obtained and remembered information was, it seems, easier to utilize by the subnormal persons for shape reproduction from memory.

Abnormalities in Processes Underlying Motor Skills Development.   However, a major unresolved issue concerns which stage or stages of processing are most impaired in retarded persons. Libkuman and Freidrich (1972) spoke of limitations in brief perceptual memory or, as Neisser (1967) called it, iconic storage. Others (e.g. Spitz and Thor 1968; Harris and Fleer 1974) have pointed to more central factors such as speed of information transfer from iconic storage to a more permanent memory system. More recently Saccuzzo, Kerr, Marcus and Brown (1979) even found results which showed deficiencies in both iconic storage and speed of processing in mental retardation. Most of these authors have also clearly demonstrated that deficits related to visual processing cannot be explained on the basis of just low mental age. Limitations in the amount of speed of information transfer would obviously limit learning as well as other cognitive variables and could have a cumulative effect in the course of development.

The speed and fluency with which children come to combine the various subunits which go to make up common, yet complex everyday behaviour may well reflect the rate at which they are able to transmit information. In addition, changes in their properties as information-handling systems are likely to affect their motor performance. A common finding is that severely subnormal people exhibit a lack of behaviour strategically directed towards the maintaining of information in memory (Zeaman and House 1963; Spitz 1966; Ellis 1970; Fisher 1970) and in particular visual information (Anwar 1981a, 1983a, b). The general problem of the severely subnormal is that they seem deficient in the repertoire of information acquisition strategies and furthermore seem unaware of the usefulness of their own knowledge system (Brown 1974).

O'Connor and Hermelin (1963) attempted to identify specific aspects of the learning process that account for the impaired performance reported for handicapped children on a variety of tasks. The *acquisition* phases of learning rather than *retention* or retrieval have also been isolated by these investigators as the phase in which most frequent deficits are observed. Within the *acquisition* phase, these investigators have done extensive examination of input coding, organization, integration and selective attention processes in a variety of diagnostic categories and propose 'inappropriate input organization and integration have significant effects on subsequent processes'. It could be assumed that inappropriate stimulus acquisition strategies may well reflect an overall structural deficit in general information organization and storage. Thus, referring back to the studies on target localization and drawing ability discussed earlier (Anwar 1981a, b), it could be argued that the better use of kinaesthetic information at the input stage in both tasks was due to the explicit nature of the perceptual 'input'; in the present case kinaesthetic knowledge of direction is thereby made explicit and potential conceptual error matched against experience.

Similarly in the drawing condition, tracing the stimulus figure explicitly forced attention on all the features of the stimulus shape, thereby forcing (explicitly) organization of information. Thus, when the person with cognitive deficit is unable implicitly to acquire and use information, then explicit organization may be imposed in the form of moving the hand to feel the extent and direction of localization error and in the form of tracing the finger around a stimulus shape in order to perceive all its characteristics. Such interaction can be effectively used by the mentally handicapped.

The organization of sensory input obviously depends in part on the clarity of memory and its accessibility. If either aspect of recall is deficient, sensory input and hence motor output may be less effectively organized or anticipated.

What these studies on motor skills have clearly shown is that persons with severe cognitive deficit are unable adequately to focus visual attention to relevant areas of a visual display.

From studies on semantic organization in memory, Spitz (1966), Jensen (1970), and Bender and Johnson (1979) have suggested that the mentally handicapped do not spontaneously organize material as well as they store it and retrieval reflects this lack of organization. Jensen (1970) maintained that the mildly retarded children lack the organizational and conceptual skills involved in using a class inclusion hierarchical system — i.e. do not cluster as much as non-retarded children. From verbal learning and picture recognition studies it has been found that, if organization is imposed, then the mentally handicapped person does make use of it and retrieval is better organized and more accurate (Bilsky, Evans and Gilbert 1972; MacMillan 1972). The results reported from target localization and drawing skill studies support this view (Anwar 1981b, 1983a, b).

The 'Accessibility' Concept

One major effect of deficits in organization and integration of information would be on the accessibility of information already acquired. The concept of *accessibility* has been central to many theories of psychology from many different experimental paradigms. According to Campione and Brown (1977), the diagnoses of severely subnormal people's learning problems based on process theories are fundamentally diagnoses of restricted access. These authors provided rich support for the hypothesis that the slow learning subjects have peculiar difficulties with second order knowledge — i.e. knowledge about what they know (reflective access) and flexible use of alternatives available to the system (multiple access). There is ample evidence to show that retarded subjects experience difficulty in transferring the results of any training to new situations. Campione and Brown proposed that cognitive development is the process of proceeding from the specific task-related rules to more generalized abstract schema.

Accessibility and Its Relevance to Motor Programming

A prevailing account of motor behaviour is in Schmidt's (1975) schema theory which suggests that the basis for action is through the representation of motor programmes in a scheme-like form. The motor schema Schmidt proposed is dependent upon two memory schemas that develop during the course of learning a movement. The *recall* schema is the set of relations built up through experience between initial conditions (e.g. position of the limbs), response specifications and actual outcomes. The *recognition* schema reflects the relation of initial conditions, response specifications and actual outcomes. Thus the schema stores any information on the relations between the various operations and new requirements are interpolated to specify a given motor programme. The generalized schema is not dependent on storing a variety of programmes for specific movements and can provide the basis for novel movements never previously realized.

Hogg (1983) drew on the motor schema theory to integrate several streams of work within an integrating framework. Brewer and Nettlebeck (1977) have shown that the mentally retarded need more time than their peers to inspect a display to which they have to respond. Similarly it could be argued that, in the target-persisting condition and the drawing condition, the mentally handicapped people could not use the visual information more adequately because they were slow (Anwar 1981b, 1983a). This delay, according to Hogg, will clearly influence development of both recall and recognition schema, as under conditions of time pressure information on initial conditions will fall short of what is recognized to effect pairings between these conditions, response specifications and outcomes on the one hand (recall) and sensory consequences and outcomes on the other (recognition).

Poor sensory discrimination will also affect schema formation through its impact on analysis of initial conditions and with respect to sensory feedback. Thus the studies discussed earlier which were conducted on visuo-motor coordination (Anwar 1981b) have demonstrated both specific problems with respect to visual information and more general difficulties with regard to certain aspects of cross-modal information covering sensory feedback, especially when memory for visual information was involved. These studies do indicate the specific impact of these factors on motor behaviour and, as proposed by Hogg, it would be anticipated that, in the light of Schmidt's theory, they would have direct consequences for the build-up of motor schemas that would have a wider debilitating effect on motor performance: Hogg (1983) also suggested that the deficit lies in the planning or programming of a motor response rather than its execution.

From experimental studies where deficits were observed either in acquisition processing or in integration of sensory information then, it could be reasonably supposed that the underlying development of schema or representation of that skill would have been retarded. However, a thesis is presented in the next section which proposes that, even when equal levels of performance on a motor task are observed, this does not necessarily imply that the underlying representation is the same in subjects with severe cognitive deficit as compared with normal children without such a deficit.

Representation of Motor Skills

A well-established notion in motor control theory posits that the successful accomplishment of purposeful movements is dependent upon some central representation of the properties of the motor system (Bernstein 1967; Paillard and Brouchon 1974; Schmidt 1975; Glencross 1980) and the representation of the properties and constraints of the physical world within which the movement is executed (Gachoud, Mounoud, Hauert and Viviani 1983). According to these authors, the latter representation is not only concerned with the immediate perception of the properties of the object *per se*; the relationship among the properties of several objects (relational schemata) is also of primary importance. It has also been suggested that both the representation of the properties of the motor system and the relational schemata and inferences concerning the external world would evolve into a fully developed perceptual-motor representation during the various stages of development. Gachoud *et al.* (1983) provided experimental evidence to show that the planning of a specific simple movement changes during maturation in normal development. These authors argued that this change is consistent with the hypotheses of an underlying evolution of the representational schemata. For example, these authors found that, whereas overt behaviour on a lifting task did not differ qualitatively in nine-year-old children and adults, the pattern of motor commands, however, as recorded by electromyographic recordings, were strikingly different. The motor strategies adapted by adults depended upon an advanced internal representation of the properties of the motor system and of size/weight covariation in natural objects. Such a representation was found not to be fully developed in nine-year-old children.

In a similar vein, Mounoud (1982) suggested that representational knowledge which provides the interface between perception and action must also undergo change in development. Thus the manner in which available data is interpreted to organize and plan actions may change/improve over normal development. It is suggested that, in subjects with cognitive deficit of the same mental age as normal children who can ostensibly do a task just as well as normal children, such representational knowledge may nevertheless be different.

It had been incidentally observed in previous experiments (Anwar 1983b) that even when adequate drawing approximations were made of simple shapes, there seemed to be no consistency in the sequential patterns to which the mentally handicapped person conformed. At times the same shape was reproduced again in a different manner from that adapted previously. A number of studies have shown that, in normal development (Goodnow and Levine 1973; Goodnow 1977), children follow a set of rules or principles that can be extended to any new shape. This incidental observation of differences in drawing strategies in normal and mentally handicapped subjects was objectively investigated subsequently.

Drawing skill for simple shapes was compared and matched in groups of mentally handicapped and normal subjects who had initially been matched for mental age (Anwar 1985, in press). These groups were then closely matched on drawing initiation and progressive rules. The results clearly showed that, when levels of drawing performance were the same, whereas normal children actively abstracted and extended general themes, the mentally retarded people were unable to do so to the same degree. Thus the same shape was initiated in a different manner on repeated trials. There were differences in progression of the drawing movement and there was little homogeneity within the group of subjects with cognitive deficit in strategies adopted. Thus, even though the mentally retarded subjects could draw equally well as compared with normal children, nevertheless the motor strategies used to initiate, sequence and complete the shape were quite different. Those with cognitive deficit were unable to abstract and extend general rules and thus provided little evidence of representational changes which would result from reorganizations and representational updating. In order to achieve this, once having attained a robust initial success, it would be important to go beyond it trying to understand why certain procedures are successful or economical in number of movements required, unpacking what is implicit in them and unifying separate instances of success into a single framework. Such representational changes would also have a direct consequence for the build-up of motor programmes in a scheme-like form or representation as proposed by Schmidt (1975). In the absence of such a framework or representation, each new motor skill will pose problems as actions could not be adequately planned in advance using predictions and inferences made on the basis of a certain number of cues or representations elaborated over development.

Summary and Conclusions

The results from a few isolated experiments on motor skill suggest that cognitive deficit has a direct implication for (1) the processing and organization of sensory information and (2) the development of motor programmes and representations elaborated in the course of development. It is quite possible the two processes are inter-related and depend on each other. Thus deficits in organizing information, i.e. properties or characteristics of the physical world, would have direct consequences for the build-up of representational knowledge or motor schemas.

In the literature on mentally retarded most of the studies on motor development have in essence been experiments of phases or levels of 'motor skill' and little is known of motor development in the presence of severe cognitive deficit. In the absence of such long-term studies of macrodevelopmental sequences where mechanisms of change may be observed, the present status of experimental data from isolated motor skills does not permit the use of an overall theoretical framework which could be used either to explain or to predict the motor behaviour of persons with severe mental retardation.

Annette Karmiloff-Smith (1983) made a good case for distinguishing between *behavioural* change and *representational change*. The results do suggest that, when comparing normal children with severely retarded adolescents, what one observes is similarities in 'behaviour' — i.e. equal ability to draw a shape from memory. However, from such observations of similarities in particular isolated skills, little insight is gained into the underlying representations in the mentally handicapped as compared with normal children. Perhaps what one observes in the mentally handicapped is procedural success where each behaviour unit is merely added to the previously learned unit and attempts are not made towards overall organization which would link behavioural units one to the other in a consistent whole.

Thus ostensibly similar skills in drawing simple shapes from memory by normal and mentally handicapped adolescents do not necessarily imply that the underlying processes have been elaborated or represented in the same manner. Whereas normal children were predictable in their choice of motor plan, i.e. rules and strategies for drawing, those with cognitive deficit were not so predictable. Such differences in the underlying representation for the same behaviour may be one of the major reasons for the delayed milestones in perceptual motor development. It would be reasonable to presume that severely mentally handicapped people are satisfied by goal attainment and procedural success (to use Karmiloff-Smith's terminology) and do not adhere to systematic organization and updating processes.

It would be of considerable interest to determine such representational differences between normal and mentally handicapped children in the development of other motor skills. Of particular relevance would be experiments designed to investigate and compare the representation of the properties of the motor system (by electromyographic recordings in the manner of Gachoud *et al.* (1983) in subjects with and without cognitive deficit. Whether or not differences are observed in either or both the representation of motor programmes (or schemas) and the motor system itself would be important to determine.

That is, if the kinematic features of the movement do not differ in the two groups on certain tasks, are the pattern of motor commands still the same or different? No doubt developmental studies of this kind in children with cognitive deficit would yield useful information for both experimental psychologists and clinicians.

References

Abercrombie, M.L.J. (1970) 'Learning to draw' in K. Connolly (ed.), *Mechanisms of Motor Skill Development*, Academic Press, London, pp. 307-324

Adams, J.A. (1971) 'A closed loop theory of motor learning', *Journal of Motor Behaviour, 3,* 111-50

Annett, J. (1957) 'The information capacity of young mental defectives in an assembly task', *The Journal of Mental Science, 103,* 621-31

Anwar, F. (1981a) 'Motor functions in Down's syndrome' in N.R. Ellis (ed.), *International Review of Research in Mental Retardation, 10,* 107-38, Academic Press, New York

—— (1981b) 'Visual-motor target localization in normal and subnormal development', *British Journal of Psychology, 72,* 43-57

—— (1983a) 'Vision and kinaesthesis in motor movement' in J. Hogg and P. Mittler (eds.) *Advances in Mental Handicap Research. Vol. 2,* Wiley, Chichester

—— (1983b), 'The role of sensory modality, for the reproduction of shape by the severely retarded', *British Journal of Developmental Psychology, 1,* 317-27

—— (1985) Representational differences in drawing skills in the mentally retarded (in press)

Bender, N.N. and Johnson, N.S. (1979) 'Hierarchical semantic organization in educable mentally retarded children', *Journal of Experimental Child Psychology, 27,* 277-85

Bernstein, N. (1967) *The Coordination and Regulation of Movements*, Pergamon Press, London

Bilsky, L., Evans, R.A. and Gilbert, L. (1972) 'Generalization of associative clustering tendencies in mentally retarded adolescents: Effects of novel stimuli', *American Journal of Mental Deficiency, 77,* 77-84

Brewer, N. and Nettlebeck, T. (1977) 'Influence of contextual cues on the choice reaction time of mildly retarded adults', *American Journal of Mental Deficiency, 82,* 37-43

Brown, A.L. (1974) 'The role of strategic behaviour in retardate memory' in N.R. Ellis (ed.), *International Review of Research in Mental Retardation, 7,* Academic Press, New York

Bruininks, R.H. (1974) 'Physical and Motor Development of Retarded Persons' in N.R. Ellis (ed.), *International Review of Research in Mental Retardation, 7,* Academic Press, New York

Campione, J.C. and Brown, A.L. (1977) 'Memory and metamemory development in educable retarded children' in R.V. Kaine and J.W. Hogan (eds.) *Perspectives on the Development of Memory and Cognition*, Lawrence Erlbaum, New Jersey, pp. 367-406

Connolly, K. (1970) 'Skill development: Problems and plans' in K. Connolly (ed.) *Mechanisms of Motor Skill Development*, Academic Press, London

Craik, K.J.W. (1947) 'Theory of the human operator in central systems I: The operator as an engineering system', *British Journal of Psychology, 38,* 56-61

—— (1948) 'Theory of the human operator in central systems II: Man as an element in a central system', *British Journal of Psychology, 38,* 142-8

Cratty, B.J. and Martin, M. (1969) *Perceptual Motor Efficiency in Children*, Lea and Febiger, Philadelphia

Ellis, N.R. (ed.) (1963) *Handbook of Mental Deficiency: Physiological theory and research*, McGraw-Hill, London

—— (1970) 'Memory processes in retardates and normals' in N.R. Ellis (ed.), *International Review of Research in Mental Retardation, 4,* Academic Press, New York

Fisher, L. (1970) 'Attention Deficit in brain damaged children', *American Journal of Mental Deficiency, 79,* 502-8

Fleishman, E.A. (1964) *The Structure and Measurement of Physical Fitness*, Prentice-Hall, Englewood Cliffs, NJ

Gachoud, J.P., Mounoud, P., Hauert, C.A. and Viviani, P. (1983) 'Motor strategies in lifting movements: A comparison of adult and child performance', *Journal of Motor Behaviour, 15,* 202-16

Gibson, D. (1978) *Down's Syndrome: The psychology of mongolism*, Cambridge University Press, Cambridge

Glencross, D.J. (1980) 'Levels and strategies of response organization' in G.E. Stelmach and J. Requin (eds.), *Tutorials in Motor Behaviour*, North Holland Publishing Company, Amsterdam

Goodnow, J. (1977) *Children's Drawing*, Open Books, London

—— and Levine, R. (1973) 'The grammar of action: Sequence and syntax in children's copying', *Cognitive Psychology, 4,* 82-98

Gubbay, S.S. (1975) *The Clumsy Child,* W.B. Saunders & Co, London

Harris, G.J. and Fleer, R.E. (1974) 'High speed memory scanning in mental retardates: Evidence for a central processing deficit, *Journal of Experimental Child Psychology, 17,* 452-9

Hermelin, B. and O'Connor, N. (1961) 'Shape perception and reproduction in normal children and mongol and non-mongol imbeciles', *Journal of Mental Deficiency Research, 5,* 67-71

Hogg, J. (1982) 'Motor development and performance in severely mentally handicapped people', *Developmental Medicine and Child Neurology, 24,* 188-93

—— (1983) *Towards a comprehensive account of motor skill in severely retarded people.* The Royal Society of Medicine, First European Symposium on *Scientific Studies in Mental Retardation.*

Jackson, C.V. (1954) 'The influence of previous movement and posture on subsequent posture', *Quarterly Journal of Experimental Psychology, 6,* 72-8

Jensen, A.R.E. (1970) 'A theory of primary and secondary familial retardation' in N.R. Ellis (ed.), *International Review of Research in Mental Retardation, 4,* Academic Press, New York

Karmiloff-Smith, A. (1984) 'Children's problem solving' in M. Lamb, A.L. Brown and B. Rogoff (eds.), *Advances in Developmental Psychology, 3,* Laurence Erlbaum, Hillsdale, NJ

Libkuman, R. and Freidrich, D. (1972) 'Threshold measures of sensory register storage (perceptual memory) in normals and retardates', *Psychonomic Science, 27,* 357-8

MacMillan, D.L. (1972) 'Facilitative effects of input organization as a function of verbal response to stimuli in E.M.R. and nonretarded children', *American Journal of Mental Deficiency, 76,* 408-11

Mounoud, P. (1982) 'Visuo-manual tracking in children from 3 to 9 years old', Paper presented at the symposium on the development of action at the Institute of Child Development, University of Minnesota, Minneapolis, October 1982

—— and Hauert, C.A. (1982) 'Development of sensori-motor organization in young children' in G. Forman (ed.), *Action and Thought: From sensori-motor schemes to symbolic operations,* Academic Press, New York

Neisser, U. (1967), *Cognitive Psychology,* Appleton Century Crofts, New York

Newell, K.M. and Kennedy, J.A. (1978), 'Knowledge of results and children's motor learning', *Developmental Psychology, 14,* 531-6

O'Connor, N. and Hermelin, B. (1961), 'Visual and stereognostic shape recognition in normal children and mongol and non-mongol imbeciles', *Journal of Mental Deficiency Research, 5,* 63-6

—— and —— (1963) *Speech and Thought in Severe Subnormality,* Pergamon/MacMillan, New York

—— and —— (1978) *Seeing and Hearing and Space and Time,* Academic Press, London

Olson, D.R. (1970) *Cognitive Development: The child's acquisition of diagonality,* Academic Press, New York

Paillard, J. and Brouchon, M. (1974) 'A proprioceptive contribution to the spatial encoding of position cues for ballistic movements', *Brain Research,* 273-84

Saccuzzo, D.P., Kerr, N., Marcus, A. and Brown, R. (1979) 'Input capability and speed of processing in mental retardation', *Journal of Abnormal Psychology, 88,* 341-5

Schmidt, R.A. (1975) 'A schema theory of discrete motor skill learning', *Psychological Review, 82,* 225-60

Spitz, H.H. (1966) 'The role of input organization in the learning and memory of mental retardates' in N.R. Ellis (ed.), *International Review of Research in Mental Retardation, 2,* Academic Press, New York

—— and Thor, D.H. (1968) 'Visual backward masking in retardates and normals', *Perception and Psychophysics, 4,* 245-6

Yarbus, A.L. (1967) *Eye Movements and Vision,* Plenum Press, New York

Zeaman, D. and House, B.J. (1963) 'The role of attention in retardates discrimination learning' in N.R. Ellis (ed.), *Handbook of Mental Deficiency,* McGraw Hill, New York

9 SENSORY HANDICAP AND COGNITIVE DEFECT

Neil O'Connor and Beate Hermelin

Introduction

The information-processing model of cognitive processing has tended to reject or perhaps it would be better to say to ignore intelligence as a concept, despite the strongly positive correlation which is always found between subtests of intelligence over a very wide range of cognitive functions. One reason for this attitude is the absence of any dynamic quality in the concept of intelligence and its assumed independence of processes occurring over time during the acquisition of knowledge. Thus no reason is ever given by those interested in intelligence levels to explain how these levels operate to advance or retard the learning process or any other cognitive process. Another reason is that those interested in information processing frequently work with subjects of normal or superior cognitive ability and show little interest in individual differences. An exception to this trend is work such as that of Hunt, Frost and Lunneborg (1973) and Hunt (1978). These authors attempt to bridge the gap between verbal intelligence level on the one hand and, for example, short-term memory function on the other, by seeking a mechanism which connects the two. One suggestion offered is that rapidity of encoding, ensured by ready verbal access, enables those of good verbal intelligence to expand their immediate memory span.

It is clear that some such bridging has to be attempted if one is to explain the way in which low intelligence can be related to deficiency of information processing, whether by extensive malfunction of each separate cognitive operation, in a linear processing chain, or through a more localized, or specific dysfunction of one link in the series.

The connection between an information-processing model and the exploration of individual differences is one important question for cognitive psychology. This is of special concern for psychologists involved with the mentally handicapped and their cognitive problems. We have tried to consider some of the problems presented on previous occasions, for example in research reported by O'Connor (1973) and O'Connor and Hermelin (1978). This research was concerned with peripheral handicaps such as blindness and deafness on the one hand and subnormality of intelligence on the other and their effects on cognitive processes. One finding which emerged was that a number of tasks involving input into a single modality channel had to be relearned when presented to another modality (O'Connor and Hermelin 1971). Another was that some types of processing inevitably occurred if input were restricted to one modality irrespective

184

of the previous experience of some subjects in other modalities (Hermelin and O'Connor 1971). In some special circumstances these modality-restricted effects were also shown by subjects of low intelligence. This finding will be discussed below. The conclusion emphasized here is that stimulus organization was determined to a large degree by the modality of input. So, at least for some forms of encoding, a strong modality dependence could be demonstrated. This finding is important, especially if the commonly used modality in any form of processing differs from the modality of input. In the discussion of these conclusions one question frequently emerged. This is the question of whether the subnormal person is capable of coding from one modality to another to an extent sufficient to enable him to match stimuli in an efficient manner? For example, if a subject must select one or two stimuli by touch, can he then recognize the previously chosen stimulus by sight? The tracing of this question in developmental psychology has been extensively researched by Birch and Lefford (1963) and more recently by Bryant (1974). Its implication for encoding processes by those of mild and severe mental handicap has been discussed and investigated by Luria (1961), O'Connor and Hermelin (1963) and Hermelin and O'Connor (1964).

The importance of this question of cross-modal coding for the study of information processing and its malfunctioning in those of low intelligence is essentially that it raises two basic issues, abstraction on the one hand and the encoding process itself on the other. By abstraction in this sense is meant the reduction of a sensory image to a minimal conventional form which might serve as an idealized representation of the object or event to which it refers. Rosch's (1973) discussion of prototypes which are representational images also made this point. The abstraction process which must be assumed to occur so that, for example, the word 'table' can be applied to 'tables' of many kinds may be subject to the same problems of identification which led Neisser (1967) to discuss questions of feature-extraction as applied to the problem of letter identification. In other words, certain aspects or features of a letter as identified in Neisser's (1967) discussion had to be present before a letter could be identified and critical discrimination from other letters made. However, at the same time any accidental aspects of the letter form could be ignored without failure to recognize and code the information. The same process is operative in relation to Rosch's prototypes. Simple template matching involving identity of size and retinal location, for example, is not essential for recognition of named equivalence. In the case in which images are encoded into words, the stripping process could be very radical or one could say complete, in so far as the word in no way resembles the object of which it is the name.

In a situation in which encoding into words of a situation appreciated initially through vision or touch, for example, proves difficult, abstraction may be difficult also. This may be because abstraction may be facilitated by verbal encoding. Such encoding allows us to carry in memory a 'disembodied "image" ' of say a table — an 'idea' of a table rather than an image of it.

When, therefore, verbalization and perhaps, therefore, abstraction are impossible because of linguistic incompetence, as in some subnormals, an image may resist abstraction and retain certain features of the modal form in which it was initially processed.

In such circumstances, mental operations might be radically altered and schema based on them changed, when encoding strongly reflects the characteristics of the input modality. In cases in which an appropriate input is for some reason not available, as in deafness for example, then an alternative modality channel will take over the input function and the characteristics of this modality may then be reflected in the encoding procedure. These characteristics will usually be different from those of the more appropriate modality. Here the word appropriate is used to convey the idea that, for certain kinds of messages, vision or hearing or touch may be more suitable. The appropriateness of a modality in this sense has been discussed elsewhere by O'Connor and Hermelin (1978) and we have summarized evidence presented by many authors, but notably by von Senden (1932), Attneave and Benson (1969) and Paivio (1971), that the perception of space depended primarily on vision, and evidence from other sources including Hirsh, Bilger and Deatherage (1956) and Behar and Bevan (1961) that temporal successive and durational judgements depended primarily on audition. It might be said that such a proposition is more or less self-evident. However, the specialization of audition for successive events can also be justified and the evidence for such a view is available at essentially two levels. Children's capacity to discriminate short intervals occurs in audition at about the age of eight years according to Bradley (1947) and these findings have been confirmed by Gilliland and Humphreys (1943) in previous studies. Conrad (1965) has examined the appreciation of succession in auditorially presented material and Gibson (1966) and Arnheim (1969) have both noted that the auditory mode is peculiarly well suited for dealing with time-distributed information. Similar modality-specific views have been advanced by Savin (1967) confirming, in this case, work by Goodfellow (1934).

Most of this work was carried out with relatively long intervals but there is another body of work with extremely short intervals, down to 2 ms, which tells a similar story. This work was initiated by Exner who found in the late nineteenth century that two visual events had to be separated by about 44 ms before they could be discriminated, whereas auditory intervals of 2 ms were detectable as two stimuli. Efron (1963) and Hirsh (1967) have taken a similar view on the basis of their own more recent work and Tallal and Piercy (1973) have confirmed this view for normal and aphasic children. With few exceptions, therefore, the conclusion has been that, in normal and in pathological development, audition is better specialized for the appreciation of succession and order than is vision.

Such work as that of Efron (1963) and Tallal and Piercy (1973) demonstrates that the development of language appreciation may depend on the rapid temporal discrimination of phonemes which may occur with considerable rapidity in any series of words forming any simple statement. Whilst arguments of this kind can be adduced to demonstrate the relevance of the appreciation of succession to the development of language, it can be shown that the simultaneous comprehension of a large number of items can only be accomplished in vision. Simultaneous integration in audition can occur as, for example, in listening to a chord in music or to a number of notes blended in an acceptable manner. However, for the most part successive sounds convey meaning by reason of their temporal order.

The problem of abstracting and encoding, therefore, may follow a different course in vision and audition if direct access to visual or auditory input is blocked. Thus, if vision is not available, simultaneity of spatial organization may be lost and, if hearing is lost, an appreciation of order or succession may be disturbed.

Mental Subnormality and Encoding

If damage to the cortex has occurred, which we know to be the case in a high percentage of those people with severe mental retardation (Crome 1960), then damage of a central character will presumably have affected judgemental and categorizing as well as association functions, but also encoding strategies and consequent schematic organization of input and recall. In a variety of studies we have made comparisons between peripheral and presumed central damage in subjects who were either congenitally blind or deaf, or severely mentally handicapped. Whilst it has been the case that these experiments have demonstrated that severe subnormality of intellect and congenital deafness may have similar consequences, no regular association could be established and the picture emerging would seem to be more complex. The role of experience in relation to cross-modal transfer and matching is also far from simple. However, it would seem that modalities play a crucial part in determining encoding strategy and their presence or absence for whatever reason is critical. The presence or absence of a modality channel is not simply a matter of the presence or absence of sight or hearing, but can also be a function of an inadequately operating central process.

This particular point will be illustrated in more detail when the experimental material is presented, but the exposition can be anticipated by making a general point. If anyone is presented with a series of auditory verbal stimuli to encode for recall, he will record them serially as they fall on his ear. If he sees a visual form of the same stimuli, he may repeat them to himself in a sub-vocal form so that he is essentially encoding the same 'auditory' input.

However, if the subject suffers from congenital deafness or severe linguistic disability, he may not automatically encode a presented input in a verbal form, but perhaps in terms of the code of some other modality, for example one derived from vision. Various consequences can arise from a different medium of encoding which may affect the form of encoding and of course the consequent output.

Modalities in other words operate according to different procedural rules and a process in one does not always appear to be identical with a similar process in another. One consequence of this state of affairs may be that automatic transfer from one modality to another may not occur.

The evidence presented in subsequent sections is offered as support for the statements made here. Exemplary illustrations of both encoding specificity and intermodality transfer block are offered sometimes in a predominantly spatial and sometimes in a temporal setting.

Encoding Specificity

By the term 'encoding specificity' we mean that the presentation of a set of stimuli to one modality determines the manner in which these stimuli will be encoded and processed. How such a modality-restricted processing operation is affected is demonstrated in an experiment in which the same motor task is carried out either with visual guidance or through the agency of touch with vision occluded. Such a task was presented to our subjects (Hermelin and O'Connor 1971) who had first to learn to respond with one of four words which were assigned to the index and the middle fingers of both hands. After training, the subject had to respond with the appropriate word when a finger end was tactually stimulated. The two fingers of each hand were laid out in front of the subject on four imaginary points running away vertically from the subject in the midline. When a criterion of successful responses had been reached (19 out of 20 correct successive responses) and a series of between 32 and 40 trials had been given, the position of the hands in relation to each other was reversed and random stimulation of the finger ends was continued as before until a further 40 trials had been concluded. In this phase of the experiment no correction was given.

The subjects carried out the task either by touch alone if they were blind or blindfold, or with vision in one special condition. The role of intelligence was also controlled for, in so far as some groups of subjects were of low intelligence whereas others, whether blind or sighted, were not. In this study, subjects' responses were found to be one of two kinds, either continuing to respond in the second part of the experiment as they had in the first — before hand reversal — or changing the response as the hands were interchanged. Thus, in the first instance response words occurred in the same absolute order, as before, irrespective of hand change, whereas in the second the word order changed, along with the change in the order of the hands.

The variable responsible for the difference in response was the presence or absence of sight. In the sighted, irrespective of intelligence level, or indeed of age, word order was preserved despite hands changes, but in the case of the blind, the dependence on touch rather than vision resulted in an order reversal corresponding to the hand position change. Thus the presence or absence of vision was critical in determining the effect of hand reversal. However, the effect occurred independently of the intelligence level of the participating group.

Another example of coding specificity depending on the presence or absence of a modality channel can be demonstrated in another experiment (O'Connor and Hermelin 1972) in which subjects had the same stimuli presented to them either visually or auditorily and were asked to make a simple judgement about them. The stimuli were three digits and, when these were presented visually, they were offered singly in temporal succession in three windows arranged in a row so that only one digit appeared at any one time and always in a temporal order which was incongruent with a left-to-right or right-to-left spatial order. When presented auditorily, the digits were presented to the subject from three loudspeakers arranged round the subject, one in front and one on each side. Once again only one digit could be heard at once and the temporal order of presentation was incongruent with a left-to-right or right-to-left spatial order.

The subjects' task was to decide, after the presentation, which of the three digits in any one presentation had been the middle one. No guidance was given in this situation as to the meaning of 'middle', and the subject was left to decide for himself whether, in the ambiguous situation of the existence of both a spatial and a temporal middle, he should choose one or the other. Of all the 80 subjects tested in this study, only two queried the intention of the experimenter. Thirty subjects took part in the visual presentation, 30 in the auditory and a further 20 in a second supplementary study. In the visual condition of the first experiment, 10 deaf and 20 hearing children, 10 of whom wore ear muffs, took part. In the auditory condition 10 blind and 20 sighted (10 blindfold) participated. All children were between 13 and 14 years of age and had digit spans of at least five.

The results showed that, independently of the ambiguity of the instruction to choose the 'middle' digit, nearly all subjects presented with visual stimuli (whether deaf or not) chose the spatially middle digit, and all who had received signals auditorily, i.e. heard the digits presented, chose the temporally middle digit. In other words, in this experiment, judgement or choice depended on modality of presentation.

To control for the fact that responses to auditory signals were verbal and those to visual signals were written because of the participation of deaf subjects, a second experiment was carried out. In this study 10 normal adults were given both visual and auditory tasks responding to half of each verbally and half in writing. Order of presentation and response was of course counterbalanced. Results were shown to be determined by input modality and not by response mode.

Although all subjects in this study were of near normal intelligence, other experiments with the mentally handicapped have yielded comparable findings. Hermelin and O'Connor (1964) demonstrated the existence of a sensory hierarchy in normal, subnormal and autistic children with a tendency to visual or light dominance or saliency. However, when deaf, blind, subnormal and normal children were given a duration discrimination task in one modality (touch) and then retested in another modality, e.g. sight or hearing, no cross-modal transfer of training effects was detectable for any of the groups (O'Connor and Hermelin 1971). This result suggests that the modality-specific encoding processes used by blind and deaf children were also used by subnormals. Thus a strong degree of encoding specificity might be said to be characteristic of all subjects tested. Demonstrably in the cases of the deaf and blind, one modality channel is blocked. In the case of normal subjects, blindfolding them or the creating of artificial deafness by ear muffling, can have similar consequences. This could be dramatically demonstrated in the case of adult sighted subjects who were blindfold and asked to carry out the first task described above which involves hand reversal. In this condition, these sighted adults immediately began behaving as if they were congenitally blind. In other words, they adopted a response strategy which ignored Euclidean space and reverted to the kind of self-referred topological space which Piaget and Inhelder (1956) have described as being characteristic of three-year-olds.

The question to be raised here is what, if anything, encoding specificity, which is clearly triggered by the presence or absence of a particular input mode, might have to do with low intelligence. Research has always shown that subnormality is frequently associated with peripheral sensory deficits (O'Connor 1957; Woodruff 1977; Ellis 1979). Thus a predisposition to additional sensory handicap can always be anticipated among the mentally handicapped. It is not this perhaps accidental association, however, with which we are concerned here, but with the effect of specificity of encoding and its causes. We need to know whether this is due to malfunction of peripheral receptors or, as we suggested above, in some cases because of dysfunction of the central analyser or associated cortical areas.

Peripheral and Central Causes of Encoding Specificity

The effects of encoding specificity have been illustrated in the previous section. However, during the course of the studies described, we have noted that not only could some encoding peculiarities result from the artifactual or long-term absence of an appropriate modality channel, but also from other conditions.

The experiment which most clearly illustrates the fact that modality specific coding can be the consequence not only of sensory but also of cognitive impairment is an extended form of the 'middle' experiment with three digits described above. In the form to be presented now, this task was not a judgemental one but required short-term recall. The task required both recall of items and recall of order. Three digits were presented to subjects in this case, i.e. in three windows arranged in a horizontal row but in such a manner that only one digit appeared at a time and so that the spatial order of presentation was never an uninterrupted linear (or left-to-right) one. This ensured that spatial and temporal order were incongruent. Subjects were requested to observe the three digits as they appeared and either to reproduce them after they had been seen or to recognize a correct display as distinct from an incorrect one. Normal hearing subjects as well as deaf and both mentally handicapped and autistic subjects of low intelligence were tested.

In this study a group difference appeared in the results. The deaf always recalled the digits in a spatial or left-to-right order whereas the normal hearing subjects recalled them in the order in which they had appeared successively or temporally. This encoding difference between the deaf and the hearing occurred despite the fact that the modality of presentation was the same for both groups, i.e. visual.

The explanation we have offered for this result is that the deaf did not rehearse the numbers sub-vocally as they were displayed, but retained a visual image of the digits with spatial reference or indexing. The hearing, however, verbalized sub-vocally as the numbers appeared and stored an encoded form of the digits in their original order.

This explanation is satisfactory so far as the deaf are concerned. However, the two low-IQ groups also gave a similar result and the explanation is less plausible in their case because both groups could hear perfectly well. However, as they do respond as if they had encoded the digits in a visual–spatial form, they must rely on this form of coding not because they cannot hear, but perhaps because they do not use implicit speech as a form of rehearsal and encoding. Such an explanation would, in the case of autistic children of low IQ be quite plausible, because their verbal IQs are even lower than their performance measures.

A subsequent study of a mentally handicapped group performing this task carried out by Miklausic (1976) has made it clear that there is a critical point in the level of verbal intelligence below which words may be understood and used in communication, but may tend not to be used as tools of thought, i.e. for encoding into memory. Both the deaf and those of low verbal intelligence may encode visually because they cannot readily encode their auditory input into sub-vocal speech for memory encoding. In the case of the deaf this may be because of hearing and speech deficits and in the case of those of low verbal IQ because their speech level is inadequate for it to act as a vehicle of thought.

Other similar studies have shown that visual encoding procedure is not obligatory for the deaf, but elective. In other words, they appear to be capable of adopting other strategies when under pressure to do so. O'Connor and Hermelin (1978, p. 96) attempted to determine the role of speech in temporal ordering by comparing material which was readily verbalizable (nonsense syllables) with other material (photographs of faces) which could not so easily be verbalized. Subjects were either deaf or hearing children aged between 11 and 13 years. The procedure, as with the three-digits experiment, was to present in this case five nonsense syllables or five faces on a linear set of display windows but in sequential order incongruent with a left-to-right or right-to-left order. After the display, two items were presented from the series just seen, but one above the other. They were used as a probe for the subject to indicate which one had come first in the series. In this study, a group by conditions interaction demonstrated that the deaf were better at recalling the order of the faces and the hearing better at the nonsense syllables. This result was interpreted as confirming the tendency of the deaf to process non-verbally and the hearing in an auditory–verbal manner. However, the overall result showed that the deaf could in fact recall temporal order when required.

The three-digit experiment demonstrated that both the deaf and those of low verbal intelligence differ from the hearing in their characteristic memory-encoding strategy. Such a modality or intelligence-dependent difference from the norm cannot be so convincingly demonstrated in relation to visual defects or blindness. This might be because vision has, unlike audition, no associated higher order signalling system. There is no comparable notational encoding process in vision as we have in audition, i.e. nothing comparable to speech which makes both communication and thought so relatively easy. Even though representational conventions in the depicting of events may be thought in some respects to correspond with the written word and may — as is assumed for instance in the pictorial story completion test, in the Wechsler scale — have some 'syntactic' rules, none the less we cannot ourselves easily use any communicable picture language, as we can use words. Perhaps for this kind of reason, one cannot so easily find parallels in coding strategies between say blind and subnormal people, as one can between the deaf and the mentally handicapped.

Our experiments with the blind as compared with the sighted have, therefore, shown results which have been more difficult to interpret and have been less effective in illustrating similarities of strategy between the blind and the mentally retarded. It seems that it is symbolic and primarily linguistic usage which is similarly handicapped by peripheral and central defects and not direct non-symbolic experience. When equivalent images can be readily and appropriately constructed in a tactile or visual form, subnormals or peripherally handicapped groups are not worse performers than normals. This result was found in a tactile–visual transfer task comparing shapes of different sizes, which was an attempt to extend Posner and Mitchell's (1967) finding with letter recognition.

In the Posner and Mitchell study letters were presented followed sometimes by identical letters and sometimes by letters of the same name, one for example lower case and one upper case. So in one condition an 'a' could be shown and followed by an 'a' and in another condition an 'a' might be followed by an 'A'. In a third condition an 'a' would be followed by a different letter, for example 'b'. In these three conditions, the subject was asked to say whether or not the two letters had the same name. Identity was recognized faster than were two letters of the same name.

We attempted to repeat this finding with some modifications using cutout shapes. Subjects who were either normal, deaf or mildly subnormal were aged 11 years. They were asked to explore a shape kinaesthetically without seeing it and this exploration was then followed immediately by a visual presentation with a shape which either shared or did not share a name with the first shape. The visually presented shapes were either identical with the tactually explored shapes, or of a different size though the same shape, or of a different shape although of the same size as the first shape. Five different shapes were presented for encoding in memory and recognition. These were a triangle, a moon or crescent, a rhombus, an ellipse and a Greek cross.

The key finding was that no difference in the speed of judgement of 'same' or 'different' in the shape comparison appeared in the results, when groups were compared. A facilitating effect of size-identity was found for the deaf and the subnormal as well as for the normal subjects. We had expected the facilitating effect of size-identity to show itself only for the deaf and the subnormal, who might rely on visual or tactile similarity rather than name identity. However, as all three groups showed the effect, we can only assume the equal availability to each group of a non-verbal tactile–visual code.

Thus subnormal children seemed to remain stimulus-bound in those instances in which the necessary recoding would have to take place in language-derived terms. A great deal of our own work as well as that of Luria (1961) lends support to such a view. There thus seems to be a fundamental difference in the relationship between mental handicap and deafness on the one hand, and mental handicap and blindness on the other. In the former case an encoding deficit can occur for different reasons in both groups giving a similar or identical outcome. In the latter case, the effects of blindness, whether congenital or artifactual, are unique and can only be brought about by the deprivation of sight.

This finding is illustrated by two experiments which were carried out with blind, blindfold and sighted subjects. One was concerned with the identification of two shapes which, if brought together, would in some instances form a square. These shapes were fixed to a background and had to be explored in situ by touch. Any bringing together of the two shapes had therefore to be in imagination. Apart from pairs of shapes which would not form a square if brought together, there were two other kinds of pairs which would do so. In one instance the two parts had only to be brought together, while in the other one part had to be rotated before being fitted with its mating shape. The task was to decide by touch whether any two shapes would form a square or not. No group differences were found in this experiment. In one condition, where sighted normal controls were allowed to do the task by sight, the level of performance was significantly improved. However, in tactile conditions the blind and the blindfold performed at the same level despite the difference in the previous visual experience of the latter. In this particular experiment no control of intelligence levels was undertaken but, for those of average ability, previous experience of sight apparently did not aid subjects in making correct decisions.

The second experiment has been described already in the section on Encoding Specificity. This was an experiment involving words as indicators of relative position but not as meaningful referents. It was the spatial task described above involving finger location and hand reversal in sighted and sightless conditions. In this case deprivation of sight, irrespective of IQ level, led to an encoding process which was quite different from that involved when sight was present. Intelligence differences again did not interact with this processing difference in this experiment. Verbal response in this case, associated with particular fingers, were simply sound-signs rather than meaningful symbols. Thus no 'secondary signalling system' to use Pavlov's (1927) phrase, in other words no meaningfully related language encoding, was involved and deprivation of sight had the direct consequence of changing the encoding strategy. No comparable phenomenon due to another cause, for example low general intelligence, was relevant in this case unlike the instance of the recall of the order of three digits visually displayed.

Inferences and Conclusions

The research reported above was concerned to estimate the extent to which subnormal intelligence had the effect of creating encoding problems which in any sense resembled those brought about by peripheral sensory defects. The reasons for this research were to make comparisons between specific defects and their consequences and the effects of general cortical damage (O'Connor 1973). The relevance of the experimental results to the present chapter is twofold, firstly demonstrating the effect of deprivation of sensory input on the encoding process, independently of the intelligence of the subject, and secondly indicating the manner in which the same encoding process can be affected, not only by sensory deprivation, but also by low levels of measured intelligence.

One conclusion would seem to be that absence of vision, independent of intelligence level, can lead to a stimulus-bound encoding strategy which, whether in relation to judgements of form, order or duration, can be sharply restricted and which does not generalize to other modalities. It is also the case that, as well as being stimulus- or modality-bound, and independent of level of IQ, the encoding capacity of tactile and motor input which is invoked in relation to the dimensions referred to is independent of previous visual experience. In other dimensions, such for example as spatial 'orientation', it seems this need not be the case, and sighted blindfold subjects may recognize a right as opposed to a left hand by touch, better than a blind person can. However, in all other dimensions which we have explored, an IQ-independent, modality-determined coding strategy is manifest, i.e. independent of experience.

Thus, so far as the mentally handicapped are concerned, blindfolding should affect them in much the same way as it affects those of normal intelligence, being forced to rely on one restricted form of input as happens with the more able. Thus, in a study of blind estimates of distance and location (Hermelin and O'Connor 1975), autistic children of low IQ who were blindfolded performed similarly to blindfolded normal children so far as these two dimensions were concerned.

However, as was shown above, a comparison of the mentally handicapped with the deaf shows that the dysfunctions or inappropriate codings which occur are not IQ-independent in the same way. Although similar coding specificity occurs in the deaf and the mentally handicapped, it is not because they are deaf or wearing ear muffs, but precisely because they are impaired in verbal coding ability.

The implications of this difference between blindness and deafness in connection with subnormality of intelligence, if verified, would be that, where verbal IQ was found to be lower than a limit yet to be determined but in the region of 60 points of IQ, subjects would have a problem of encoding in an appropriate modality when given problems involving ordering, whether these problems were of a temporal, or perhaps of a meaningful nature. However, in cases relying on visual or tactile encoding or their interaction, we would not expect low IQ to play a complicating role. The reason for the difference would appear to lie in the peculiarly symbolic character of language and also in its availability for the secondary purpose which Vygotsky (1962) noted, namely that it could be used not only as a means of communication with others, but also as a tool of thought. When verbal symbols which may have completely different characteristics and appearance from the things and events which they represent, are used as memory-encoding devices, they may constitute in this function a language system with a syntactic structure different from the events they represent, or be only encodable in a different way. Our experiments have indicated the existence of such a different encoding medium and the consequences for memory encoding when it does not function because of peripheral or central handicap.

References

Arnheim, R. (1969) *Visual Thinking*, Faber and Faber, London

Attneave, F. and Benson, L. (1969) 'Spatial Coding and tactual stimulation', *Journal of Experimental Psychology, 81*, 216-22

Behar, J. and Bevan, W. (1961) 'The perceived duration of auditory and visual intervals: crossmodal comparisons and interaction', *American Journal of Psychology, 74*, 17-26

Birch, H.G. and Lefford, A. (1963) *Intersensory development in children.* Monographs of the Society for Research in Child Development, 28,5 (whole No. 89)

Bradley, N.C. (1947) 'The growth of the knowledge of time in children of school age', *British Journal of Psychology, 38*, 67-78

Bryant, P. (1974) *Perception and Understanding in Young Children*, Methuen, London

Conrad, R. (1965) 'Order error in immediate recall of sequences', *Journal of Verbal Learning and Verbal Behaviour*, *4*, 161-9

Crome, L. (1960) 'The Brain and Mental Retardation', *British Medical Journal, i*, 897-904

Efron, R. (1963) 'Temporal perception and aphasia and Deja Vu',*Brain, 86*, 403-24

Ellis, D. (1979) 'Visual Handicaps of Mentally Handicapped People', *American Journal of Mental Deficiency, 83*, 497-511

Gibson, E.J. (1966) *The Senses Considered as Perceptual Systems.* Houghton-Mifflin, Boston

Gilliland, A.R. and Humphreys, D.W. (1943) 'Age, sex, method and interval as variables in time estimation', *Journal of Genetic Psychology, 63*, 123-130

Goodfellow, L.D. (1934) 'An empirical comparison of audition vision and touch in the discrimination of short intervals of time', *American Journal of Psychology, 46*, 243-58

Hermelin, B. and O'Connor, N. (1964) 'Crossmodal transfer in normal, subnormal and autistic children', *Neuropsychologia, 2*, 229-35

—— and —— (1965) 'Visual Imperception in psychotic children', *British Journal of Psychology, 56*, 455-60

—— and —— (1971) 'Spatial coding in normal, autistic and blind children', *Perceptual and Motor Skills, 33*, 127-32

—— and —— (1975) 'Location and distance estimates by blind and sighted children', *Quarterly Journal of Experimental Psychology, 27*, 295-301

Hirsh, I.J. (1967) 'Information processing in infant channels for speech and language: the acquisition of serial order of stimuli' in F.L. Darley (ed.), *Brain Mechanisms Underlying Speech and Language*, Grune and Stratton, New York, pp. 21-38

—— Bilger, R.C. and Deatherage, B.H. (1956) 'The effects of auditory and visual background on apparent duration', *American Journal of Psychology, 69*, 561-74

Hunt, E. (1978) 'Mechanisms of verbal ability', *Psychological Review, 85*, 109-30

Hunt, E.B., Frost, N. and Lunneborg, C.E. (1973) 'Individual differences in cognition. A new approach to intelligence' in G. Bower (ed.), *Advances in learning and motivation, 7*, Academic Press, New York, pp. 87-122

Luria, A.R. (1961) *The Role of Speech in the Regulation of Normal and Abnormal Behaviour*, (J.Tizard, ed.), Pergamon Press, London

Miklausic, K. (1976) 'The Spatial or Temporal Organization of Short Term Memory in the Severely Subnormal', unpublished dissertation, University College London

Neisser, U. (1967) *Cognitive Psychology*, Appleton-Century-Crofts, New York

O'Connor, N. (1957) 'Imbecility and Colour Blindness', *American Journal of Mental Deficiency, 62*, 83-7

—— (1973) 'Psychological Studies in Subnormality', *Psychological Medicine, 3*, 137-40

—— and Hermelin, B. (1963) *Speech and Thought in Severe Subnormality*, Pergamon Press, London

—— and —— (1971) 'Inter and Intra-modal transfer in children with modality specific and general handicaps', *British Journal of Social and Clinical Psychology, 10*, 346-54

—— and —— (1972) 'Seeing and Hearing and Space and Time', *Perception and Psychophysics, 11(1A)*, 46-8

—— and —— (1978) *Seeing and Hearing and Space and Time*, Academic Press, London

Paivio, A. (1971) *Imagery and Verbal Processes*, Holt, Rinehart and Winston, New York

Pavlov, I.P. (1927) *Conditioned Reflexes*, Oxford University Press, London

Piaget, J. and Inhelder, B. (1956) *The Child's Conception of Space*, Routledge and Kegan Paul, London

Posner, M.J. and Mitchell, R.F. (1967) 'Chronometric analysis of classification', *Psychological Review, 74*, 392-401

Rosch, E.H. (1973) 'On the interval structure of perceptual and semantic categories' in T.M. Moore (ed.), *Cognitive Development and the Acquisition of Language*, Academic Press, New York

Savin, H.B. (1967) 'On the successive perception of simultaneous stimuli', *Perception and Psychophysics, 95*, 285-9

Senden, M. von (1932) *Raum und Gestalt. Auffassung bei operierten Blindgeborenen vor und nach der Operation*, Barth, Leipzig

Tallal, P. and Piercy, M. (1973) 'Defects of non-verbal auditory perception in children with developmental aphasia', *Nature, 241*, 468-9

Vygotsky, L.S. (1962) *Thought and Language*, MIT Press and Wiley, New York

Woodruff, M.E. (1977) 'Prevalence of visual and ocular anomalies in 168 non-institutionalized mentally retarded children', *Canadian Journal of Public Health, 68*, 225-32

PART FOUR

ASSESSMENT OF SENSORY FUNCTIONS

10 METHODS OF OBJECTIVE ASSESSMENT OF VISUAL FUNCTIONS IN SUBJECTS WITH LIMITED COMMUNICATION SKILLS

Janette Atkinson

Introduction

There are now a number of new methods and techniques available for measuring various aspects of vision in infants, young children and those with limited communication skills because of mental handicap. Most of these new methods have been devised by researchers interested in the course of visual development. The techniques have usually been carried out by personnel familiar with the limitations of the tests being used and with the difficulties of testing the young such as changes of state or mood and the importance of rapport and encouragement. Once norms have been established for these tests many clinicians feel that the tests should be standardized for use in hospital clinics: sometimes this has been successful, whereas at other times it has led to unreliable and variable results together with a general disenchantment concerning the test. Sometimes this is because of the sheer impossibility of transposing a laboratory test to a busy out-patient clinic, where the clinical personnel do not fully understand the psychological and technical requirements for using particular techniques and methods.

In this chapter I will describe some of the techniques and tests we have used and found valuable in assessing some aspects of vision in young children in the Visual Development Unit (VDU). Because there are many questions still to be answered in the field of visual development, our assessments cannot always be complete; they contain information concerning certain aspects of vision such as spatial detail and binocularity but may not be able to say very much about the visual perceptual world for the child. For many questions concerning perception and cognition in children future research and testing is required before we can give paediatricians and teachers of the handicapped a clear idea of what vision is like for the partially sighted. For the moment it would seem best to keep research of visual development in close contact with assessment of vision, so that the assessment procedures can be updated and modified, in line with new research developments. Whenever possible in this chapter I will give some indication concerning the difficulty of using a particular test. It is hoped that it will give general information for those who know nothing about vision tests; for those interested in the details of particular tests, specific references are given in each section.

Accurate information on functioning vision makes an important contribution to the treatment and rehabilitation of infants and children with a visual problem. However, such an assessment is not a substitute for the assessments and examinations already made by ophthalmologists and paediatricians, but a supplement to them, giving a more complete picture of the visual functioning of the child.

The procedures we use are outlined in Table 10.1. Each part of the assessment will be briefly described with references to research results relating to particular techniques and methods. Other methods, not regularly used in the VDU, are also described when they would be an appropriate substitute or additional test. However, before describing the particular tests, it is important to consider the general requirements for carrying out visual assessments and in particular the testing environment.

The Psychological Environment for Visual Assessment

It is of prime importance when assessing vision in infants and young children to have an atmosphere that is comforting, friendly and visually exciting. The domestic needs of young children and their families must be accommodated together with adequate technical facilities for accurate testing. These requirements are often unavailable in hospital out-patient clinics rendering them unsuitable for visual assessment of the young. Infants and young children can very quickly build up an aversion to a clinic if their experience of the place is frightening and boring; they will also pick up any anxiety that is experienced by their care-givers, which may lead to difficulties in assessing their vision and underestimates of their ability. Assessment of vision in young children is exacting, time-consuming and therefore costly, but the cost in time and effort can be greatly reduced by choosing the right times for testing. We have found that, in general, we get better results and waste less time if we run a very 'loose' appointment scheme, having several children and their parents in the nursery/play area of our Unit at the same time. The testing rooms are separate from the nursery; each child is taken to be assessed from time to time, with frequent breaks between tests. Some of the informal tests can be given in the nursery with encouragement being given to care-givers to tell us about the child's

Table 10.1: Clinicial Assessment of Vision

1.	Discussion of child's medical history/family history of visual problems.
2.	Observation of general visuo-motor behaviour.
3.	Orthoptic tests.
4.	Acuity assessment (preferential looking (FPL), Stycar balls test, Sheridan–Gardiner, 'Crowding').
5.	Photorefraction and retinoscopy.
6.	Binocular vision — monocular optokinetic nystagmus (MOKN). — binocular visual evoked potentials (BVEP).
7.	Discussion of results.

behaviour. It is also important to know whether the child's behaviour in the nursery is 'typical' for that particular child. For many children with a visual handicap their progress will depend very largely on the help and support they are given by parents and other close care-givers. It is, therefore, of prime importance to discuss the child's vision and the assessment in detail with the parents and teachers, so that they have some idea of what vision is like for the child in everyday situations.

Many people underestimate the skill involved in testing infants and young children (both normal and handicapped). A combination of apparent informality of manner towards both parents and children and a rigorous approach to the scientific tests is essential for successful assessment. At present no specific training schemes exist for sensory assessment in any discipline and so testers generally learn while carrying out the tests rather than having any formal training. Hopefully this lack in training schemes might be remedied in the future. In the meantime it is hoped that this chapter will be some help to those faced with assessment. One fallacy that remains is that it is solely the job of the ophthalmologist to assess visual function. Indeed it is highly desirable for any visual assessment to involve the skills of an ophthalmologist in detecting any retinal pathology. This, however, will not answer the question 'what does this child see?' or 'is the visual perception of this child normal?' A whole team of people, besides the ophthalmologist, from different disciplines is needed to tackle this broad question. We have found in our group that among those who have proved most useful in assessment are (1) the psychologists and paediatricians (for looking at global visual behaviour); (2) the orthoptists (for looking at abnormalities of eye movements and binocular vision), and (3) scientists (in electronics and computer science) for devising new and accurate labour-saving ways of testing and analysing results, and for coping with the many technical demands involved in these tests. Communication between members of the team carrying out the assessment is essential, so time should be allowed for this during the assessment. We have found that a simple form listing the tests is essential for assessment. It reminds the testers as to what is to be done, and gives a brief summary of results.

Medical and Family History

While watching the child's visual response to the new environment in our nursery, a careful medical history concerning the child's sight and that of the family should always be taken. In cases of handicap it is often important to know about any medication and to take this into account when assessing the visual alertness of the child. For some conditions there is clearly a higher risk of visual abnormality if it is also found in a first-degree relative (for example, strabismus) and so it is important to make the questions as clear and unambiguous as possible, often asking the same questions in a number of different ways. The word 'squint' is very ambiguous, as is 'lazy' eye. In general, if a parent says that someone in the family had a lazy eye, we try to ascertain details as to the age, circumstances and treatment surrounding the condition. If an accompanying relative has an apparent visual problem, we often carry out informal vision tests on the adult to ascertain a little more about his or her particular condition.

Informal Observation of Visual Behaviour

As a crude measure of visual attention, it is often valuable to find out how much the child scans the visual world and whether his or her visual attention can be directed to particular objects. Any visually guided reaching or grasping is noted while the child is playing; small toys are presented to the child by either the tester or the parent and the response noted. We usually carry out some informal field testing by seeing whether the child moves his or her head and eyes to fixate a moving, silent, visually conspicuous toy, which is moved into the child's field of view laterally from the side to the child's midline. In this way any gross asymmetries of the visual field can be assessed (which may be particularly important in hemiparesis). When perceptual rather than sensory defects are suspected, the child's level of object permanence and visual recognition should be assessed. We have found stacking Russian Dolls, Fisher Price Zoo animals or small clockwork toys, when hidden under cups, particularly useful for these informal tests. If a child is incapable of the hand and arm movements necessary to remove the cup, then simple disappearance/appearance toys such as a Jack-in-the-Box can be substituted.

Standard Orthoptic Examination

The role of the orthoptist (who is a member of the paramedical staff associated with ophthalmology) is to assess the presence of binocular vision (i.e. both eyes working together to provide single vision) and to diagnose and assist in the management of abnormalities of binocular vision, such as in the case of a squint or strabismus. The tests used require specific training, so it is in general undesirable for non-orthoptists to use them. In the case of infants and young children where co-operation may be limited, the results of these tests are in general less quantitative than when used with co-operative adults. Four tests are routinely used.

Hirschberg Test.   Here the orthoptist shines a small pen torch into the pupils and compares the position of the corneal reflections within the two eyes. Any sustained asymmetry of the reflexes indicates a manifest squint.

Assessment of Ocular Movements.   The orthoptist observes the child's eye movements in following a light from the straight ahead position into the right and left fields, upwards and downwards and where possible into the oblique positions. In young infants it is often difficult to observe the eye movements made upwards and obliquely, without the child moving the head instead of the eyes. Limitations of eye movements may indicate neurological disorder. Additionally, convergence to an approaching target should also be assessed for symmetry of the eye positions.

Cover Test.   This test is used to detect a manifest squint. One eye is occluded momentarily by the orthoptist's hand or a small piece of card. The orthoptist talks to the child to maintain attention on the face (or small torch held in front of the face) and watches the position of the unoccluded eye before, during and after occlusion. Any movement of the unoccluded eye indicates a squint. The test can also be used to indicate a tendency towards squinting by observation of the occluded eye, but with young children it is often difficult to get unambiguous results with this part of the test.

Prism Test.   A prism (15 or 20 prisms dioptres strength) is placed in front of each eye in turn, and each time the fellow eye is observed by the orthoptist. The prism induces double vision by displacing the image laterally in the eye covered by the prism. To eliminate double vision the fellow eye must make a compensating eye movement. Thus the test is used as a test of binocular vision.

It is sometimes difficult to test the second eye with infants because of lack of sustained concentration. It is usually better not to keep retrying the test as the child will obviously become bored and may not co-operate with later tests.

Acuity Assessments

The commonest measure used to specify the quality of vision is the measure of *visual acuity*, that is, a measure of the finest detail that can be resolved.

Forced-choice Preferential Looking.   Acuity is usually measured in infants by us using the forced-choice preferential looking procedure, or FPL (for example, see Teller 1979; Atkinson and Braddick 1981a; Atkinson, Braddick and Pimm-Smith 1982; Atkinson and Braddick 1983a). The method depends on 'preferential looking' where the infant prefers to look at a striped pattern rather than a blank screen of matched mean luminance (see Figure 10.1). A staircase procedure to adjust the stripe width and hence determine an acuity threshold is used, with observations being recorded by a 'blind' observer (who does not know on which of the two screens the striped pattern is displayed). The full staircase procedure works well for infants under 9 months (or children of mental age under 9 months), but can be used on older infants and children in an abbreviated form giving a valuable estimate of acuity. One trick we have found that works well for two to three-year-olds is to ask them to point a finger at the stripes to 'switch them off'.

The acuity value obtained using FPL will depend on a number of stimulus variables such as screen size and eccentricity. At present it is necessary for anyone using this procedure to devise their own norms on normal children, although one simple approximation might be that the expected acuity for a child would be their age in months in cycles/deg. visual angle, i.e. a one-month-old has an acuity around 1 cycle/deg., a three-month-old 3 cycles/deg. and a twelve-month-old 12 cycles/deg. It is likely that FPL underestimates the acuity of older infants, but gross deviations from this norm can be a useful indicator of visual loss.

Tracking Tests.   In a few cases where motor control is very poor (for example, in a child with choreoathetotic syndrome), and for a number of

Figure 10.1: Assessment of acuity using the forced-choice preferential looking procedure (FPL). The child fixates a striped pattern rather than a blank screen matched in mean luminance. The screen sizes are identical, although in this photograph they appear to look different because of the camera angle.

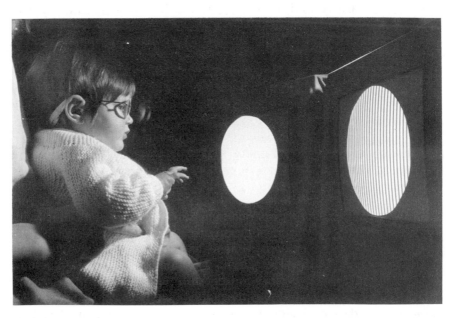

older children with very limited attention span, it has been possible to gain a qualitative idea of acuity only by using the mounted STYCAR balls at 1, 2 or 3 metres. Because these tracking tests such as Catford Drum (Catford and Oliver 1973) and STYCAR balls (Sheridan, 1976) are tests of detection of a single object against the background rather than true tests of resolution, they can never give accurate measures of acuity (Atkinson, Braddick, Pimm-Smith, Ayling and Sawyer 1981). For emmetropic individuals the Catford Drum overestimates acuity by a factor of 4 and for some myopes the overestimation may be 10 times the true value. However, the STYCAR balls test can be used to give some indication of the distance over which a child will attend visually and can also be used to give a very appropriate measure of visual acuity if other tests are not possible.

Operant Methods. With some children of over three years mental age we use an operant alley-running technique (Atkinson, French and Braddick 1981), where the young child has to choose between two gratings of different orientations and a reward is hidden under a consistent orientation of grating, e.g. a sweet is always placed under the cube with the vertical grating on it (see Figure 10.2). As well as grating targets, modifications of Sheridan-Gardiner letter optotypes can be used in this test (see Figure 10.3). In this task the child has always to pick the cube with the letter '0' on it. This allows the assessment of visual 'crowding' (Atkinson, Pimm-Smith, Evans, Harding and Braddick, in prep.) which may reveal visual problems that are not apparent from a grating or single optotype test. We have also designed, and are currently evaluating, a 'crowded' version of the standard single optotype Sheridan–Gardiner test for use with three to five-year-olds. It is hoped that this will be equivalent to acuity obtained with adults on a Snellen Chart.

In a prevous publication we have discussed clinical assessments using FPL (Atkinson, Braddick and Pimm-Smith 1982). In general we have found that FPL is a robust technique for use with a wide range of infants and children (particularly the mentally handicapped). However it does require highly trained observers to get the 'best' results out of this age group. In most handicapped children recently assessed by our team it has been used with very few failures. The procedure utilizes specialized laboratory equipment including oscilloscopes and micro-computer to allow automatic presentation of the stimuli and analysis of the results; consequently this procedure should not be used without reasonable technical knowledge concerning the equipment.

Optokinetic Nystagmus. In a recent series of assessments on two infants no evidence of visual behaviour was seen in either the children's general behaviour, in FPL, or in the STYCAR balls test. In such cases we have been particularly concerned as to whether there is any vision at all, so have tested for optokinetic nystagmus (repetitive following eye movements

Figure 10.2(a): Assessment of acuity in the alley-running task. The barrier separates the two cubes which display the stimuli. The child has to choose between the vertical stripes and the horizontal stripes.

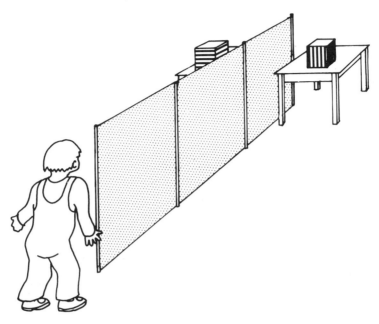

elicited by a large area of moving patterns) with a visual stimulus consisting of a large area of moving randomly spaced dots. The infant is seated close to the screen of moving dots. The dots are made up of a film loop of Letratone texture which moves in front of a small projector and is back projected on to a large screen (see Figure 10.4). For the stimulus to be effective the field has to cover a wide area of the child's visual field (approximately 120° visual angle), so that the child is unable to inhibit OKN by fixating an edge or stationary contour. The speed of movement can be varied, but we usually use a velocity of around 20-30 deg./sec. with infants and young children. OKN for binocular viewing can be taken as an indicator of at least a functioning subcortical visual system. Both infants who did not respond using FPL, when tested with the OKN stimulus showed binocular OKN, although neither of them showed spontaneous shifts of visual attention. Both children were thought to have extensive cortical damage from previous neurological examinations.

The binocular OKN test is relatively easy to use as long as the screen is of adequate size filling the infant's field of view. However, one difficulty that has been encountered is to get the observer's view as close to the baby's eyes as possible, while not providing the baby with a fixation point (the observer) or blocking the infant's view of the stimulus. Some have felt that this difficulty warranted EOG recordings rather than direct

Figure 10.2(b): When the child has made a choice, he or she looks under the cube for the reward.

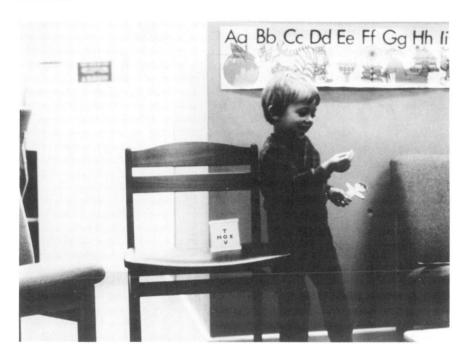

Figure 10.3: Types of display used to assess 'visual crowding'.

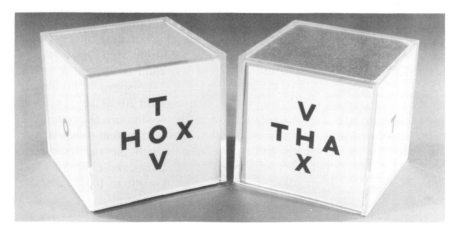

observation. We have tried both methods and in general find that the discomfort to the observer (sometimes, for example, lying on the floor looking up at the infant's eye) does not outweigh the difficulty of fixing electrodes close to the eyes of an alert manipulative infant!

Figure 10.4: Infant looking at a large field of randomly arranged blobs which move laterally by means of a motorized film loop, to elicit OKN.

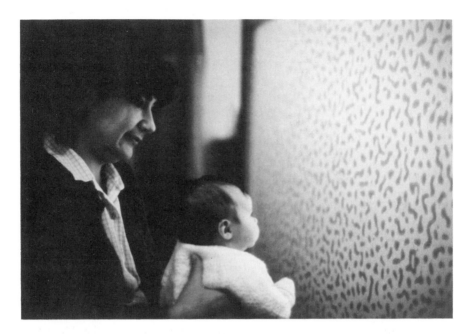

Visually Evoked Potentials. It is also possible to estimate visual acuity and contrast sensitivity using measurement of visual evoked potentials or VEPs (for example, Harris, Atkinson and Braddick 1976; Marg Freeman, Peltzman and Goldstein 1976; Pirchio, Spinelli, Florentini and Maffei 1978; Spekreijse 1978; Atkinson, Braddick and French 1979; Sokol and Jones 1979; Tyler 1982). Either latency or amplitude measurements can be made. We have used phase reversing grating patterns with high temporal reversal rates (between 2Hz and 10Hz) to measure the amplitude of the VEP which is time locked to the contrast reversal of the visual stimulus. In general, estimates of visual function by means of the VEP have not been used routinely by us for these clinical assessments, because of the requirement for rapid testing procedures and the need for good co-operation on the part of the child for electrode attachment and noise-free recordings. However, under certain circumstances the measurement of the VEP can provide additional information which is not available from other tests. For example, in the case of children with suspected cortical damage, whose eye-movement control is very poor, the measurement of VEPs for estimating acuity can sometimes be used when other behavioural methods are limited or inappropriate. For example, one recent case assessed by us had extensive 'fitting' from two months of age and under subsequent necessary medication showed excessive random eye movements and lack of eye-movement control. These effects reduced with reduced medication but were never completely eliminated. FLP and OKN did not give extensive quantitative reliable results so VEP pattern measures were undertaken. The first pattern used (pattern appearance) rendered a normal VEP, typical of a subcortical visual response. However no orientational response to pattern changes was found in the child, indicating extensive cortical damage or cortical involvement in fitting. It seemed likely that the child while in this state was unable to use vision at all normally or 'see' or 'interpret' changes in patterned stimuli. Under such circumstances VEP measurements may be essential, but they involve highly specific technical skills and experience together with extensive knowledge of infant behaviour. As such they should not be lightly undertaken and do not usually form part of our routine visual assessment.

Photorefraction and Retinoscopy

Statements about refraction and refractive errors usually refer to the focusing power of the eye when accommodation is completely relaxed, for instance by a cycloplegic drug. Where the eyes are actually focused in normal vision, however, depends not only on whether the eyes are myopic (short-sighted), emmetropic (no refractive error) or hyper metropic (long-sighted) when relaxed, but also on the degree of active accommodation.

Photorefraction is a technique developed originally by the Howland brothers (Howland and Howland 1974) for photographically observing the plane of focus of the two eyes. The original technique using an orthogonal photorefractor has been used to find out about the development of focusing (active accommodation) in infants (Braddick, Atkinson, French and Howland 1979) and for looking at astigmatism (differential defocusing of the eye along different meridians) in infancy and its disappearance with age (Howland, Atkinson, Braddick and French 1978; Atkinson, Braddick and French 1980). Several years ago a new device called the isotropic photorefractor was developed by us in Cambridge and used to look at both active accommodation and cycloplegic refractions in infants and young children (Atkinson, Braddick, Ayling, Pimm-Smith, Howland and Ingram 1981; Atkinson and Braddick 1983b). In our clinical use with this device, video photographs are taken with a flash delivered through a fibre-optic light guide centred in the camera lens. Three different settings of focus are used with a wide aperture lens, attached to the camera. By alternation of the camera focus we can tell from the amount of light returning to the camera whether the infant is focused in front or behind the camera and whether both eyes are focused in the same plane (see Figure 10.5). Figure 10.6 shows an infant where there is a large difference in focusing between the eyes (anisometropia). Photorefraction has been calibrated against conventional retinoscopy (Atkinson, Braddick, Ayling, Pimm-Smith, Howland and Ingram 1981; Atkinson and Braddick 1983b; Atkinson, Braddick,

Durden, Watson and Atkinson 1984) so that the method can be used to measure refractions. It is a particularly useful method for cases where little co-operation is given by the child, because the procedure only requires the child to look at the camera for very brief periods, with the operator at some distance from the child.

Figure 10.5: Focused illuminated pupils, using the photorefractor. Note the symmetrically placed corneal reflexes in each pupil, indicating that the child is *not* strabismic.

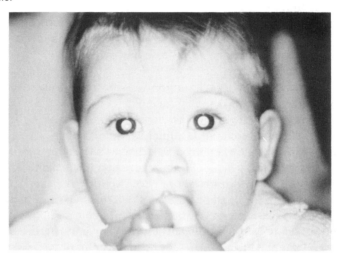

Figure 10.6: Deliberately blurred photograph using photorefraction, showing an infant with a difference in focusing between the eyes. The bright blur circle in the right eye shows a smaller refractive error than the completely blurred out image in the left eye.

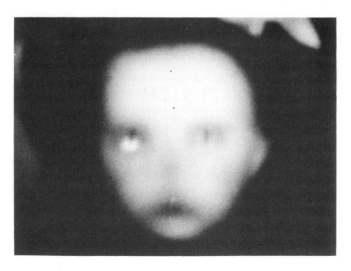

We routinely use photorefraction to assess active accommodation which provides a valuable measure of visual attention as well as a pointer to refractive errors.

In most clinical assessments we also photorefract the child under cyclopentolate hydrochloride 1 per cent (Atkinson and Braddick 1983b). A retinoscopic refraction when possible is carried out by a skilled paediatric retinoscopist in parallel with photorefraction. However, in quite a number of infants and children accurate retinoscopy is not possible because of the lack of co-operation on the part of the child. In such cases photorefraction provides a valuable tool for estimating refractive errors. A good indication of any astigmatism is given from the photorefraction pictures. An astigmatic refractive error is shown in Figure 10.7, where the blur is elongated to an ellipse along the axis of astigmatism. At present we are investigating yet another modification of photorefraction (eccentric photorefraction) which might make it possible to measure even very large refractive errors from the video photograph, with accuracy and ease (Bobier, Braddick, Atkinson and Wattam-Bell 1984).

As a method used in visual assessments, photorefraction has proved to be the most universally useful of our techniques. However, its use can clearly not directly answer the question 'what does the child see?' as it does not indicate anything about acuity or contrast sensitivity, but merely indicates how well the eyes are focused and are able to change focus. It is, however, an important result for allowing the tester to eliminate the possibility of poor vision being merely a consequence of refractive error. If, for example, a child is found without any apparent vision on behavioural tests such

Figure 10.7: Deliberately blurred photograph, using photorefraction, showing an infant with an astigmatic refractive error. Each eye shows a blurred ellipse, the long axis (close to horizontal) of which has a larger refractive error than the short axis.

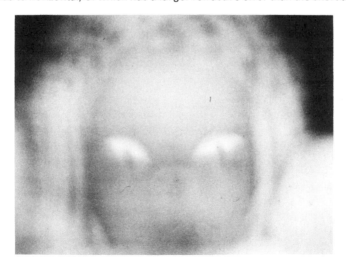

as FPL, nor was any significant refractive error indicated from cycloplegic photorefraction, then it is possible for the tester to say that no simple refractive problem is preventing the child 'seeing'. It is likely that the defect in the visual system is due either to retinal pathology or to neurological problems in the optic nerve or higher nervous system. This type of pattern of behaviour is often found in handicapped children with extensive cortical damage. However, it is necessary at this point in assessment for the oph-thalmologist to examine the finding and check for any retinal abnormality before cortical problems can be indicated.

A new development in photorefraction which may become available in the near future is a device to allow calibration of the video images obtained in photorefraction, so that the tester will be provided automatically with an estimate of refractive error. This device, involving interactive dialogue with a microcomputer, will tell the tester the estimated refraction, specifying the bandwidth of refraction rather than an exact measurement. The device should speed up photorefraction considerably and give the tester instant results, so that the possibility of refractive correction can be considered.

With certain categories of children with mental and physical handicaps photorefraction is often more successful than retinoscopy, for example, in testing older mobile infants, hyperactive children or children with Down's syndrome. However, with some physically handicapped children, with restricted head postures and eye movements, it may be easier for the retin-oscopist to get the retinoscope on the child's visual axis rather than adjust a camera to the correct position. Also, because of limited arm movements, it is often not possible for these children to remove lenses held in front of the eyes. However, under these circumstances it is often necessary for the retinoscopist to carry out the test rapidly to avoid boredom and frustration to the child due to the physical strain of maintaining an upright body and head posture.

Test of Binocularity

Besides the orthoptic checks for strabismus already discussed there are two specific tests that have been used in the VDU as indicators of functioning cortical binocularity.

Symmetrical Monocular Optokinetic Nystagmus (MOKN).   Asymmetries of OKN in the two directions with monocular stimulation is an indicator of lack of binocularity (Atkinson 1979; Atkinson and Braddick 1981b); directional asymmetries found in one eye may be a sign of lateralized occipital cortical damage. (The same stimulus described above for eliciting OKN is used for testing MOKN, with the infant wearing a patch or occluder on one eye.)

Binocular Visual Evoked Potentials (BVEP). A VEP specifically related to binocular vision can be elicited in infants with normal visual development after the age of three months (Braddick, Atkinson, Julesz, Kropfl, Bodis-Wollner and Raab 1980; Braddick and Atkinson 1983). We have not yet used this method (or the psychophysical analogue) for clinical assessment, but similar behavioural tests are being developed and used in a number of laboratories (e.g. Fox 1981). A number of these techniques are likely to become widespread in assessments in the next few years.

In general, such a visual assessment involves each child being in our Unit between 30 minutes and $1\frac{1}{2}$ hours, although actual testing only occupies a fraction of that time. While demanding in resources (both techniques, personnel and time), it provides information on children's visual capabilities which is useful to parents and to the clinical team and makes an important contribution to the child's treatment and rehabilitation.

In our experience, success in these assessments depends on several factors, *besides* the technical facilities and experience in infant vision testing. Among these factors are (1) a separate position from, but in close contract with, both paediatricians and ophthalmologists; (2) an appropriate atmosphere including flexibility in scheduling to fit the changing state of young infants and sufficient time and close contact to allow observation of the child's visual behaviour in an informal setting; (3) care to inform parents of the nature of the tests and the implications of the findings and an attempt to answer any queries or problems presented by the parents.

Summary

Even a relatively successful visual assessment made on a child using both technical and psychological expertise cannot answer all the questions concerning the child's vision. It is often frustrating to have to admit to parents that, although there is no fundamental sensory defect in the child, the vision of the child is not normal. Sometimes the tester is left with rather weak and vague statements to the parents concerning 'lack of visual attention' or 'lack of perceptual skills', where no clear-cut decisions can be made and no obvious immediate treatment is available. To this extent the field of visual assessment is in its own infancy, with many gaps in our knowledge concerning the normal state of affairs for infants and children. It would seem better at present to admit that current medical knowledge in this field is at its limit to parents of handicapped children, so that they do not feel that some simple remedy such as the wearing of spectacles is being denied their child because of other physical and mental handicaps. Perhaps, when this chapter is rewritten in ten years' time, we will be able to discuss in more concrete terms tests for visual perceptual functions such as attention and recognition. For the present a great deal could be put into action to look at the more basic aspects of visual sensory assessment. It is the joint task of scientists and clinicians to do this efficiently and as soon as possible.

References

Atkinson, J. (1979) 'Development of optokinetic nystagmus in the human infant and monkey infant: an analogue to development in kittens' in R.D. Freeman, (ed.), *Developmental Neurobiology of Vision*, Plenum Press, New York

—— and Braddick, O.J. (1981a) 'Acuity, contrast sensitivity, and accommodation in infancy' in R.N. Aslin, J.R. Alberts and M.R. Peterson (eds.), *Development of Perception: Psychobiological Perspectives, Vol. 2: The Visual System*, Academic Press, New York

—— and —— (1981b) 'Development of optokinetic nystagmus in infants: An indicator of cortical binocularity?' in D.F. Fisher, R.A. Monty and J.W. Senders (eds.), *Eye Movements: Cognition and Visual Perception*, Lawrence Erlbaum, Hillsdale, NJ

—— and —— (1983a) 'Assessment of visual acuity in infancy and early childhood', *Acta Ophthal., Suppl., 157*, 18-26

—— and —— (1983b) 'The use of isotropic photorefraction for vision screening in infants', *Acta Ophthal., Suppl. 157*, 36-45

——, ——, Ayling, L., Pimm-Smith, E., Howland, H.C. and Ingram, R.M. (1981) 'Isotropic photorefraction: a new method for refractive testing of infants', *Doc. Ophthal. Proc. Series 30*, 217-23

——, ——, Durden, K., Watson, P.G. and Atkinson, S. (1984) 'Screening for refractive errors in 6–9-month-old infants by photorefraction', *Brit. J. Ophthal., 68*, 105-112

——, —— and French, J. (1979) 'Contrast sensitivity of the human neonate measured by the visual evoked potential', *Invest. Ophthal. Vis. Sci., 18*, 210-13

——, —— and —— (1980) 'Infant astigmatism: its disappearance with age', *Vision Res., 20*, 891-3

——, —— and Pimm-Smith E. (1982) '"Preferential looking" for monocular and binocular acuity testing of infants', *Brit. J. Ophthal., 66*, 264-8

——, ——, ——, Ayling, L. and Sawyer, R. (1981) 'Does the Catford Drum give an accurate assessment of acuity?' *Brit. J. Ophthal., 65*, 652-6

——, French, J. and Braddick, O.J. (1981) 'Contrast sensitivity function of pre-school children', *Brit. J. Ophthal., 65*, 525-9

——, Pimm-Smith, E., Evans, C., Harding, G. and Braddick, O.J. *Visual Crowding in Young Children* (in prep.)

Bobier, W., Braddick, O.J., Atkinson, J. and Wattam-Bell, J. (1984) 'Eccentric and isotropic photorefraction: applications to infant accommodation', *Perception, 13*, A 27

Braddick, O.J. and Atkinson, J. (1983) 'The development of binocular function in infancy', *Acta Ophthal., Suppl. 157*, 27-35

——, ——, French, J. and Howland, H.C. (1979) 'A photorefractive study of infant accommodation', *Vision Res., 19*, 1319-30

——, ——, Julesz, B., Kropfl, W., Bodis-Wollner, I. and Raab, E. (1980) 'Cortical binocularity in infants', *Nature, 288*, 363-5

Catford, G.V. and Oliver, A. (1973) 'Development of visual acuity', *Archives of Disease in Childhood, 48*, 47-50

Fox, R. (1981) 'Stereopsis in animals and human infants' in R.N. Aslin, J.R. Alberts and M.R. Petersen (eds.), *Development of Perception: Psychobiological Perspectives, Vol. 2: The Visual System*, Academic Press, New York

Harris, L., Atkinson, J. and Braddick, O.J. (1976) 'Visual contrast sensitivity of a 6-month-old infant measured by the evoked potential', *Nature, Lond., 264*, 570-1

Howland, H.C. and Howland, B. (1974) 'Photorefraction: a technique for study of refractive state at a distance', *J. Opt. Soc. Am., 64*, 240-9

——, Atkinson, J., Braddick, O.J. and French J. (1978) 'Infant astigmatism measured by photorefraction', *Science, 202*, 331-3

Marg. E., Freeman, D.N., Peltzman, P. and Goldstein, P.J. (1976) 'Visual acuity development in human infants: evoked potential measurements', *Invest. Ophthalmol., 15*, 150-3

Pirchio, M., Spinelli, D., Florentini, A. and Maffei, L. (1978) 'Infant contrast sensitivity evaluated by evoked potentials', *Brain Res.*, *141*, 179-84

Sheridan, M.D. (1976) *Manual for the STYCAR vision tests*, NFER Publishing Company Ltd, Slough

Sokol, S., and Jones, K. (1979) 'Implicit time of pattern evoked potentials in infants: an index of maturation of spatial vision', *Vision Res.*, *19*, 747-55

Spekreijse, H. (1978) 'Maturation of contrast EPs and development of visual resolution', *Arch. Ital. Biol.*, *116*, 358-69

Teller, D.Y. (1979) 'The forced-choice preferential looking procedure: a psychophysical technique for use with human infants', *Infant Behav. and Devel.*, *2*, 135-53

Tyler, C.W. (1982) 'Assessment of visual function in infants by evoked potentials', *Devel. Med. and Child Neurol.*, *24*, 853-5

11 METHODS OF OBJECTIVE ASSESSMENT OF AUDITORY FUNCTION IN SUBJECTS WITH LIMITED COMMUNICATION SKILLS

Ivan Tucker and Michael Nolan

Introduction

Many research reports highlight the fact that there is a higher incidence of deafness in the mentally handicapped population than in the normal population. Researchers in our own department have reported this (Nolan, McCartney, McArthur and Rowson 1980; Cunningham and McArthur 1981) and there are excellent reviews and discussions of the subject in Lloyd (1970), Davies and Penniceard (1980) and McCartney (1984).

In light of the above research findings it is imperative that every effort is made to identify and quantify the hearing problems of mentally handicapped people. A survey by Whelan and Speake (1977) of 305 ATCs in England and Wales asked ATC staff how many times they had had contact with a range of professionals thought to be of potential benefit to the centres. Speech therapists came top of this list, but audiologists were not included on the list. The result indicates the concern felt by ATC staff over the communication difficulties of trainees in their care. But clearly little thought was given to the very real possibility that lack of hearing may have been contributing to this poor speech and language development.

There appears to be a general lack of audiological services available to both mentally handicapped adults and children. This fact has been noted by Tempowski, Felstead and Simon (1974), who suggested that one in three of the deaf mentally handicapped presently in hospital do not require permanent care and that services for the mentally handicapped must be improved to reduce the numbers placed inappropriately in mental handicap hospitals.

Audiological Services for Mentally Handicapped People

The National Development Group for the Mentally Handicapped report (1978) emphasized the fact that audiological services should be made available to both mentally handicapped children and adults and we see this as a vital step if real progress is to be made in helping mentally handicapped people to realize their full potential. We most certainly do not agree with the view held in some quarters that there is little point in attempting to assess hearing ability in mentally handicapped people because they are untestable and only rarely have hearing difficulty. Clinically we know they are testable and research has shown us they are more prone to problems with hearing than the normal population.

Many mentally handicapped people have difficulty with both receptive and expressive aspects of spoken language (Whelan and Speake 1977). Our aim as audiologists must be to provide those people with the best possible experience of the sounds of spoken language, so ensuring that it is not a lack of exposure (as may arise with hearing-impairment) that is creating or adding to the already existing physiological anomalies.

The audiologist, when he is attempting to assess the auditory function of such patients, has two major aims in mind. Firstly, he wishes to quantify the hearing levels across the speech range of frequencies, and secondly he wishes to establish the site of the problem and therefore the possibility of improving the hearing levels. Figure 11.1 illustrates where the two main types of hearing problem arise, those of the outer and middle ear which are termed conductive and those of the inner ear, the cochlea and retro-cochlear pathways, which are called sensori-neural. The former are often amenable to medical or surgical intervention, whilst the latter are not and if significant in level will require the fitting of suitable hearing aids.

When writing about assessment it is usual to distinguish screening from diagnostic procedures, but it is our considered opinion that, where the subjects are known to have or are suspected of having other handicaps, and especially mental handicap, then diagnostic procedures should apply and the subject should be seen by audiologists for full assessment.

The point of major issue in this chapter will relate to how far one might possibly expect mentally handicapped subjects to co-operate in conventional testing and how informative newer electrophysiological and other more 'objective' tests can be. It is important at this point to highlight the fact that much resorting to electrophysiological technique is resultant upon

Figure 11.1: The Peripheral Hearing Mechanism

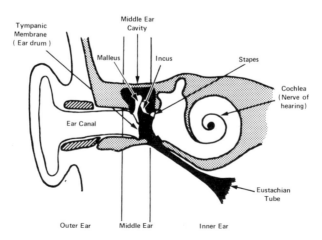

lack of experience, or training, or skill of clinicians involved. It is most important that audiological clinicians experienced in working with children test mentally handicapped subjects and it is well worthy of note that in the Nolan *et al.* (1980) study 87 per cent of the mentally handicapped subjects were testable by play audiometry and other behavioural techniques. It is highly likely that audiologists will be prepared to:

1. adapt conventional techniques, for use with mentally handicapped subjects;
2. use techniques designed for babies on young mentally handicapped children; and
3. use techniques designed for testing normal children on mentally handicapped adults.

There will, however, be a small proportion of subjects so handicapped that they require testing in a way in which no co-operation is required, possibly under anaesthetic or sedation. These methods will be described shortly. The behavioural tests of hearing which are used with children and which can be used or adapted for use with mentally handicapped subjects include the Distraction Test, the Co-operative Test, the Performance Test and Pure-Tone Audiometry (see also Chapter 6, this volume). The above tests were designed to relate to the developmental stages of normal children and therefore the paediatric audiologist should be able to relate test procedure to a particular mentally handicapped subject's level of development, rather than merely basing the test on age.

Behavioural Tests of Hearing

The Distraction Test (6-18 months)

The test stimuli used are of the 'meaningful' kind, since research and experience have shown babies to be most responsive to this approach (Taylor 1964); for example, the human voice and the sounds of rattles are used. However, whilst the test seems very simple, the stimuli are carefully controlled. For example, the low-frequency signal is a voiced sound such as the vowel 'oo' (as in shoe), rhythmically presented.

One of the high-frequency signals is the consonant 's' (air is gently blown over top of tongue and between teeth — with no voicing) rhythmically presented, and another is the Manchester high-frequency rattle specially developed in our department and used by many health visitors and audiologists throughout the country.

A spoon is usually gently scraped against the side of a cup as an arousal item, but this is not frequency specific (Nolan and Tucker 1981) and, whilst most normally hearing children respond very readily to the sound, it is not counted as a test item. The stimuli are presented first at minimal levels and then raised in steps until the subject responds by turning to locate the source of the sound. The signal level is measured on a sound-level meter and then recorded.

The arrangement of the test in the clinic is that the baby sits on his mother's knee. Therefore the child should have good back and head control. The baby sits slightly forward on the knee and is supported only at the waist. One audiologist attracts the baby's attention to the front, perhaps using a small toy. He will have nothing very elaborate because he wants to attract attention without getting the child so fixed to the front that he will not turn to the quiet sounds. Whilst the attention is to the front, the second audiologist moves into position at the rear. At the front the interest factor will be reduced — perhaps by hiding the toy — and at that instant the sound is made three feet from the child's ear and slightly behind so that he cannot see the tester. The child is distracted by the sound and must respond to two low-, two mid-, and two high-frequency 'minimal' signals to each side to pass the test. Great care needs to be taken to ensure that it is only sound to which the child is responding and not vision (e.g. the tester's head coming into the child's line of vision), or smell (e.g. the tester wearing perfume), or vibration (e.g. a tester moving carelessly on a hard floor).

Where this test is appropriate for the cognitive level of the subject but the subject cannot satisfy the postural (i.e. back and head support) and motor (i.e. turning response) requirements, certain modifications to the test can be acceptable, e.g.

1. use of baby relax chair or support cushions for postural difficulties;
2. acceptance of repeatable eye movements to the sound stimuli where head turning is impossible;
3. adjustments to signal distance;
4. adjustments to signal duration;
5. changes in the order of signal intensity.

All of the above changes to standard procedure should only be made by a qualified audiologist and as part of a test battery. For example, at this stage of cognitive development electric response audiometry may provide useful additional information.

Co-operative Tests (18–30 Months)

Children who are tested at this age are able easily to inhibit (ignore) the distraction type of test item, so use is made of the normally hearing child's growing understanding of spoken language. Rapport is gained by playing with some toys with the child and then the tester moves into a routine of asking the child to do things with the toys in response to very quietly spoken commands; for example, with a bus and 'play people' the child would be asked to 'put the man in the bus', give 'one to mummy', 'put one on the table', etc. Simple sentences such as these would be spoken very quietly at a distance of three feet from each ear.

The child's ability to hear high frequencies would be tested as in the distraction test using the high-frequency rattle or the high-frequency consonant 's'. The child's ability to locate sounds at distance is checked using a chime bar or other noise maker. The child's attention is first drawn to some toys so that he cannot anticipate where the test sound is being produced.

At this time age is not as important as stage. Some children of 18 months may not be able to understand and follow commands in the way described above, so the test for an earlier age would be carried out. This does not imply that the child is backward, it implies that the test range is wide. Clinicians are also aware of the negativistic stage which occurs in many children around two years of age. This is where the polite request for the child to do something is met with a firm No! There are times when the co-operative aged child is anything but co-operative, but the skilled clinician will usually be able to complete a test.

This test can be very useful in highlighting the functional hearing capacity and can demonstrate for the benefit of teachers and family the extent of any hearing impairment in functional terms. The test can easily be manipulated in order to cater for subjects with appropriate cognitive development, but who lack the necessary motor skills.

Performance Tests (about 2½-3½ Years)

By the time the child is around two and a half years old, he is usually able to wait, listen for a sound signal and make a response. We frequently use a wooden boat which has positions for eight men to sit. We often start the test using the mother. 'Mum, you listen and when I say "go" you put the man in the boat ... go!' Then the child's mother demonstrates and the child imitates. 'Go' tests low frequency. The signal is again given very quietly at three feet from the ear, and out of vision of the child. The high-frequency signal is the consonant 's' and the child responds again by performing some action each time the signal is given.

The skills involved in the performance tests are similar to those required to undertake pure-tone audiometry which is described later. The child shows the ability to wait, and hear a quiet signal and then indicates he has heard by making a defined response.

Again this test is adaptable; for example, it is possible to say with some subjects 'when I say go you put the little man in the boat', with others this can be reduced to a simple training of response to one word, i.e. 'go', without any other verbal instruction. In subjects with severe physical handicaps any reliable motor response can indicate perception of the test stimuli, e.g. eye blinks, finger lifting, knocking blocks off a table.

Pure-tone Audiometry

Diagnostic tests of hearing that are normally used with children up to three years of age have been described. Once a child reaches the age of three to three and a half years the pure-tone test of hearing will be attempted. This test is very similar in format to the performance test. However, in the pure-tone test the child is conditioned to respond to a whistle of a particular pitch (frequency) rather than to 'go' or 's' as in the performance test. Initially, using a portable audiometer, the clinician will demonstrate to the child what he is expected to do. The audiometer produces tones in the speech frequency range (125 Hz-8,000 Hz). The child is trained to 'put a man in a boat' or 'a ball in a box' each time he hears a tone. Once the clinician has satisfied himself that the child is capable of waiting until a tone is produced before completing the task, he will proceed to the pure-tone audiometric test. This involves the child wearing a pair of headphones. Many children find this exciting though some do require careful handling to encourage them to wear them. The headphones are connected to an audiometer.

Each ear is tested separately and the child's hearing thresholds are measured for a number of different pure-tone frequencies in the speech frequency range. The threshold is the level of the quietest signal the child can hear. The information from this test tells the clinician what the child's hearing levels are and how they compare with the normal population. The test using the headphones is known as a test of pure-tone audiometry for air conduction. This means that it is a measure of the child's total hearing. The sounds travel through the whole hearing system from the headphones, down the ear canal, are transmitted through the eardrum, across the middle ear cavity via the ossicles to the nerve of hearing.

Another test that employs the same procedure, from the child's point of view, is the test of pure-tone audiometry for bone conduction. In this test a small vibrator is placed on the mastoid bone behind one ear. Pure tones, the same as those used for headphone testing, are directed from the audiometer to the bone vibrator on the mastoid. New hearing thresholds for these signals are measured and recorded (Tucker and Nolan 1984).

The bone conduction signals effectively bypass the middle ear system. They make the skull vibrate and this stimulates the nerve of hearing directly. A normally hearing person will hear the air and bone conducted signals at the same level on the signal level dial of the audiometer; i.e. air conducted level OdB HL, bone conducted level OdB HL.

If a child shows a loss for air conduction and normal levels for bone conduction, the indications will be that the pathway to the brain centre for bone conduction is normal and not damaged. Hence, the inner ear is normal. As the air-conduction level is abnormal, the loss must lie in the outer or middle ear, so the loss must be conductive in nature.

If a child shows an equal loss for air- and bone-conducted signals, indications would be that there must be damage in the inner ear pathway (because the bone conduction sensitivity is depressed) and the outer and middle ears must be normal. This loss would be sensori-neural in nature.

If a child shows a loss for air- and bone-conducted signals with a greater loss for the air-conducted signals, a mixed loss is indicated. This means a loss resulting from a problem in the outer or middle ear which affects the air-conduction level but not the bone-conduction level; and an added loss resulting from a problem in the inner ear, affecting air- and bone-conduction levels equally (see example in Table 11.1).

The bone-conduction test of hearing is a very useful aid in helping to identify the nature of a hearing problem. However, it is only one of a number of tests that will be applied during the diagnostic session, and the clinician will consider the results of all tests before coming to a firm decision. One of the limitations of the bone-conduction test with young children is that it cannot be applied unless they are developmentally mature enough to carry out a pure-tone audiometric test. The majority of children under the age of three years will not be tested by this technique. In such cases it will be necessary to rely more heavily on the results of other tests.

Another problem of testing by bone conduction is that the bone conductor sets the whole skull into vibration, and both ears are stimulated at the same level regardless of the position of the vibrator on the head. This means that the clinician cannot put the vibrator behind the right ear and test this ear, and then repeat for the left ear as is possible in the headphone testing.

So a technique known as masking has to be employed in order to determine the bone-conduction levels of each ear. This involves introducing a continual noise into one ear while the test signal is introduced in the other ear (test ear) in the normal manner. Young children find this procedure very difficult and many are unable to perform reliably on this test until the age of seven years.

Masking is also necessary in air-conduction testing if there is a significant difference between the hearing levels of the two ears. This is because for high signal levels it is possible to hear the signal in the opposite ear to that being tested. If the difference between ears is greater than 40 dB, the clinician will have to apply masking to the better ear so as to ensure

Table 11.1: Example of how Different Hearing Losses Result

	Outer–middle ear loss	Inner ear loss	Total loss
Air conduction	a	b	a + b
Bone conduction	—	b	b
Normal hearing	a = 0	b = 0	
Conductive loss:	a = 30 (e.g.)	b = 0	
	Air conduction =	30dB	
	Bone conduction =	0dB	
Sensori-neural loss:	a = 0	b = 40 (e.g.)	
	Air conduction =	40dB	
	Bone conduction =	40dB	
Mixed loss:	a = 20	b = 40	
	Air conduction =	60dB	
	Bone conduction =	40dB	

that this ear does not hear the signal and so confuse the results for the poor ear (see Brasier 1974).

Thus, although pure-tone tests are extremely useful with young children, they are sometimes limited in their effectiveness by the maturational development of the child. This point is very significant in relation to mentally handicapped subjects some of whom may never reach the cognitive level required to co-operate with masking procedures. This can, therefore, limit our information on both type and degree of loss and therefore highlights the need for 'objective' measures in the overall test battery. Although there is agreement among larger sample studies as to the incidence of hearing impairment in the mentally handicapped population, some writers have questioned such findings and have suggested that pure-tone audiometry is not a reliable and valid estimate of the retardate's auditory acuity (see Lloyd 1970). A variety of tests in addition to those already described, e.g. speech testing, electroacoustic impedance bridge measurements, reflex measurements and electric response measures, may therefore be applied.

Speech Tests of Hearing

Appropriate speech tests prove useful in assessing the likely hearing difficulty that subjects experience at normal conversational voice level while providing a further measure of the reliability of the hearing test. Examples of commonly used speech tests include:

Closed-circuit Speech Test (taped AB)

In this test the patient is presented via headphones with taped lists of monosyllabic words (Boothroyd 1968). The intensity level of the words is set by the tester and the patient is requested to repeat each word of the list of ten words as they are presented. The patient's response is scored phonemically and a measure of discrimination score as a function of intensity is obtained for each ear. This test is normally applied to children from the age of seven years and will therefore be beyond the capabilities of many mentally handicapped subjects. As it requires a verbal response, it is not suitable for subjects with poor speech production. A simpler test which does not require a verbal response is the Manchester Picture Test, devised by Thomas Watson and standardised by Fraser (1971).

The Manchester Picture Test

The Manchester Picture Test comprises eight sets of 10 picture cards. Each card contains pictures of four objects, and the child is asked to point to one specified object on each card. This test may be applied to children from the age of approximately four years. It is designed to test a child's ability to discriminate specific vowel and consonant sounds of speech. Each set of 10 cards tests the child's ability to hear five specific vowel sounds and five spe-cific consonant sounds. If, for example, the vowel sound to be tested is 'e', as in the word well, the test card will contain pictures of a ball, a wall, a doll and a well. The child would have to hear 'e' in order to identify the well, because this vowel sound occurs only in this picture on the card.

If the consonant sound being tested is 'd', as in dish, the test card will contain pictures of a tin, a pin, a dish and a fish. Here again only the test word contains the required 'd' consonant sound. Hence the child would have to hear 'd' in order to identify the dish.

The tester will apply the test for certain fixed voice levels (measured on a sound level indicator), and monitor the child's performance with change in voice level. If voice level has to be raised to a high level before the child scores accurately on the test, the results will support a diagnosis of hearing impairment. An even simpler test, again not requiring a verbal response from the subject, is the Kendall Toy Test (Kendall 1957).

Modified Kendall Toy Test (KT)

In this test a selection of toy items which should be familiar to most three-year-old normally hearing children is used. The test is not used in its original form (Kendall 1957) as a screening procedure, but rather as a modified form of speech audiometry. The aim of the test is to have the subject point to the items named by the tester. The subject is not required to name the items, but simply to give evidence of recognizing the names by pointing to the toys. The toy items are grouped according to the vowel sounds, because subjects with hearing losses frequently confuse words such as 'cup' and 'duck', hearing only the low-frequency vowel. The subject is scored on the number of items identified correctly, and the voice level at which words are presented is measured by means of a sound level meter. It is therefore possible to measure the voice level at which accurate responses are consistently recorded. Further details of this test are given in Nolan, Tucker, McArthur and Fulbeck (1979).

Electroacoustic Impedance Bridge Measures

A major advance in recent years in respect of identifying or confirming the site of the hearing problem, has been the widespread use of the electro-acoustic impedance bridge. This machine provides the clinician with much valuable information on whether a subject has a conductive component in the hearing loss. The machine tells the clinician whether the middle ear is functioning normally. The measurements made are objective (the test only requires the passive co-operation of the patient) and are very easy for the clinician to interpret in terms of normality or abnormality.

The machine consists of a probe unit with a small rubber tip attached to its end. This tip is placed in the subject's ear canal such that an airtight seal is produced. The probe unit comprises three tubes. One of the tubes is connected to a 'sound generator' and a low-frequency tone is fed down the tube towards the ear drum. The second tube is connected to a tiny microphone. This microphone is able to measure the amount of sound being reflected from the ear drum. The third tube is connected to a pump and therefore enables the clinician to apply small amounts of pressure on to the outer side of the ear drum. Thus the clinician can vary the stiffness of the drum by varying the air pressure.

In a normal ear sound travels down the ear canal, passes through the ear drum and is conveyed across the air-filled middle-ear cavity by the ossicular chain to the nerve of hearing. (This is the conductive mechanism of the auditory system.) Very little sound is reflected in such cases from the ear drum, because it is flexible and relaxed and therefore able to transmit sound extremely well.

If a problem exists anywhere along the conductive mechanism such that the ear drum becomes stiffer than normal, the result will be that more sound will be reflected than happens normally. Hence, less sound will cross to the nerve of hearing and a hearing loss results.

The electroacoustic impedance bridge is able to measure how much sound is reflected from the drum and therefore how efficient the middle-ear mechanism is at passing sound to the nerve of hearing. With this information the clinician can decide whether or not a conductive loss is present.

The measurement of middle-ear function by means of the electro-acoustic impedance bridge is a quick and easy test to perform. It may be carried out on children of all ages and, as already suggested, requires no co-operation from the child other than that he sits reasonably still. In the clinics in our department the test is used routinely on children from a few months old and few children object so violently that the test cannot be carried out. No discomfort is caused but occasionally the child will object to anything being put in the ear. It will be useful to consider how the impedance bridge test is carried out and what information is recorded.

Children would normally be seated on the parent's knee. The child's ear is examined to check that the entry to the ear canal is not full of wax which can block up the probe. A suitable sized probe tip will be selected and pushed on to the end of the probe unit. This unit is often incorporated into a headset. If so, this is positioned over the top of the child's head. The probe is carefully placed in the ear canal and a check is made that an air-tight seal has been obtained. The clinician will then perform the test, the results being recorded on an automatic chart recorder.

The machine measures the amount of sound reflected back from the eardrum when the drum is subjected to differing amounts of pressure. This is achieved by use of the three tubes incorporated into the probe that we described earlier. The shape of the pattern recorded on the chart recorder indicates to the clinician where, if any, a problem exists in the conducting mechanism.

There are various patterns produced. One is consistent with a normal conductive mechanism while other patterns are associated with known disorders. See Figure 11.2.

Once this information has been obtained the clinician will consider it along with information from the other test procedures, particularly those which relate to the extent of the loss. This is so since the most severe conductive loss can only be approximately 60dBHL so, if the patient has abnormal impedance but a very severe loss, say 90dBHL, then some element of the loss must be sensori-neural. Without pure-tone air- and bone-conduction audiometric results the extent of the sensori-neural and conductive components of the loss will not be clear. However, if information on the overall severity of loss is available, it would be likely that the clinician would decide that an Ear, Nose and Throat (ENT) investigation was urgently necessary, that the subject should have a hearing aid and that, following any ENT medical or surgical treatment, the hearing levels would be reviewed and modifications to amplification made resultant upon any improvement in the middle-ear component of the hearing loss. The point regarding the fitting of hearing aids, where a significant hearing loss exists, is very pertinent in relation to mentally handicapped subjects. It has been suggested that there is a feeling among certain clinicians that retarded children do not benefit from wearing hearing aids (Davies and Penniceard 1980). It is our experience that many mentally handicapped

Figure 11.2: Normal and Abnormal Patterns of Middle-ear Function Measured Using the Impedance Bridge

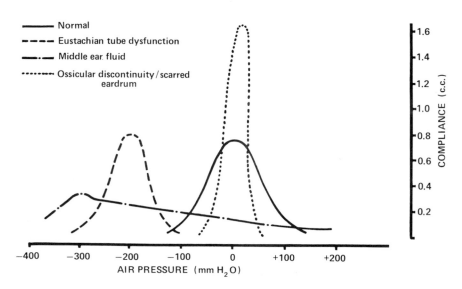

subjects who are given the opportunity of using hearing aids use them very successfully. This view is supported by the work of Balkany, Downs, Jafek and Kragicek (1979).

The Stapedial (or Acoustic) Reflex

The middle ear includes two muscles — the tensor tympani and the stapedius. The latter is considered as responding to sound stimulation, contraction occurring at levels of 70-90dB above threshold in normals (Anderson, Barr and Wedenberg 1970; Liden 1970; Borg 1972; Chiveralls and Fitzsimons 1973). The muscle is attached to the posterior crus of the stapes and is innervated by the VIIth cranial nerve (facial nerve). The reflex contraction occurs bilaterally and produces an increase in the stiffness of the middle ear. These changes are measured on the electroacoustic impedance bridge.

It is possible for the acoustic reflex to be obscured from detection. It has been found that it may be absent in many conductive disorders as well as in various types of sensori-neural loss. In fact the reflex is unlikely to be observed in an ear with anything but the slightest conductive lesion apart from some cases of ossicular discontinuity (Chiveralls, Fitzsimons, Beck and Kernohan 1976). Even normally hearing subjects can show an absence of the reflex — it has been suggested that this may be as high as 10 per cent. It is unlikely that the reflex will be observed in the neonatal period by means of a conventional impedance bridge. A probe tone of 800Hz or higher is needed to indicate its presence in such cases (Wetherby and Bennett 1979).

It has been suggested that the reflex could be used as an estimate of hearing level. Various approaches to predicting an audiogram from reflex thresholds to pure tones and noise have been put forward (Popelka 1981). Such methods tend to be prone to inaccuracy and, while a recent method based on single frequencies seems to be more accurate, it does appear to be impractical for general clinical application (Sesterhenn and Brueninger 1977).

Stapedial reflex testing with mentally handicapped subjects can prove to be very difficult. Whereas it is possible to obtain tympanometric information on a crying or restless subject, it is not so easy to observe reflex contraction in such cases. A considerable amount of time, effort, patience and skill in handling such subjects will be needed if the measure is to be successful.

The presence or absence of the reflex is not indicative of anything when taken in isolation. However, when put together with other diagnostic findings, it can prove to be useful. In particular, it can help to identify and pinpoint the location of an ossicular disruption. It can be taken as a very strong indicator, when present, of normal middle-ear function (with the exception noted earlier). It can help to draw attention to a hearing-impaired subject who may have loudness tolerance problems. This is particularly important when standard 'upper limits of tolerance' tests are difficult to apply.

Other Objective Measures

Another group of tests which may be loosely described as 'objective' has evolved and is continuing to be developed. Many of these tests are intended as a means of identifying children as 'at risk' with regards hearing very early on in life (neonatal period). These tests are not as widely practised or (for certain tests) as practical to use for mass screening. However, the most recently developed computer-based 'crib' approaches which are still undergoing validity trials may find more general application as part of an ongoing audiological screening programme. None of the tests in this category can be considered truly objective because of the subjectivity in test design and in the interpretation of the test results. Furthermore, subjectivity on the part of the baby also plays a significant role. This is particularly relevant to handicapped babies. It has been found that there is a much higher false positive detection rate for deafness in sick new-borns than in 'well' babies when physiological reactions to sound are used as the identifying medium (Blair-Simmons, McFarland and Jones 1979).

Neonatal Screening (Objective Tests)

Testing the baby at birth might be regarded as the optimal situation, since the great majority of babies are born in maternity wards and are thus captives there for at least two or three days following birth.

The cluster of physiological responses provoked in a new-born baby (neonate) by a sudden sound involves changes in heart beat rate, respiration rate, head movement, body activity, muscle tone, head jerk and eye blink. These responses have been advocated for use as a means of screening hearing in new-borns.

Before the development of microprocessors the tests were administered by one or two clinicians. One clinician, the operator, administered the test stimulus (usually a relatively loud 90dB SPL sound) while the other acted as observer and noted the baby's response (eye blink, limb movement, etc.) to the stimulus (Redell and Calvert 1969).

Test Pitfalls

It is relatively simple to get inter-observer agreement on what is considered to be a response to sound. Unfortunately, the baby has all the possible patterns in its natural behaviour. The basic problem is distinguishing genuine from spontaneous responses. Furthermore, testing time required of personnel may be long and impractical in a busy hospital nursery. Clearly, trained personnel are required to apply such tests and as a result the efficiency of the test will depend on the skills of the observers. Obviously, additional handicaps make the business of test interpretation more difficult.

Recent developments of this principle have allowed automated recording of motor responses in babies.

Microprocessor-based Systems

It has proven possible to replace the operator and observer in neonatal testing by microprocessor-based auditory cradles or cribs. These devices seek to screen hearing on the basis of physiological reactions to sound in much the same way as the 'clinician'-applied test. The most appropriate time to apply this type of test is about three to four days of age.

The Crib-o-gram.   The Crib-o-gram system employs a motion-detecting transducer attached to each crib or cot. The baby is stimulated by bursts of 92dB SPL narrow band (2-4kHz) noise and a microprocessor-based decision analysis system assesses motor activity from the highly sensitive motion detector in response to a series of 30 stimulus trials. Testing time is quoted as averaging $2^{1}/_{2}$ hours but interruptions are permissible without affecting the screening process. The signal is delivered by a loudspeaker situated at the end of the child's cot (Blair-Simmons *et al.* 1979).

Auditory Response Cradle.   The Auditory Response Cradle (ARC) is a microprocessor-controlled system which seeks to examine a baby's head turn, startle or headjerk, body activity and respiratory signals in response to sound stimulation. The system is automatic and takes three to ten minutes to complete a screen. The baby lies in the cradle which incorporates the non-contacting head turn, startle, body activity and respiratory sensors. Ear probes are used to deliver the test sound — a high pass broad band noise at 85dB SPL acts as test stimulus (Bennett 1979).

High pass noise is considered optimal for screening purposes because the vast majority of congenital deafness involves high frequencies.

Early results from ongoing validity trials of these systems with 'well' babies are encouraging (Bennett and Wade 1980; McFarland, Blair-Simmons and Jones 1980; Telesensory Systems Inc. 1982). Many clinicians, however, have reservations as to the usefulness and reliability of such measures when applied to handicapped new-borns.

It is important to remember that all of the neonatal tests described are screening tests. There is no quantification of hearing capacity nor determination of the site of the problem if one exists. Furthermore, for a variety of reasons, there will be some degree of false negativeness in such testing, i.e. hearing-impaired babies passing the test criteria — perhaps because of a very moderate degree of hearing loss or the phenomenon of recruitment (abnormal growth in loudness) with a more severe hearing loss, which enabled the babies to exhibit 'normal' responses to sound stimulation. As a matter of interest, the minimal hearing loss detected by the Crib-o-gram is reported as 45dB HL (McFarland *et al.* 1980). There will, as mentioned earlier, be some degree of false positiveness, whereby normally hearing babies will fail the test criteria. This will be a function of the baby's condition at birth and may rise to 20 per cent in 'sick' newborns. This is of particular relevance to the mentally handicapped population. While microprocessor-based tests in particular have potential for identifying hearing impairment early in the life of some children, they will only prove effective if, and in many cases when, the subsequent follow up *diagnostic* programme is efficiently organized and appropriately staffed.

Reflex Responses

A very commonly observed reflex response to sound is the auropalpebral reflex (APR) or eye blink response. This reflex was first noted by Wedenberg (1956) after tests on 20 children aged one to ten days. All normally hearing children in his sample exhibited the reflex in the frequency range 500-4000Hz to pure tones of 105-115dB SPL.

The auropalpebral reflex (APR) shows similarity with the stapedius reflex threshold and anatomically there are similarities between the two. The afferent part (n. acusticus) and the efferent part (n. facialis) of the reflex arc are common to both, though the reflex centre of the stapedius is at a lower level of the brain stem (Pons) than the APR (Formatio Reticularis). More recently a very large investigation by Froding (1960) on 2,000 subjects all under the age of 30 minutes showed the APR to be a reliable response. Those who consistently failed to exhibit the APR were found to be neurologically impaired.

In view of the fact that eye blinks occur frequently anyway, it might be thought that clinically it would be difficult to distinguish random from stimulus-based responses. In fact, it has been suggested that spontaneous 'responses' giving a false positive can occur in up to 20 per cent of tests and there is a high rate of false negatives necessitating repeated testing (Bench and Boscak 1970). Despite this many centres do make use of this reflex. Such centres use at least two clinicians to observe the subjects response either to a voiced plosive-vowel 'ba' signal or to intense sound from a signal generator. The subject (who could be a mentally handicapped adult) is usually in a relaxed state when the signal is delivered at a fixed screening level of, for example, 90dBA for plosive vowel 'ba'. Such a test is, therefore, relatively easy to apply with mentally handicapped subjects and very useful.

Electric Response Audiometry (ERA)

Electric response audiometry is a term that is used to encompass a collection of testing procedures that involve the recording of tiny electrical responses (potentials) that occur along the auditory pathway in response to acoustic stimulation (Gibson 1978). There are, in fact, many different responses and each is classified according to the 'time after the stimulus' at which it occurs. This parameter is known as the latency. While many of these tests are particularly applicable to adults for identification of neurological disorders and objective measurement of hearing, some have been advocated for use in screening and diagnosis of hearing impairment in children. They, therefore, have relevance in testing hearing of the mentally handicapped.

Such testing warrants the use of relatively sophisticated and expensive equipment operated by specially trained technicians. As a result it is not normally available for routine screening and is more usually found in specialist audiology centres where it may be employed in diagnostic procedures following screening failure or in assessing difficult-to-test children.

There are four widely used tests (Gibson 1978), that involve the recording of tiny electrical potentials that occur in the auditory system in response to sound stimulation:

1. electrocochleography (E.Co.G; E.Coch.G);
2. brain-stem electric response audiometry (BSER);
3. post-auricular myogenic response (PAM);
4. slow vertex cortical potential.

Electrocochleography

E.Co.G. is an invasive procedure — a needle electrode normally being placed through the eardrum on to the promontory of the cochlea. This means that the subject will require a general anaesthetic for the measure to be made. Very short sharp sounds (clicks) are used to elicit the response which are usually detected by an averaging computer to within 15dB of subjective threshold. The test involves the recording of electrical activity within the cochlea and auditory nerve close to the cochlea. Information is only provided on the subject's hearing for high frequencies (greater than 2kHz). It will be clear that damage more central than the cochlea will not be detected by this test. Three electrodes are used to recover the characteristic waveform of the E.Co.G. This involves, in addition to the needle electrode (the active electrode), two surface electrodes — earth on forehead, reference on ear lobe — which are attached to the subject.

As this response is not influenced by anaesthesia, it is possible to apply it with the mentally handicapped 'difficult-to-test' subjects who can undergo a general anaesthetic. Normally this would have to be done in a General Hospital. It is, therefore, not particularly practical for mass application. A more appropriate test practically speaking for many such subjects is the brain-stem evoked response audiometry.

Brain-stem Evoked Response Audiometry (BSER)

The BSER response test involves recording from the scalp of tiny electrical potentials that are generated in the cochlear nerve and the auditory pathway up to the inferior colliculus in response to sound stimulation. In order to 'recover' the potentials from the ongoing random noise of the brain, it is necessary to deliver a large number of sound impulses in a relatively short time period. Clicks are therefore used to elicit the response. The potentials are recovered by three electrodes, placed on forehead (earth), vertex and behind each ear on the mastoid process. It is, therefore, a non-invasive procedure. The information from the electrodes is processed by an averaging computer and the response appears on a visual display as a char-acteristic multi-wave complex. The test is applied with the subject sitting on a sun lounger-type chair on mother's knee or more appropriately with young babies, during natural sleep — the subject *must* be quiet and relaxed. The signal is presented via a circumaural headphone held against the ear. The response is not affected by natural sleep or sedation (Sohmer, Gafni and Chisin 1978) and is therefore particularly appropriate for many 'diffi-cult-to-test' mentally handicapped subjects. The information on hearing is limited to the high frequencies.

Attention has been drawn to a relatively small group of children in the 'difficult-to-test' category who produced discrepancies between BSER and impedance thresholds (Mokotoff, Schulmann and Galambos 1977) or BSER and E.Co.G. measures (Ryerson and Beagley 1981). Both studies recommended a thorough assessment of these children using other objective measures before firm conclusions were made about hearing levels. This is one reason why BSER information must be considered together with other information of the diagnostic investigation before any firm conclusions are drawn. The main limitation as regards management on the basis of BSER information relates to the fact that the test only provides threshold information for higher speech frequencies. Information on which to base a hearing-aid prescription will therefore be very limited.

Research has shown that the BSER in young babies differs from normal adult response (Mecox and Galambos 1974). The amplitude of the response is smaller, the wave complex is less well defined with only two or perhaps three waves, instead of the full five-wave complex being present, and the waveforms occur slightly later in time. The response is present at 26 weeks gestation and then undergoes maturation process so that by about 18 months of age the normal adult latencies are present. Application of the test and in particular interpretation of test results requires the experience and expertise of specially trained staff.

The Post Auricular Myogenic Response (PAM)

This response is a reflex response to sound of the muscle behind the pinna (Kiang, Christ, French and Edwards 1964). It is characterized as having a latency of about 15msecs and a large amplitude.

As with all electric response audiometry measures, measurement is facilitated by placement of three tiny electrodes, in this case one on the forehead, one on the scalp and one behind the ear on the mastoid bone.

These electrodes sense the tiny electrical signals from the muscle in response to sound stimulation and a computer sorts and averages the results.

This is not generally considered as a sufficiently sensitive measure for diagnostic purposes; however, in light of the recent development of a portable screening instrument based on the PAM response (Flood, Fraser, Conway and Stewart 1982) it may have some value in helping to identify subjects requiring more detailed audiological investigations.

Testing, using this instrument, may be carried out in any room with low background noise. The test is non-invasive, placement of the three electrodes on the head being the only contact with the subject. The subject is seated on a chair or on the mother's knee and the sound (clicks) is delivered from a loudspeaker built into the test unit. Testing time is approximately ten minutes.

The PAM response is myogenic and, because of this, it is necessary for the subject to have a high degree of muscle tone. This is why the optimal test position is upright on a hard chair or mother's knee. It may often prove possible to test restless subjects because the muscle tone will be achieved fairly easily.

The main drawbacks of this approach relate to the variability in PAM response as a function of neck muscle tension. It can prove difficult to obtain even in subjects who have been instructed to tense their neck muscles. Absence of response is not therefore necessarily abnormal. It is not possible to obtain the response in sleeping subjects. The response provides no information on the subject's cortical response to sound.

Cortical-evoked Response Audiometry

This measure, which is also known as ERA or the slow vertex response, is the response of the cortex to any form of sensory stimulation. It is the only one of the four tests for which pure tones may be employed as the stimulus. This test is not considered appropriate for use in assessing hearing in the mentally handicapped. It is a relatively long test in comparison to the other three tests. It requires the subject to be alert throughout and is very strongly influenced by arousal, attention to the sound stimulus and medication. This test was at one time the most commonly used electric response measure. However, with developments of other measures, particularly BSER and E.Co.G, it is now rarely used in diagnostic practice.

Decision-making

Once the diagnostic procedures have been completed, the clinician will consider the results of all the tests. If both the conventional hearing test and a speech test have been applied, for instance, the clinician will check for consistency. The impedance bridge measurements will aid in deciding on whether there are any conductive problems that should be dealt with before any sensori-neural ones are tackled. By this time the clinician should have a reasonably clear picture of both degree and nature of the loss. This information will be fundamental to the management programme.

If there is a conductive element in the hearing impairment, the first thing the clinician should do is arrange for an otologist to perform an ENT examination. Subjects must be reviewed routinely following ENT treatment so as to determine whether improvement in hearing has taken place.

In cases where sensori-neural problems are indicated, the clinician will probably inform the parents of the position, discuss the implications and arrange for immediate help from the support and guidance service. In cases of children this should involve educational services while adults should receive help from hearing therapists and audiological technicians. Ideally an interactive service of teachers and therapists for all age groups would be ideal. Although such arrangements are made (McCartney 1984), workload tends to make this very difficult and in some cases impractical. During the short interim period between the diagnostic session and the first follow-up appointment, the clinician will be organizing the hearing-aid prescription and earmould provision and will be briefing the guidance team, in particular the visiting teacher of the deaf or hearing therapist, about the subject.

The diagnostic tests should continue to be applied to a mentally handicapped subject as part of the management programme. This is crucial because more comprehensive information will be obtained as the subject matures. Such information can have a critical effect on factors such as hearing-aid prescription. Such prescription must therefore be very flexible and amenable to change — should change be indicated from information from the ongoing diagnostic tests.

Conclusion

The importance of applying routine checks on sensori-neural hearing-impaired subjects cannot be over-emphasized. It has been reported that the incidence of middle-ear effusion in the mentally handicapped population is very high (Brooks, Wooley and Kanjilal 1972; Davies and Penniceard 1980). Subjects with sensori-neural impairments simply cannot afford to be 'carrying' an overlying conductive problem. For this reason regular checks, perhaps as part of the management sessions, should be carried out.

The present authors believe that there are many cases where mentally handicapped subjects can be greatly helped by audiological support services and, if such people are to be aided to achieve their full potential, then they must be brought under the umbrella of these services. The expertise in assessment is available in major centres, though there is need for resource expansion in some parts of the country. There is also a clear need for more liaison between specialist educators of the deaf and those who provide the educational support for mentally handicapped subjects.

References

Anderson, H., Barr, B. and Wedenberg, E. (1970) 'The early detection of acoustic tumours by the Stapedial Reflex test' in G.E.W. Wolstenholme and J. Knight (eds.), *Sensori-neural hearing loss — Ciba Foundation Symposium*, J. and A. Churchill, Edinburgh

Balkany, T.J., Downs, M.P., Jafek, B.W. and Kragicek, M.J. (1979) 'Hearing Loss in Down's Syndrome. A treatable handicap more common than generally recognized', *Clinical Paediatrics (Phila)*, *18*, 116

Bench, R.J. and Boscak, N. (1970) 'Some Applications of Signal Detection Theory to Paedo-audiology', *Sound*, *4*, 693

Bennett, M.J. (1979) 'Trials with the Auditory Response Cradle, I: Neonatal responses to auditory stimulation', *British Journal of Audiology*, *13*, 125

—— and Wade, H.K. (1980) 'Automated newborn hearing screening using the auditory response cradle' in I.G. Taylor and A. Markides (eds.), *Disorders of Auditory Function III*, Academic Press, London

Blair Simmons, F., McFarland, W.H. and Jones F.R. (1979) 'An automated hearing screening technique for newborns', *Acta. Otolaryngol*, *87*, 1

Boothroyd, A. (1968) 'Developments in Speech Audiometry', *Sound*, *2*, 3

Borg, E. (1972) 'On the change in the acoustic impedance of the ear as a measure of middle ear muscle reflex activity', *Acta. Otolaryngology*, *74*, 163

Brasier, V.J. (1974) 'Pitfalls in audiometry', *Public Health, London*, *89*, 31

Brooks, D.N., Wooley, H. and Kanjilal, G.C. (1972) 'Hearing loss and middle-ear disorders in patients with Down's Syndrome', *Journal of Mental Deficiency Research*, *16*, 21

Chiveralls, K. and Fitzsimons, R. (1973) 'Stapedial reflex action in normal subjects', *British Journal of Audiology*, *7*, 105

——, Fitzsimons, R., Beck, G.B. and Kernohan, H. (1976) 'The diagnostic significance of the stapedial reflex', *British Journal of Audiology*, *10*, 122

Cunningham, C. and McArthur, K. (1981) 'Hearing loss and treatment in young Down's syndrome children', *Child: Care, Health and Development*, *7*, 357

Davies, B. and Penniceard, R.M. (1980) 'Auditory function and receptive vocabulary in Down's syndrome children' in I.G. Taylor and A. Markides (eds.), *Disorders of Auditory Function III*, Academic Press, London

Flood, L.M., Fraser, J.G., Conway, M.J., Stewart, A (1982) 'The assessment of hearing in Infancy using the post auricular myogenic response', *British Journal of Audiology*, *16*, 211

Fraser, J.C.L. (1971) 'Validation of the New Manchester Picture Test', Unpublished dissertation for the Diploma in Audiology, University of Manchester

Froding, C.A. (1960) 'Acoustic Investigation of Newborn Infants' *Acta. Otolaryngology* (Stockholm), *52*, 31

Gibson, W.P.R. (1978) *Essentials of Clinical Electric Response Audiometry*, Churchill Livingstone, Edinburgh

Kendall, D.C. (1957) 'Mental development of young children' in A.W.G. Ewing (ed.) *Educational Guidance and the Deaf Child*, Manchester University Press

Kiang, N.Y.S., Christ A.H., French, M.A. and Edwards A.G. (1964) *Quarterly Progress Report*, Laboratory of Electronics, Massachusetts Institute of Technology, *28*, 218

Liden, G. (1970), 'The Stapedius muscle reflex used as an objective recruitment test: A clinical and experimental study' in G.E.W. Wolstenholme and J. Knight (eds.), *CIBA Symposium on Sensori-neural Hearing Loss*, J. and A. Churchill, London

Lloyd, L.L. (1970) 'Audiologic Aspects of Mental Retardation' in N.R. Ellis (ed.), *International Review in Research in Mental Retardation*, Academic Press, London

McCartney, E. (1984) *Helping Adult Training Centre Students to Communicate*, British Institute of Mental Handicap, Kidderminster, England

McFarland, W.H., Blair Simmons, F. and Jones, F.R. (1980) 'An automated hearing screening technique for newborns', *Journal of Speech and Hearing Disorders*, *45*, 495

Mecox, K. and Galambos, P. (1974) 'Brainstem auditory evoked responses in human infants and adults', *Archives of Otolaryngology, 99,* 30

Mokotoff, B., Schulmann, C. and Galambos, R. (1977) 'Brain-stem auditory evoked responses in children', *Archives of Otolaryngology, 103,* 38

National Development Group for the Mentally Handicapped (1978) *Helping Mentally Handicapped People in Hospital,* DHSS, London

Nolan, M., McCartney, E., McArthur, K. and Rowson, V.J. (1980) 'A Study of the Hearing and Receptive Vocabulary of the Trainees of an Adult Training Centre', *Journal of Mental Deficiency Research, 24,* 271

—— Tucker, I.G. McArthur, K. and Fulbeck, C. (1979) *Testing the Hearing of Young Children,* National Deaf Childrens' Society, London

—— and —— (1981) *The Hearing Impaired Child and the Family,* Human Horizon Series, Souvenir Press, London

Popelka, G.R. (1981) *Hearing Assessment with the Acoustic Reflex,* Grune and Stratton, New York

Redell, R.C. and Calvert, D.R. (1969) 'Factors in Screening Hearing of the Newborn', *The Journal of Auditory Research, 3,* 278

Ryerson, S.G. and Beagley, H.A. (1981) 'Brainstem Electric Responses and Electro-cochleography: a comparison of threshold sensitivities in children', *British Journal of Audiology, 15,* 41

Sohmer, H., Gafni, M. and Chisin, R. (1978) 'Auditory nerve and brain-stem responses: comparison in awake and unconscious subjects (normals)', *Arch. Neurology, 35,* 228

Sesterhenn, G. and Brueninger, H. (1977) 'Determination of hearing threshold for single frequencies from the acoustic reflex', *Audiology, 13*(3), 201

Taylor, I.G. (1964) *Neurological Mechanisms of Hearing and Speech in Children,* Manchester University Press

Telesensory Systems Inc. (1982) *Crib-o-gram Validation Study. A Summary of Results,* Telesen Palo Alto, California

Tempowski, I., Felstead, H. and Simon, G.B. (1974) 'Deafness and the Mentally Retarded', *Apex, 2*(2), 4

Tucker, I.G. and Nolan, M. (1984) *Educational Audiology,* Croom Helm, London

Wedenberg, E. (1956) 'Auditory tests on newborn infants', *Acta Otolaryngology* (Stockholm), *46,* 446

Wetherby, L.A. and Bennett, M.J. (1979) 'The neonatal acoustic reflex', *Scand. Audiology, 8*(4), 233

Whelan, E. and Speake, B. (1977) *Adult training centres in England and Wales. Report of the First National Survey, Manchester,* Hester Adrian Research Centre, NATMH, University of Manchester

12 COLOUR-VISION TESTS FOR MENTALLY HANDICAPPED PEOPLE

Robert J. Fletcher

Reasons For Testing

Among the population of the United Kingdom some 8 per cent of men and rather less than 1 per cent of women have imperfect colour vision. The popular term 'colour blindness' hardly does justice to the variety of conditions which occur; confusions of colour are experienced (usually between olive and beige colours). It is well known that red and green can be confused by such people but this is likely only in the more severe cases. There are distinct types of colour vision deficiency, as summarized in Table 12.1, and within the two common types there are subdivisions of severity. The *protanope* (sometimes described as 'red blind') has reduced sensitivity to red lights such as stop or warning lights in transport and is liable to dangerous errors. However, the most prevalent form of defect is *deuteranomaly,* a non-extreme condition where green perception is diminished and where orange may be confused with green or certain colours may appear colourless.

Table 12.1: Main Types of Colour-vision Defect

Type	Subtype	Per cent in Britain		Confusion colour for grey	Specific colours confused
		Male	Female		
Red perception deficiency	protanopia	1	0.02	red or blue–green	brown & red orange & green blue & purple
	protanomaly	1.5	0.03	pale red or pale blue–green	yellow & orange also pale colours as for protanopia
Green-perception deficiency	deuteranopia	1	0.01	reddish-purple or some greens	green & tan olive & beige brown & red
	deuteranomaly	5	0.4	pale colours as for deuteranopia	pale versions of deuteranopia confusions
Blue-perception deficiency	tritanopia	very small	very small	violet or yellow	green & blue
	tritanomaly	very small	very small	pale colours as for tritanopia	pale versions of tritanopia confusions
	most of the acquired defects	?	?	as for tritanopia	as for tritanopia
Total colour deficiency	achromats of several types	very small	very small	all	all if equally bright

Almost half of these people suffering from colour-perception deficiency (known as 'Daltonism' in the romantic languages) are able to manage everyday colour discrimination. Under favourable circumstances they do not show their deficiency, but when colours are pale, 'desaturated' (mixed with white) or when the coloured objects are small, they may make distinctive errors. Therefore, those colour-vision tests which are difficult to pass (such as the very common Ishihara book of coloured dots arranged as symbols) and which operate on a 'go — no go' basis, tend to fail subjects even if they are only mildly defective and even if they have few practical difficulties.

The Inherited Deficiencies

A sex-linked recessive mode of X-chromosomal inheritance accounts for most of the cases, that is the *protan* and *deutan* types. Sometimes colour-vision defects can be used as markers in a genetic study, such as may be indicated when another sex-linked condition is suspected in a family (see Kalmus 1965).

Figure 12.1 illustrates an imaginary family tree in which five groups of siblings appear. Those in families A and E are all normal with respect to their colour vision. Family B was started by the (unlikely) combination of a Daltonic male and a carrier with the same sort of 'abnormal' genes; their two daughters are shown as one carrier and one Daltonic. Family B could have comprised all normal sons but the daughters would have to be either carriers or Daltonic. In the siblings at C two carriers appear, family E is as unaffected as family A but the trait appears in one of the sons of family D and could be transmitted by one of the daughters, who happens to have become a carrier by receiving her mother's affected X chromosomes.

Clinical workers interested in genetic 'peculiarities' associated with 'colour blindness' will find useful descriptions and references in Walls's (1959) paper dealing with irregular colour deficiency in unusual subjects. He proposed that the incidence of Daltonism in 'intersex' conditions should be expected to equal that in normal people with the same number of X chromosomes. Irregular colour defects (not those expected in males, from the same genes) in 'female' patients can be related to heterozygotes (XX) or to hemizygotes (XO or XY). Daltonism has been used for study of some chromatin negative Turner's syndrome cases, perhaps suggesting fathers whose sperms lacked a sex-chromosome element.

Börjeson's syndrome and more common types of institutionalized mental conditions are X-linked (McKusick 1962). This experienced geneticist pointed out the advantages of establishing the actual *types* of colour-vision defects, that is whether *deutan* or *protan* and, possibly, the extent as far as differentiating between dichromats and anomalous trichromats. Such details can be used for X-linkage studies. He showed

Figure 12.1: Examples of Inheritance Patterns Resulting in Colour–Vision Deficiencies

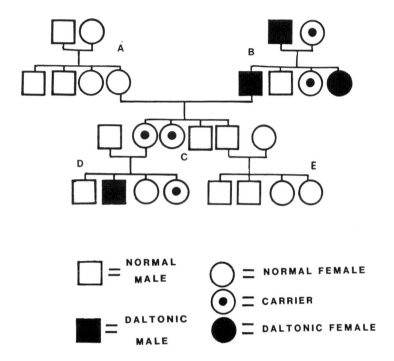

how testicular feminization may be independent of the appearance of 'colour blindness'; see also Walls (1959).

Acquired Defects

Acquired defects of colour vision have become well documented since the beginning of the century. In some cases they appear as unwanted effects of medication, usually as disturbances of 'blue–green' differentiation or as what are commonly called *tritan* (blue–yellow) deficiencies. Some diseases disturb colour vision, often as an early symptom, and there is the possibility of inherited bodily conditions being related to one or more varieties of abnormal colour vision. Consequently colour-vision testing offers an opportunity to estimate the progress or regress of a malady or the effect of a prescribed drug on a vulnerable part of the nervous system. The chloroquine and quinine types of drugs, some anti-epileptic agents, some sedatives and hypnotic preparations may sometimes cause colour-vision defects. Largactil, a tranquillizer (or hypnotic), and Melleril, another tranquillizer, related to Chlorpromazine, have been considered to have effects on colour vision.

Damage to optic nerve fibres is one source of the trouble, for example in the long-term use of anti-tuberculosis, cardiac and anti-inflammatory drugs; to a lesser extent anti-depressants such as hydrazines or analgesics can do this. It is important to test each eye separately, a fact which tends to be overlooked, since one eye is usually affected more.

Ethambutol disrupts function of intermediate retinal neurones, where colour coding normally takes place. Vitamin-A deficiency or liver disease, diabetes and several other conditions are likely to disturb blue-yellow perception by damage to the cone receptors, which rely on different opsins for their functions. Various colour-vision disorders can be found among alcoholics; methyl and ethyl alcohol tend to poison the conducting paths used in colour vision so both red–green and tritan tests may help in detecting relatively early conditions. There is evidence that alcoholic cirrhosis lowers the rate of replacement of retinal pigments (Cruz-Coke 1972).

For detailed descriptions papers by Francois and Verriest (1961), and by Pinckers (1976) can be consulted; these and a monograph by Voke (1980) describe specialized test methods.

Mentally Retarded People and Colour Vision

A normal child can be expected to show characteristic development of colour perception, starting with real preferences for some hues at about one year. Early colour vision is now known to be considerably better than was believed to be the case some decades ago, just as the perception of form is now known to be almost 100 per cent by an age of one year (Bornstein, Keffea and Weiskopf 1976; Chase 1937). Colour perception, the learning of colour terms and the ability to express these tend to reflect education and experience so that a peak of skill in this field is reached about age 20. After this a decline in physiological function (offset to some extent by further experience) reduces ability with colours. This decline is attributable to changes in the crystalline lens, in the retina and in perceptual processes. Since multiple handicap is common, it may be assumed that people with mental handicap are more likely than usual to have abnormal colour vision.

Archer (1964) and Krause (1967) did suggest prevalences of 30.9 and 22.3 per cent for such males, with 26.1 and 21.5 per cent respectively for females. We must take into account the types of tests used and the modes of their administration. Kratter (1957) gave a figure of 10 per cent for 'feeble-minded' male adults and O'Connor (1957) reported a prevalence of 13 per cent. A test using symbols (the HRR plates, now out of print) enabled Courtney and Heath (1971) to examine the colour vision of about 200 retarded or 'disturbed' children; they found between 4.3 and 9.7 per cent of the males to be colour deficient and this figure has distinct credibility.

Patients with multiple handicaps should experience progressive improvement of quality of life as each difficulty is identified and as alleviation is attempted. The 'mental patient' who responds to visual correction by spectacles is well recognized, as are some difficulties in maintaining the correction. So it is with hearing. Likewise 'being stupid about colour' may be the manifestation of a benign condition rather than an intellectual shortcoming.

Test Methods

Two approaches must be differentiated. Screening for the identification of any colour defect is not the same as a careful detailed examination; the latter should identify both the type and extent of the deficiency. Common screening methods (such as the use of Ishihara plates) have advantages, particularly if further examination of 'positives' is done. There are disadvantages, such as the restriction of detection to red-green disorders and the likely grouping of all grades of defect into a single 'fail' category.

There is considerable choice of colour-vision tests, but seldom will any two of these test the same thing in the same way. Conceptual, skill and mechanical factors vary between tests and the application of most to subjects with mental handicap is questionable, hence the different estimates of incidence of defects reported above. Salvia and Ysseldyke (1972) used five tests, of different types, with 90 boys each with some mental handicap. Their results ranged from 11 per cent failure to 40 per cent, according to the test. Using HRR plates Salvia and Ysseldyke (1972) had already found similar difficulties and the reasonable conclusion is that the tests presented problems in application. Alexander (1975) looked at the range of tests likely to be used for normal young children and suggested that in most there were cognitive demands which rendered the test unsuitable. Tests developed for children have often failed on this score or on account of bad choice of colours. Even tracing the pathways or identification or orientation of 'E' used in some 'pseudoisochromatic' tests presents difficulty and with children and the mentally retarded adult the question of soiling or destruction of delicate printed material arises. It might be thought that simple colour-matching tests can be home made but the complexity of controlling the colours is beyond this sort of approach. Lanterns and colour-mixture instruments such as anomaloscopes have specialized use in colour-vision investigation but these are not recommended for subjects likely to have difficulty in comprehension and co-operation.

Specific Tests in Mental Handicap

In order to evaluate the relative merits of different tests of colour vision in mental hospital residents, a small sample of 60 residents was used at a long-stay institution for mentally handicapped people (Leybourne Grange, Kent). The patients assessed included several with Down's syndrome, while some cases of epilepsy, 'primary amentia' and depression were included. The study made 146 separate attempts to administer different tests, drawing upon a range of tests as appeared most suitable in each situation. Only five complete failures were experienced as a result of complete lack of co-operation. This shows the advantage of having alternatives available.

About a third of the residents produced at least one result which was either unacceptable or unintelligible with at least one of the tests; no definite pattern of reasons is clear. Ten residents could not be tested using numeral-based plates of the 'pseudoisochromatic' type (e.g. Ishihara) and seven did not respond to the fact that three wooden blocks shown included two red and one green. Results otherwise were as follows:

PIC tests: 21 of 38 attempts were at least 'acceptable';
CUT test: 8 of 9 attempts were at least 'acceptable'.
(These attempts were limited to residents unlikely to spoil the paper surfaces.)

SCVT-type mosaics: 32 of 49 attempts were acceptable;
SCVT-type 'matches': 8 of 9 attempts were acceptable.
(These attempts were usually good rather than merely acceptable.)

These experiences support the general view that more than one mode of testing is best, even for routine screening. If a careful choice of items is made, so that a minimum of testing elements is involved, it is possible to test a co-operative subject in as little as four minutes; see Fletcher (1981b).

Personal experience and preference (also long traditions!) tend to dictate which tests are used, or not used. The literature offers guidance sometimes too simplified and sometimes full of complexities. The book by Kalmus (1965) is a good example, but useful up to a point, and most more recent texts are anything but concise. Papers by Taylor (1975) and Voke (1980) will be found to be helpful. A textbook to be published in 1985 is intended to be used by a variety of readers needing the theory and practice of colour blindness presented in sections (Fletcher and Voke 1985).

Conventional tests must really only be used in good daylight or (better still) with controlled artificial light. Most light sources, including most fluorescent tubes, do not give suitable colour rendering and introduce spurious results (see Fletcher 1981a). For example, Ishihara plates are easier to pass if unfiltered tungsten light is used. The present writer prefers an ordinary slide projector, adapted by placing a small piece of Chances OB 8 glass (about 2.5 mm thick) over the projection lens. The light is then deflected by a small (handbag-type) mirror on to the test plates. In this system the projector is mounted about 40 cm above the table top on a box.

Methods To Be Chosen

Thought must be given to the choice of a good test battery. Even subjects with no mental handicap often give conflicting results if two tests are given, thus three or four should be available. Repeating one test can give another result. It is essential to use at least parts of several tests so that a consensus can be interpreted and this actually simplifies the decisions in most cases.

Fletcher (1979, 1980a, 1982) introduced 'childproof' tests comprising mosaics of selected coloured plastics, dominoes and other modes of presentation. To use the fact that one approach is often better than another for an individual, two concepts were involved. These were (1) similarity of colours and (2) detection of colour differences. Some of these are made by Hamblin Instruments, London (Fletcher 1984). This Simplified Colour Vision Test (SCVT) has been designed for use with unfiltered light from an ordinary 100 Watt bulb. It has two 'units' for the detection of most 'red–green' deficiencies and one for 'blue' defects, the last one mentioned using relatively subtle colours. While the 'red–green' errors which are revealed are most likely to be made by those with fairly marked or extreme conditions, in some cases very slight degrees of anomaly can be shown up. Two of the 'units' are each made up of 16 small coloured squares in which there are some obvious colour contrasts (i.e. seen by all) and some confusion colours which are missed by the Daltonic. The third 'unit' requires a choice of an approximate colour match for a 'model' isolated coloured square, the choice being made from four other squares; two of these are actually confusion colours, while one is the most obvious choice for normals (Figures 12.2, 12.3 and 12.4 illustrate this test).

The City University Test (Keeler Instruments, London) can be used in many cases. It comprises a series of page-sized plates each showing four spots of colour arranged around a fifth coloured spot (see Figure 12.5). One of the four has to be chosen as the 'best colour match' for the central colour and the hues are based on the likely colour confusions of the three types of defect, plus a suitable choice for normal subjects. If the usual approach proves to be conceptually difficult for a patient or a child, it is useful to ask for a colour name for each of the five spots, which often reveals the information required. Figure 12.5 illustrates this test.

Colour-vision investigation must be preceded by building rapport, perhaps by some simple games, with which the possibility of co-operation can be estimated. Two red cards and one green card can be used, but the reds must be identical. With these cards the patient is asked to name colours and to identify a difference or similarity of colour, as appropriate. Then, without undue hurry, the first three or four plates of an Ishihara Test and some of the City University Test plates can be presented. Since the CUT shows only 'significant' degrees of defect and the Ishihara Test is very sensitive to slight red–green defects, the combination gives an idea as to the actual severity of defect in an individual. Ishihara Tests do not attempt to show up *tritan* or blue deficiency.

Figure 12.2: The Fletcher–Hamblin Simplified Colour Vision Test (Hamblin Instrument Company, London) being used by a young subject. The light from a Tungsten bulb is throwing a shadow and decisions would be made with the mosaic flat on the table.

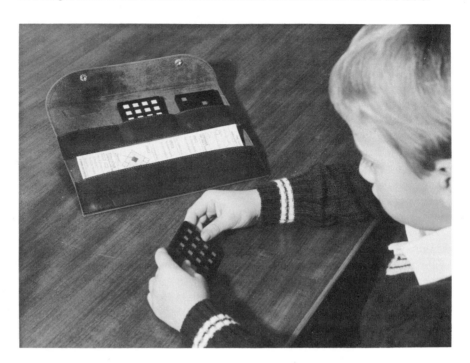

Figure 12.3: One Unit of the Fletcher–Hamblin Simplified Colour Vision Test

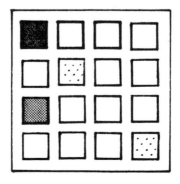

Figure 12.4: Record for the Fletcher–Hamblin Simplified Colour Vision Test

---

THE FLETCHER – HAMBLIN
SIMPLIFIED COLOUR VISION TEST

RECORD FOR . . . . NAME

MALE . . . . FEMALE . . . . SCHOOL

☐　　　　　　　〇

CONDUCTED BY . . . .

AT . . . .

DATE　　/　　/

REMINDER
USE ONLY TUNGSTEN LIGHT BULB

UNIT 1

NUMBER SEEN 　{ 4 . . . . . 〇 　"PASS "

AS DIFFERENT 　{ 2 . . . . . 〇 RED/GREEN
　　　　　　　　　　　　　　　　ERROR

ALTERNATIVE RESPONSE 　〇 QUERY ??

UNIT 2

NUMBER SEEN 　{ 4 or 5 〇 　"PASS"

AS DIFFERENT 　{ 2 or 3 〇 BLUE/YELLOW
　　　　　　　　　　　　　　　ERROR

ALTERNATIVE RESPONSE 〇 　QUERY ??

UNIT 3

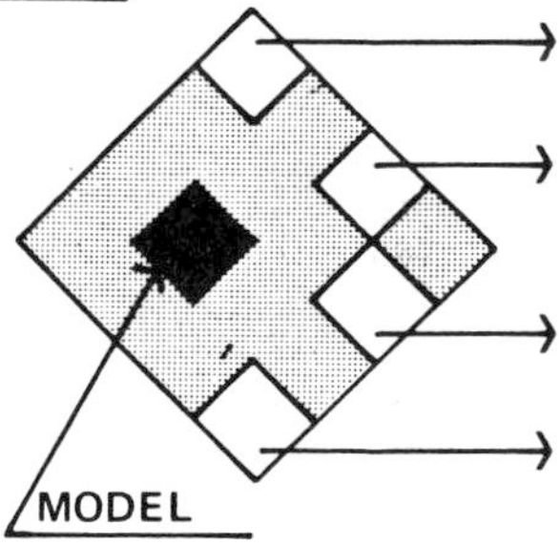

NONSENSE 〇

R/G
ERROR 〇

NORMAL
PASS 〇

R/G
ERROR 〇

MODEL

EVALUATION
(UNDERLINE ONE REQUIRED)

|PASS| |R/G| |B/Y| |MIXED| |QUERY|

RETEST INDICATED ? 　NO 〇 YES 〇

COMMENT '.'. . . . .

ACTION TAKEN . . . .

SIGNED 　　　　　DATE 　/　　/

HAMBLIN (INSTRUMENTS) LTD. 　　©

Figure 12.5: The City University Test

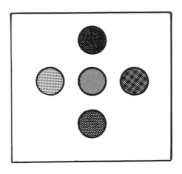

The SCVT mosaics are used in addition or as an alternative approach, particularly where soiling of paper plates is a risk from careless or inquisitive patients.

In testing in this manner it must be stressed that subjects with mental handicaps often perform better on some days, usually on retesting, so it is not always necessary to regard a resident as untestable.

One other very sensitive plate, the F2 plate described by Farnsworth [1950] is useful for tritans and for most protans and deutans. It is delicate and out of print but by laborious personal construction, following instructions given by Taylor (1975), it can be produced. The significant cost of the special papers and the time involved are drawbacks.

Possible Actions

Once a colour-vision defect has been detected, with the type and extent determined as far as possible, the next step is to consider possible actions. Where there is a suspicion of an acquired defect, the implications involve assessment of likely diseases and treatment. A congenital (or inherited) deficiency must be taken in the context of a person's needs and occupations; more guidance as to choices of colours in daily life and dress may be needed, with suitable explanations.

Within limits, colour discrimination in Daltonism can be assisted by the prescribing of filters (usually in plastics material) which give altered colour contrasts and thus extra clues to colours found in food and foliage; these can help in painting, etc. Such methods have been described by Fletcher (1980b). It is seldom appropriate that such filters (magenta or red, as a rule) should be worn permanently. They are often used in a small mount such as a colour slide or a perforated top of a dropper bottle, so that the person peeps through the filter when making a particular colour judgement and the operation is inconspicuous.

Patients' records should have details of the results of colour-vision tests entered, with the dates and enough interpretative notes to convey the practical implications.

References

Alexander, K.R. (1975) 'Colour testing in children: a review', *Amer. J. Optom. and Physiol. Opt.*, *52*, 332-7

Archer, R.E. (1964) 'Colour discrimination and association of educable mentally retarded children', Doctoral dissertation, Colorado State College

Bornstein, M.H. (1976) 'Infants are trichromats', *J. Exp. Child Psychol.*, *21*, 425-45

——, Keffen, W. and Weiskopf, S. (1976) 'Colour vision and hue categorization in young human infants', *J. Exp. Psychol.: Hum. Percept. and Performance*, *2*, 115-29

Chase, W. (1937) 'Colour vision in infants', *J. Exp. Psychol.*, *20*, 203-22

Courtney, G.R. and Heath, G.G. (1971) 'Color deficiency in the mentally retarded: prevalence and a method of evaluation', *Amer. J. Ment. Def.*, *76*, 48-52

Cruz-Coke, R. (1972) 'Defective color vision and alcoholism', *Mod. Prob. Ophthal.*, Karger, Basel, *11*, 174-7

Farnsworth, D. (date uncertain but circa early 1950s) *F2 plate for colour vision testing*, Published by US Navy E. London Submarine base

Fletcher, R. (1979) 'Investigating juvenile Daltonism', *The Optician*, *178*, 9-12

—— (1980a) 'Testing the Daltonic Child', *Col. Vision Deficiencies*, *5*, 204-6

—— (1980b) 'The prescription of filters for Daltonism', *The Ophthalmic Optician*, *20*, 334-40

—— (1981a) 'The illumination of colour vision tests', *The Optician*, *181*, 11, 12 and 32

—— (1981b) 'Colour test decisions in practice', *The Optician*, *181*, 17-18

—— (1982) 'Children's tests — further applications', *Docum. Ophthal. Proc. Series.*, *33*, 189-190

—— (1984) *The Fletcher–Hamblin Simplified Colour Vision Test*, Hamblin Instruments, London

—— and Voke, J. (1985) *Defective Colour Vision*, Adam Hilger, Bristol

François, J. and Verriest, G. (1961) 'On acquired deficiency of colour vision', *Vision Res*, *1*, 201-19

Kalmus, H. (1965) *Diagnosis and genetics of defective colour vision*, Pergamon, London

Kratter, F.E. (1957) 'Color blindness in relation to normal and defective intelligence', *Amer. J. Ment. Def.*, *62*, 436-41

Krause, I.B. (1967) *A study of the relationship of certain aspects of colour vision to educable mentally retarded children*, U.S. Office of Educ. Grant OEG2-6-088526-1953

McKusick, V.A. (1962) 'On the X chromosome of man', *Quart. Rev. Biol.*, *37*, 69-175 (see pp. 107 and 142)

O'Connor, N. (1957) 'Imbecility and color blindness', *Amer. J. Ment. Def.*, *62*, 83-7

Pinckers, A. (1976) 'An analysis of acquired disorders of color vision with a view to distinction from hereditary ocular anomalies', *Ophthalmologica*, *173*, 221-6

Salvia, J.A. and Ysseldyke, J. (1972) 'Criterion validity of four tests for red/green color blindness', *Amer. J. Ment. Def.*, *76*, 418-22

Taylor, W.O.G. (1975) 'Constructing your own P.I.C. Test', *Brit. J. Physiol, Opt.*, *30*, 22-4

Voke, J. (1980) *Colour Vision Testing in Specific Industries and Professions* Keeler Instruments, London

Walls, G.L. (1959) 'Peculiar color blindness in peculiar people', *Arch. Ophthal.*, *62*, 13-32

PART FIVE

ASSESSMENT OF PSYCHO-SOCIAL FUNCTIONING

13 PSYCHOEDUCATIONAL ASSESSMENT OF VISUALLY IMPAIRED STUDENTS WITH ADDITIONAL HANDICAPS

M. Beth Langley

Introduction

The multiplicative and pervasive effects sensory impairments impose on development, learning and integration of experience necessitate the use of a variety of approaches and instrumentation for assessing the developmental performance of a child who is sensorily impaired with additional handicapping conditions. The educational assessment of a multi-handicapped sensorily impaired youngster must have as its core purpose the delineation of the level of integration of sensory and perceptual processes, the influence of the visual impairment on all developmental domains, and a hypothesis regarding why gaps or deficits have emerged within the child's repertoire of adaptive behaviours. Once these variables are identified, they should serve as the foundation for integrative developmental intervention strategies and formulation of an educational plan.

Each multi-handicapped visually impaired (MHVI) student will exhibit skills and deficits unique to his own degree of sensory impairment and type and extent of additional handicaps. An individual student is as unique as the battery of assessment instruments and processes will need to be. Because no single measurement tool will appropriately identify how a specific child will best be taught, the evaluator of MHVI populations must know the array of assessment possibilities that exist and how and when to select and apply them.

DuBose, Langley and Stagg (1977) proposed that the assessment of a child with multiple handicapping conditions be a multi-factored process which must include specific assessments of each of those handicaps as well as of development and learning. While it is highly desirable to use instruments with standardization data on sensorily impaired populations, such instruments are, indeed, in the minority (Stillman 1978; Reynell 1979; Langley, in press). The variability that exists among MHVI children makes it most impractical to compare such a student's performance with that of another student. Since the primary purpose of assessment is to assist in designing intervention strategies, a functional assessment must be a process-orientated approach tailored to the general level of functioning of the child, his response mode and comprehension level, his chronological age, the purpose of referral, the environment in which he will function, and the most realistic approximation of his needs upon graduation from school. When a child is so severely impaired that his ability to respond to standard assessment items is restricted to very subtle behaviours, the evaluator must

253

have behavioural observation skills of physiological state, of physical handling skills, and of procedures for conducting a test–teach–test model of assessment. The evaluator must operate on the premiss that every child is testable and, therefore, that every child is 'teachable' on some level.

Ideally, an assessment of a MHVI student will incorporate both formal and informal assessment procedures, direct observation of the child in daily life settings and routines, the administration of standardized instruments, when possible, and opportunities to engage the child in a test–teach–test situation. An approach to assessment which deviates from the traditional orientation is the process-orientated, test–teach–test model (Schucman 1957; Haeussermann 1958; Fuerstein 1970; Budoff 1973; Dunst 1981; Lidz 1983). Because the evaluator is frequently presented with a student who exhibits a limited behavioural repertoire, the evaluator must test the limits of those behaviours and push to elicit responses that can be observed over time to note change or adaptation as intervention is introduced. This type of assessment identifies how the student approaches and processes stimuli, the types of conditions, environments, materials and personnel that elicit maximum responses and an estimate of learning rate. These are the essential foundations for an instructional programme. The thrust of such approaches (e.g. Piagetian, diagnostic/prescriptive, and process orientation) is on the quality of responses to assessment tasks and stimuli and the subsequent programming that can ensue from analysing the quality of the cognitive, motor and sensory components in the student's behaviours. Perhaps the most advantageous outcome of an assessment is an estimation of the child's potential to continue developing rather than a summary of unsuccessful behaviours.

Section 121 a.532 of the Education for all Handicapped Children Act of 1975 (Public law 94-142) of the United States emphasizes:

> Tests are selected and administered so as best to ensure that when a test is administered to a child with impaired sensory, manual, or speaking skills, the test results accurately reflect the child's aptitude or achievement level or whatever other factors the test purports to measure, rather than reflecting the child's impaired sensory, manual, or speaking skills (except where these skills are the factors which the test purports to measure).

Griffiths (1954) posed a realistic challenge when she asked: 'How can we give enough weight to those directions in which [the child's] effort is unimpaired, and be in a position to assess the effect of specific disabilities on the total test result?' This is the challenge the evaluator of the visually impaired student with additional handicaps must face when performing a psycho-educational assessment.

The multifactored assessment approach ensures that a student's full range of abilities has been tapped. Although there may be an overlap of items, more often data obtained from the student's performance on multiple items from an array of assessment instruments will complement and support other student data. Multiple sources of data will aid in understanding why a student functions as he does. Discrepancies in a student's performance across a variety of assessment items purported to assess a similar skill or process may be due to the conditions surrounding how the item is administered, performance expectations and scoring procedures (Simmeonson, Huntington and Parse 1980). Additionally, multivariant assessment of the MHVI child permits data to be collected from parents, teachers, medical and educational diagnosticians, medical eye personnel, and psychologists, as they view the student in different environments and situations. The results should immediately identify learning, reflect style intervention priorities, and suggest instructional methodologies and personnel which will optimize a student's potential.

The disadvantages of multivariant assessment encompass a number of variables. The assessor must be very familiar with normal development processes and sequences and expected patterns of parallels to, and divergences from, that normal developmental process that sensory impairments impose. Thorough knowledge of the tools available and specific items within those tools which are appropriate for use with students with impaired sensory systems is essential. Even more important is the ability of the evaluator to understand sensory, physical, emotional and psychological constructs tapped by each item, the inter-relationship of items, and the interpretation of the student's performance elicited by assessment items. Very few teachers and psychologists have been trained to analyse assessment items, much less in their interpretation when applied to a sensorily impaired youngster who has additional handicaps! Adaptation of items to the comprehension and response mode of the student further complicates the interpretation process.

The time needed for a process-orientated assessment of the MHVI student is a second major disadvantage. It is not unusual for a school psychologist to have 3,000 students on his caseload or for the teacher of the MHVI student to have responsibility for ten to twelve students in a single class. Affording time to perform a detailed analysis of a single student is neither time- nor cost-efficient. The complexity of planning an appropriate developmental programme for the MHVI student, however, warrants the expenditure of assessment time. Solutions to the time problem have included specialized training of an individual to serve all the MHVI students in a county, the training of a regional team of experts based in a specific locale and students transported to that locale, and the similar development of a specialized team who travelled to students. Local school funds, state grants and specialized federal, state and local monies have been allocated to support these special systems. Professionals on the team vary, but generally include a teacher of the visually impaired, a psychologist, an occupational or physical therapist, an ophthalmologist or optometrist, and an audiologist.

Assessment Environment and Equipment

Understanding why the child functions as he does should evolve from observations of how the child adapts to unfamiliar demands and settings and how he functions in routine activities and familiar surroundings.

Observations of the child participating in self-care routines provide supplementary data on cognitive, language and fine motor skills and yield insight into adaptive behaviour skills. Structured checklists, such as in Table 13.1, can organize observations done informally and often help to pinpoint abilities not seen in a more formal assessment environment. For example, a child who demonstrates object permanence may search around his plate for his spoon when he did not lift a cup to obtain a block during a standardized test. He may reverse his carton to pour milk when he refused to rotate a small bottle to dump its contents. Additionally, direct observations will yield a much more valid estimate of the child's skills. Relying on teacher or care-giver report (Fewell, Langley and Roll 1982), usually obtained with interview scales (e.g. Preschool Attainment Record, the Vineland, and the Maxfield Buchholz 1957), often leads to inflated scores and inappropriate expectations and programming strategies.

When the evaluator attempts to elicit specific, more standard expected behaviours from a student, he should have access to an area set away from auditory and visual distractions. One-way mirrors are highly desirable to permit parents, care-givers and the professionals to observe the student's performance without distracting him. Lighting and seating arrangements should afford the student alignment, security and support for his feet, and the working surface should allow him comfortably to rest his arms at his sides and his forearms on the surface. Tables that can be easily adjusted to accommodate a student's height are invaluable. An adjustable table should be able to lower to a child who is more comfortable on the floor as are many young and multi-handicapped children. Inexpensive plastic children's play desks are quite serviceable with smaller children as are highchairs, and Tri-wall, a 5/8" cardboard material, can be used to construct the surface used with a child on the floor, or to make an adjustable table. A variety of positioning apparatus should be available, such as corner chairs, bolster chairs, standing frames, and wedges of various heights and lengths. The child who has a customized wheelchair may function more optimally in his chair.

Essential in the assessment of the child with visual impairment is some form of flexible stand which holds materials such as diagrams, pictures, books and reading items at an angle for better viewing. The stand serves the purpose of keeping visual material at an even focal level and enhances more optimal head and trunk posture. A metal cookie sheet and magnets that hold pictures on the sheet can be used to place materials on a vertical plane. The stand designed by Haeussermann (1958), an invaluable aid, is a three-tiered wooden stand which can be tilted manually to angle so that it

Table 13.1: Developmental Differences Seen in Visually Impaired

---

Birth to 4 months

    Smiles to parent's voice
    Fails to turn head to sound or from side to side
    Dislikes the prone position
    Doesn't clear head well from surface

4-8 months

    Differential vocalizations
    Differential responses to holding in relation to stranger vs. parents
    Exhibits difficulty integrating new textures during the feeding process
    Hands held at shoulder level
    Hands may still be fisted
    Doesn't bring hands to midline
    Doesn't engage in finger play
    Accidental encounters with objects give the impression that objects appear from nowhere
    Toy touched to hand activates a grasp
    If a toy removed, hand performs action
    Sound of toy elicits alertness
    If toy removed from grasp, rudimentary search occurs
    Hand may move across surface where lost touch with toy but search brief
    Child may roll from supine to prone prior to supporting self on forearms and elevating head
    Exhibits definite preference for certain toys
    Encounter with toy elicits grasp
    Sits alone momentarily
    Righting reactions may not be fully developed for forward extensor thrust or for protective
       reactions

8-12 months

    Sits alone steadily
    Begins to reach for toys
    Reacts to stranger's voice or touch
    Demonstrates affection to 'give Mummy a hug'
    May be delayed in extending arms to be picked up
    Demonstrates delays in showing toys to adults
    Reaches in locale where toy lost from grasp
    Fingers move in response to sound from familiar toy
    Can locate toy through sound source
    Babbling and jargon match that of sighted child but first words may be delayed until the
       next six months period
    Begins to integrate auditory and tactile information for functional use
    Raises self to sitting
    Transfers objects from one hand to the other
    May retain a raking grasp in order to maintain contact with small objects
    Smiles begin to take on mature expression in spontaneity rather than to voice or tactile
       stimuli
    Difficulty in understanding relationships between objects
    Difficulty in locating and understanding the functional side of objects
    Difficulty in understanding means–ends relationships
    May experience difficulty in understanding own limitations
    Bridges on hands and knees
    Cruises around furniture

12-18 months

    Attributes properties to toys independent of self
    Begins to show readiness for chewing
    Experiences difficulty in scooping but may feed self with spoon
    Finger feeds readily
    Gestural imitation skills emerging once child is guided through task
    Begins to search for object in place where last experienced the interaction
    Reaches directly to sound cue if in diagonal or lateral planes
    Begins to pursue toy on sound cue when toy is out of direct reach
    Creeps independently
    Pulls to stand

Table 13.1 continued

Stands independently
Begins systematically to explore new toys and objects and uses familiar objects and toys
    appropriately

18-24 months
    Does not offer examples of domestic mimicry
    Cannot represent self through doll
    Can point to facial features on self and other people but not on doll
    Drinks from a cup
    Object permanence fairly well established
    Begins to use first two words
    Walks unsupported
    Can begin to make tactual associations with familiar objects: cups, spoons, shoes, cookies
    Small objects (miniature) have no meaning for child
    Recognizes grossly different tactual input but does not scan for a match

24-30 months
    Begins to use two-word phrases

3-4 years
    Begins to represent self in play
    Begins to make the distinction between pronouns 'I' and 'you'

---

can be used with a child who is supine. A work tray with a raised edge such as those produced by American Printing House for the Blind is most helpful for providing structure and organization and tangible spatial limits for the visually impaired child. When working behind the child, use a mirror to monitor how the child is using his eyes. If a mirror is too distracting, the one-way observation glass can also be used or the mirror can be mounted out of the child's view and angled to allow visibility of the child.

Preparing For the Assessment

Prior to the assessment the evaluator will need to review child data and select assessment tools and materials. Information which will influence the process of assessment, the selection of a battery and the child's performance can usually be obtained from previous records or from interviewing teachers and parents. Ideally, the evaluator should informally observe the child briefly to enhance his preparation of the assessment milieu.

Questions to be answered include:

1. *Purpose of assessment:* is there an identified or suspected problem in a specific area for which additional data are needed or will the child's placement in a specific programme depend on assessment data?
2. *Chronological age:* if an older multi-handicapped child, what assessment tools will provide information on potential for pre-vocational training and daily living skill independence?

3. *Child's developmental functioning level*: what scales incorporate items appropriate for a child functioning at the 3-6 month level, the 22-30 month level, etc.?
4. *Specific handicapping condition(s)*? How will the child process assessment items (visually, auditorily, tactually?) and how will he respond (e.g. by eye-pointing, manipulating, verbalizing?); what is known about visual fields, visual acuity, illumination needs, range of motion, and auditory localization and thresholds that will affect the positioning of materials and presentation of items?
5. *Medication*: will it affect alertness, are there side-effects that will influence performance, have dosage levels recently changed?
6. *Child's typical schedule or routine*: when does he sleep, eat, when is he most likely to perform optimally?
7. *Specific fears or sensitivity problems*: is he afraid of certain sounds or pictures, people, clothing (e.g. white lab coats) equipment (stop-watches, buzzers, pens that resemble syringes), environments (bright lighting, darkness, etc.) or temperatures?
8. Should any specific communication or behaviour management system be followed throughout the assessment? Will the child respond via a Blissymbolics or manual sign system? What reinforces the child and what behaviours have been discouraged in home and school settings?

Selection of Assessment Battery

The evaluator should review the purpose of assessment and the student's records before designing an assessment battery. The evaluator, however, must address the essential components of a functional assessment:

1. He must understand the purpose for the referral.
2. He must understand the content areas to be assessed in order to specify types of information needed and the procedure for acquiring it.
3. He must be able to analyse, consolidate, integrate and synthesize results from various sources into learning patterns, strengths and weaknesses of the student's performance.
4. He must demonstrate the influence of the visual impairment on development and learning.
5. He must translate results from the assessment into functional developmental and academic learning strategies.

A comprehensive psychoeducational report should include information about the student's sensory and physical functioning, cognitive abilities, means of communicating, level of independence in skills of daily living, and social and emotional well-being. The evaluator must present a representative sample of both the student's performance and communication abilities. It is not unusual to find that visually impaired students have not been presented with manipulative tasks of any nature during previous assessments and results have reflected only one aspect of a student's abilities. Dependence on verbal responses alone may lead one either to underestimate or to overestimate student expectations.

The selection of assessment instruments, developmental scales and subtests should be based on as many of the following variables as appropriate for the unique needs of each student:

1. the student's chronological age;
2. the student's approximate developmental range of abilities in the domain(s) being addressed;
3. whether reliability and validity data are available: does the tool selected measure what it purports to measure and can it be reliably administered by various examiners and across a variety of settings?
4. whether visually impaired students have been included in the standardization sample;
5. whether specific items or subtests will be biased by the visual impairment;
6. selecting instruments which are minimally influenced by timed items;
7. selecting instruments and subtests that tap the full range of the student's abilities;
8. selecting instruments that easily accommodate to a student's visual status and response mode to reduce the necessity for adaptations;
9. selecting instruments and subtests that afford overlap in concepts and abilities tapped to provide opportunities to observe similar behaviours with a variety of materials and to differing situations;
10. selecting instruments, scales, and subtests that can be used for re-evaluation. The same conclusions cannot be inferred when using two different sets of tasks to assess whether change has occurred.

More specific information regarding behaviours to target and the types of assessment instrument available for collecting data are detailed later in this chapter.

Item Adaptation

Any alteration of the original form of an assessment scale, whether its method of administration, materials or response mode, threatens the integrity of the assessment tool. The foremost rule in any adaptation is that the integrity of the item construct be maintained. Essential to the process of altering any tool is considerable familiarity with the assessment scale and anticipation of the response needs of the visually impaired student. Strategies for modifying assessment scales for MHVI students can be grouped into categories: altering the administration of the item; the materials; the response mode; child variables, and scoring procedures. Each adaptation, recombination of items, and unique management of the child and his response must be carefully documented and considered when interpreting assessment results. Specific suggestions for adaptation strategies follow.

Administration

The most common means of altering a test item for a visually impaired child is to present the item verbally. However, verbal stimuli alone often have very little meaning for the MHVI student. More relevant may be administering the item within a functional context. If the student is uninterested in searching for a cube under a cup, object permanence concepts may be elicited by observing whether the student searches for his cup moved from where he placed it during snack or mealtime (see the example in Table 13.2). The evaluator may wish to alter a test by administering all the items involving the manipulation of specific materials in succession (i.e. blocks, pictures, formboards). A means of alleviating the student's confusion over how to respond is to group all tasks from various scales or within one instrument that assess specific concepts such as 'classification'. Observing the student as he interacts with tasks grouped in this manner will yield data on optimal learning conditions. Additionally, combining multiple measures that sample similar behaviours increases performance reliability as well as the scope of conceptual mastery. Rearranging the order of item presentation may be beneficial when the evaluator anticipates that items usually administered at the end of a test will be more difficult than items at the beginning. The evaluator may choose to omit entire tasks believed to penalize the student as a result of the impairment, or substitute a similar conceptual task from another scale to sample the targeted behavioural domain. If the student's residual vision enables him to see only outlines of one-dimensional figures, the picture-matching task on the Learning Accomplishment Profile, Diagnostic Edition (Sanford 1975) may be replaced with the Decroly game from the Merrill Palmer (Stutsman 1931) and a behaviour of similar difficulty level can still be elicited.

Materials

Substituting a concrete object for a picture or enlarging a picture may not facilitate optimal performance as anticipated when the student is visually impaired. Because visually impaired students have difficulty with miniature objects (Fraiberg 1977), objects used as substitutes for pictures must be as natural and realistic as possible. When enlarging pictures to help the student focus on detail, the evaluator must remember that increased magni-

Table 13.2: Assessment of Developmental Skills During Lunchtime Activities

COMMUNICATION BEHAVIOURS

Moves/looks in direction of appropriate
locale when directed/cued by
    context
    visual cues
    sign
    gesture
    verbal direction

Discriminates appropriate object needed for
lunchtime activities
    bib
    cup
    spoon
    plate

Responds when asked if ready for lunch
    body movement
    facial expression
    gesture
    sign
    vocalization
    label

Directs attention by pointing

Requests help by
    reaching
    tugging
    pulling
    vocalizing
    gesture
    verbal label
    sign

Indicates preferences by
    turning head
    closing mouth to refuse
    pushes away
    shakes head
    spits out

Labels lunchtime items
    bib
    cup
    spoon
    milk/juice
    more
    foods (list)

Indicates when finished
    refuses more food
    takes off bib
    pushes plate/hand away
    throws spoon/cup

Opens mouth when approached with
    cup
    spoon

Requests foods/more by
    reaching
    leaning forward
    handing empty plate and/or cup
    gesture
    sign
    vocalization
    label

FINE MOTOR BEHAVIOURS

Hand to mouth

Maintains grasp on adapted spoon/eating
utensil

Prefers hand for eating
    right
    left
    neither

Grasp on utensil
    palmar
    dagger
    extended forefinger
    mature grasp

Supinates wrist

Approach to food
    slides
    scoops
    stabs

Holds cup
    right
    left
    both
    hand over hand

Passes cup/spoon from one hand to the
other

Stabilizes cup/spoon with one hand and
uses other hand to feed/drink

Pours from carton while holding

Releases spoon or cup voluntarily

Pokes food

Finger thumb opposition when finger
feeding
    palmer
    radial palmer
    scissors
    radial digital
    interior pincer
    pincer

COGNITIVE BEHAVIOURS

Object permanence
   looks for food
   looks for dropped spoon/food
   recognizes milk, cup, spoon when
      partially or completely covered
   recognizes that milk or juice is inside
      carton

Spatial relationships
   recognizes when food is on spoon
   recognizes correct end/side of eating
      tools
   recognizes when to stop pouring.

Means–ends
   selects spoon or fork as functional from
      other objects
   pulls table cloth or tray to obtain food
      out of reach
   uses all eating tools functionally

Causality
   uses dominant procedure to reinstate
      activity
   hands back/pushes plate or cup toward
      teacher for more food or drink

EATING/FEEDING/ORAL MOTOR BEHAVIOURS
(consult with occupational and speech therapist)

   length of time required to eat
   amount of food eaten at meal
   types of food eaten/consistency
   position in which the child is fed

Oral motor

   tongue thrust
   jaw thrust
   bite reflex
   jaw clenching
   grades opening of mouth for cup and
      spoon
   voluntarily releases bite on spoon when
      in mouth
   removes food from spoon with lips
   lip closure on spoon/cup
   suckles food from spoon
   swallows with tongue in mouth
   lateralizes tongue to move food to side
      and back molars
   jaw is stable
   swallows with head in line with trunk
   exhibits munching pattern
   bites off bits of food

Self-feeding
Self-feeds with adapted equipment
   bowl
   non-slip matting
   spoon
   hand over hand
   assistance at elbow
   cues to initiate scoop
   independent

Returns spoon to plate
   hand over hand
   cues at elbow
   cues tactually
   visual cues
   independent

Picks up cup
   hand over hand
   assisted at elbow
   tactual cues
   independent

Takes cup to mouth
   hand over hand
   assisted at elbow
   tactual cues
   independent

Returns cup to table
   hand over hand
   assisted at elbow
   tactual cues
   independent
   maintains non-dominant hand in lap or
      stabilized on tray or table

---

fication decreases visual field (Faye 1970). Multi-handicapped visually impaired students frequently lack integrative processes needed to piece together fragments of visual information gathered when scanning enlarged pictures or photographs. Very frequently, the stimulus value of materials in standardized assessment kits is unappealing to MHVI students. Colour, texture, novelty and even familiarity are variables to consider when making material adaptations. The MHVI student may be more motivated to imitate or copy designs when provided with scented, colourful felt-tipped markers than when expected to use a pencil. The evaluator must try to avoid shiny reflective surfaces that will distract or impede performance of the MHVI student. Providing a good contrast between materials and the surface is critical. Yellow against black offers the highest colour contrast, although blue against orange has also been suggested (Griffiths 1954). Print materials can be enlarged with special duplicating machines (Xerox) or via use of a closed circuit television, although MHVI students have difficulty relating to an image on a television screen. Black felt-tipped markers are effective for darkening materials and mimeograph stencils of blue, green or purple hues may be darkened by overlaying them with sheets of yellow acetate. Placement of materials to accommodate the student's visual and/or physical abilities will be imperative. It may often be necessary to reduce the number of objects or pictures presented simultaneously to avoid penalizing the student for restricted visual fields and/or physical range of motion.

Response Mode

Perhaps the most difficult variable to control is obtaining a reliable response from the student. When a student fails to respond or responds erratically to tasks, the evaluator must determine whether the student understood what was expected of him or whether the concept being tapped is not within the student's repertoire. In such instances the opportunity to expose the child to the concept, provide him with a means of responding and then observe whether he can succeed with another set of materials becomes an invaluable assessment measure. Due to the meaningless, echolalic verbal characteristics of many MHVI students, non-verbal means of responding may be needed. While verbal responses may offer insight into how the student perceives or into specific deficit areas, a verbal response from the MHVI student may be more reflective of the handicap than of the student's ability. Thus, matching or pointing responses may be more appropriate. It has also been effective to have a student release a token of some form on to the picture or object of choice. Many times, a MHVI student will reach for an appropriate item rather than place the stimulus item in an expected locale. If the student communicates in sign or gesture, the evaluator must be aware of, and consistently employ, that system. It is more characteristic that a student who exhibits both visual and auditory impairments will demonstrate more functional visual than verbal skills.

When the student is physically impaired, eye-pointing may be the most appropriate response mode. The evaluator must place materials to allow optimal use of visual field and focal length. Very often, the position of the child's head will significantly affect the position and function of the eyes. The athetoid student may often use his eyes more efficiently when his hands and arms are stabilized beneath his tray or in some other way. The cerebral palsied child often exhibits better vision at far point. The use of switches and other augmentative aids should always be investigated when no other reliable response can be elicited.

Child Variables

Deviations from standard administration procedures many times involve non-traditional management of the child. Better control over assessment milieu and student may be obtained by working directly beside and behind the student. Distractibility, behavioural outbursts, attempts to throw materials or to leave the assessment situation can often be minimized by this orientation. Guiding the blind student hand-over-hand through an expected response or to explore task materials is more naturally accomplished from this position than from a frontal or a perpendicular relationship to the student.

Positioning the student to enhance his ability to attend visually and respond physically will be essential when severe physical impairment accompanies the sensory impairment. Often positioning the student on his side will allow optimal integration of eyes and hands for interaction with task materials. Physically stabilizing the student's shoulder, abducting his arm, and allowing him to guide the evaluator's hand to point, write or manipulate materials are alternative means of enabling a physically involved student to express his potential. Consultation with a physical and occupational therapist will be essential prior to the assessment.

The student's alertness will aid in discriminating when to pick up or slow down the pace of item presentation, when to allow breaks and when to terminate sessions. The attention span, alertness level and frustration tolerance threshold of the student may necessitate several assessment sessions spread throughout the day or over a span of several days.

Scoring Procedures

Modifying the scoring procedure by reducing number of items presented to establish a ceiling may preserve the student's energy level and perseverance for other tasks. If there is doubt whether the student would accomplish tasks within the ceiling range, the evaluator can return to those items later. Time limits frequently penalize the sensorily impaired and the motorically impaired student. How the student approached or solved the timed task is far more meaningful than whether he could meet the time demands of a specific item. When presenting items under standardized conditions, the evaluator may feel that the student would succeed with a third trial when only two are permitted. If the student accomplishes the task on the third trial, that item is scored as *failed*, but the evaluator will have valuable data regarding the student's rate of learning. A final note on scoring: extreme caution must be exercised when interpreting a single score (i.e. 13 months). While individual scores may be useful for pre- and post-measures of skill development, those scores cannot be assumed to represent the quality and integration of performance that would be demonstrated by a normal child of 13 months. For programming design, a range of performance (12-18 months) is far more indicative of learning style and mastery.

Knowledge of Developmental Trends of Visually Impaired Students

The most complex task facing the evaluator is knowing the types and ranges of behaviours that characterize a sensory impairment. Understanding the growth and developmental patterns of visually impaired children is imperative to appropriate interpretation of assessment results and, consequently, to effective intervention strategies. As Miller (1977, p. 152) so aptly stressed: 'Research on the early cognitive development of congenitally blind children is central to understanding how such children come to be the persons they are later in life.' The sensory impairment should not be the primary focus of attention but, rather, how it affected other developmental aspects of the child. Vander Kolk (1977, p. 161) explained: 'It cannot be concluded that blindness in itself is intellectually handicapping but rather, when damage to the central nervous system includes loss of vision, impairment of intellectual functioning may also occur.' Freedman (1964), Burlingham (1965), Faye (1970), Adelson and Fraiberg (1974), Fraiberg (1977) and Stephens, Fitzgerald, Hitt and Grube (1980) have provided a wealth of information on developmental patterns of visually impaired children and youth. More recently, Bower (1977), Scott, Jan and Freeman (1977), Warren (1978) and Reynell and Zinkin (1979) have supplied additional developmental data on visually impaired children. Hart (1978), Mori and Olive (1978) and Langley (1980a,b) have discussed the combined effects of visual impairment and other handicaps on development and intervention.

It will be necessary to identify whether the student is congenitally or adventitiously visually impaired and to have some knowledge of the extent and range of experiences to which the student has had exposure. Also helpful is an awareness of care-giver expectations of, and limitations on, the sensorily impaired student. Miller (1977, p. 151) reminded us that 'for congenitally blind persons much of what may have been learned was insufficient, superficial, or had little relevance to their own limited experiences'. Hill, Rosen, Correa and Langley (1984) found that delays in movement and in cognitive development could often be attributed partially to parental overprotectiveness and/or anxiety regarding how to handle and what to expect of their visually impaired children.

Of greatest concern in the assessment of deaf—blind students is the efficiency with which the evaluator can communicate with the child. Vernon (1967), and Sullivan and Vernon (1979) warned against the use of responses elicited and reported by an interpreter. Evaluators must be aware that a non-verbal test may not be appropriate for hearing impaired students because they require verbal directions. Many tests designed for a non-verbal response rely heavily on detailed, visual formats and responses are dependent on well-integrated visual perceptual abilities. Such abilities frequently are significantly impaired in mentally handicapped and multi-sensorily disabled students.

Hearing aids must be checked for any shorts in the wiring, for working batteries, for fit (earmoulds), and volume levels immediately prior to the assessment to ensure optimal alertness of the student. Lighting must avoid glare on the materials and the evaluator's mouth and face. The evaluator should be cautious in his manipulation of concrete materials as all movements will be amplified if the student is wearing a hearing aid or auditory training system. Sullivan and Vernon (1979) also warned that the student should be asked to repeat his response if initially unintelligible, to ensure reliability and to establish trust.

Behavioural Domains Relevant to Assessment of the Visually Impaired

Imperative to further assessment of the MHVI student is knowledge of the degree of functioning, intactness and integration of the primary sensory mechanisms of sight, hearing and touch.

Vision

An understanding of the student's visual aetiology will give some indication as to visual field intactness, illumination needs and, in some cases, focal length. Students who are shunted for excess cerebral spinal fluid may exhibit fluctuations of both acuity and fields and their vision should be continuously monitored. The evaluator should note the physical appearance of the eyes, whether the child's exhibits a preference for one eye, how he holds his head to obtain optimal viewing, the range of eye movements, near- and far-distance abilities, whether visual field deficits are present, sizes, colour and forms the student is able to perceive, and any difficulty with muscle imbalance or depth perception. If the student is very low functioning, the evaluator should observe subtle behavioural responses indicating the presence and degree of any functional vision (Langley, in press). Resources for assessment of vision in a multi-handicapped child are the comprehensive STYCAR Battery (Sheridan 1973), the Functional Vision Inventory for the Severely Impaired (Langley 1980b) and the Denver Developmental Eye Screening Test; of these, only Langley (1980b) recommends goals, objectives and specific intervention strategies in seven areas of visual functioning. The Diagnostic Assessment Procedure (Barraga and Morris 1978) is appropriate for children functioning approximately from age three and also has extensive training activities.

Audition

How the child localizes, the level of intensity of the stimulus to which the child attends, abnormal head postures, and preference for one ear or specific frequencies should all be noted when observing for auditory intactness. Northern and Downs (1978) provided an excellent summary of the stages of sound localization that are critical when designing programming strategies for the child with severely limited vision. The Auditory Assessment of Deaf–Blind, Multi-handicapped Children (Kukla and Connolly 1978) assesses auditory awareness, attending, localizing, reception, comprehension and association. The manual offers excellent training activities and lists commercially available toys and estimates of their decibel levels. Also included is a list of common environmental sounds and estimates of their approximate decibel levels. The Haeussermann (1958) manual offers excellent, practical means of assessing a child's auditory abilities during other screening procedures. A sample of the types of tasks used to screen for auditory intactness is included in Table 13.3.

Tactual

The hand of the MHVI student is an essential tool for reaching out, exploring, perceiving and communicating. Well-integrated proprioceptive kinaesthetic abilities are basic to the development of orientation and mobility skills.

For the severely visually limited child it may be the only means of establishing contact with his environment and the level of integration of tactile information will significantly affect cognitive, linguistic and movement planning, and spatial relationship abilities.

Deaf–blind and other multi-sensorily disordered children have been described as being very tactually defensive. They are not eager to explore new textures and resist tasks that involve manipulating clay, finger-paint, or any unusual art media. They avoid furry textures and objects that have finely constructed protrusions that 'tickle'. This tactile-defensiveness even affects eating skills. Multi-handicapped visually impaired learners, including the deaf–blind, generally dislike lumpy or grainy foods or foods that need intensive chewing. They dislike extremes in temperatures. Danella (1973), in a study of twelve multi-impaired Rubella children's preference for tactile stimuli, found a significant attraction to vibration while fur and yarn were by far the least preferred. Danella (1973) explained the deaf–blind learner's defensiveness toward fur and yarn as an adaptive response but indicative of an immature tactile system:

> The literature on tactile defensiveness as proposed by Ayers suggests that a protective withdrawal response is often elicited by light touch and hair displacement that is not *seen* or anticipated. Therefore, these stimuli are often avoided. However, pressure, such as rubbing with a rough

cloth, is accepted and appears to have an integrating effect, particularly when it is followed by an adaptive motor response (p. 1459).

Ohwaki and Stayton (1976) found that mentally retarded adults preferred vibratory over visual stimuli. Responses to vibration of subjects functioning below 24 months consisted of smiling, laughing and vocalizing. More significant was the discovery that vibration decreased self-stimulation activities such as rocking, head- and hand-waving, and shaking.

The evaluator must determine whether the student still functions at a protective level or at a discriminative level of tactual processing. Mullen, Danella and Myers (1977) state that tactile–kinaesthetic skills are indicators of central nervous system integration. Observe whether the student processes equally well with both hands, whether he discriminates the object held in his hand without looking (stereognosis), and whether he discriminates among shapes, sizes, temperatures and textures. Items for assessing tactual skills may be extracted from the Vulpe Assessment Battery (Vulpe 1977), the Haeussermann (1958) manual, the Reynell–Zinkin Scales (1979), and from the Psychological S/R Assessment (Mullen, Danella and Myers 1977). The Tactile Differentiation section from the Psychological S/R test is extremely well organized and very comprehensive. It assesses sequentially such tactual processes as generalized localization to specific finger identification, two-point discrimination, proprioceptive and kinaesthetic awareness, stereognosis, graphesthesia and intersensory integration. The Miller Assessment of Pre-schoolers (Miller 1982) also provides excellent activities for assessing the student's tactual skills as well as proprioceptive and kinaesthetic abilities.

Screening

An initial screening of the student will enable the evaluator to plan the most appropriate battery of assessment tools. The screening should alert the evaluator to the type of media to which the student best responds, to which sensory modalities are functional, to the student's response mode, to the student's general developmental level, and to the types of professionals to be involved in the assessment process.

Formal Assessment Instruments

• *The Developmental Activities Screening Inventory II (DASI)*

The DASI (Fewell and Langley 1984) was designed specifically to screen the developmental abilities of deaf–blind, visually impaired and non-verbal children.

Developmental Ranges.　Birth to 60 months.

Table 13.3: Developmental Tasks for Screening Auditory Functioning

Test	Developmental Level	Item/Procedure
Sheridan	Neonatal	Blinks eyes or opens widely to sudden sound. May 'corner' eyes towards nearby source of continued sound. Startle reaction to sudden sounds. Freezing reaction to sudden loud sounds.
	1 month	Startled by sudden noises; stiffens; quivers; blinks; screws up eyes; extends limbs; fans out fingers and toes; and may cry. Movements 'frozen' when small bell rung gently 3-5 inches from ear for 3-5 seconds with 5-second pauses. May move eyes and head towards sound source. Stops whimpering and turns towards sound of nearby soothing human voice.
	3 months	Sudden loud noises still distress (child) provoking blinking, crying and turning away. Definite quieting or smiling to sound of mother's voice before she touches him/her. Quietens to sound of rattle of spoon in cup or if small bell rung gently out of sight for 3-5 seconds, with pauses of 3-5 seconds at 6-12 inches on level with ear. May turn eyes/head towards sound source; brows may wrinkle and eyes dilate. May move head from side to side as if searching for sound. Shows excitement at approaching footsteps, running bathwater.
	6 months	Turns immediately to mother's voice across room. Responds to voice, rattle, cup and spoon, paper and bell when activated at $1\frac{1}{2}$ feet on ear level right and left by correct visual localization.
	9 months	Eagerly attentive to everyday sounds, particularly voice. Immediately responsive to rattle, cup and spoon, voice, paper, and bell at 3 feet from ear above and below ear level but not in midline.
	12 months	Knows and immediately turns to own name. Immediate response to bell, voice, cup and spoon, rattle, and paper at $3\text{-}4\frac{1}{2}$ feet but rapidly habituates.
Koontz	1 month	When confronted with sudden noise, vibration, or bright light, child reacts with entire body. When sound is presented outside range of vision, child responds with a blink and a frown.
	2 months	Child gives evidence of listening to adult talking to him.
	5 months	Child responds by turning towards sound (no visual stimulation associated). Child responds to voices by turning head and eyes (no visual stimulation associated).
Learning Accomplish Profile (LAP)	1 month	Responds to sound of rattle. Responds to voice.
	2 months	Responds to bell.
	3 months	Looks at examiner's face.
	4 months	Turns to voice.
	6 months	Locates source of sound.
	9 months	Activity stops when hears 'no-no'.
	12 months	Responds to own name.

Test	Developmental Level	Item/Procedure	Response
Bayley	0.1 month	Examiner rings bell gently 12 inches from child's ear; few seconds later, rings on other side.	Child may blink, startle, frown, increase activity, cease activity, or cry.
		Examiner shakes rattle, three rapid shakes, at distance of 4 inches from child's ear. Repeats on other side several seconds later.	Any response as suggested above.
		Examiner makes three rapid clicks of light switch about 3 inches from child's ear. Repeats on other side several seconds later.	Any response as suggested above.
	0.7 months	Examiner stands behind and to one side of child and speaks. May repeat at intervals two or three times.	Head turning, vocalization, cessation of activity, changing facial expression.
	2.2 months	Prop child's head in midline while he/she lies supine. Stand at head of bed out of direct line of vision and ring bell or shake rattle, first to one side, then the other, at about 2 feet from his/her ear.	Child moves eyes in apparent search of sound from bell or rattle.
	3.8 months	Child sits on mother's lap, facing her. Examiner rings bell opposite each ear first one and then the other, 14 inches from his/her ear and out of his/her range of vision.	Child turns head towards sound source.
	3.9 months	Repeat with rattle using procedure described above.	Child turns head towards sound source.
Denver DST	Birth to 1 month	Examiner holds bell to the side and little behind child's ears and rings it quietly.	Child shifts eyes to sound, changes breathing rate or exhibits any other change in his/her activity.
	4-8 months	Examiner approaches child from behind as he/she sits on parent's lap facing parent. Examiner whispers child's name within 8 inches of either ear.	Child turns in direction of voice.
Brigance	4 months	Child turns eyes and head toward a sound such as a rattle or squeaking toy 3 feet to the side of him/her.	
	7 months	Child responds in some way when his/her name called.	
	9 months	Child listens to the tick of a watch when it is held to the ears.	
Griffiths	1 month	Mother asked whether child starts at sudden noises in house or on street.	Child startled by sounds.

Table 13.3 continued

Test	Developmental Level	Item/Procedure	Response
		When child is crying, mother or other adult speaks to child.	Child is quieted by voice.
		Examiner talks to baby to attract attention.	Child looks at examiner.
	2 months	Examiner/mother talks to child.	Child smiles.
		Examiner rings small handbell once beyond child's field of vision and 1½ feet away from the right ear. Repeated on left side.	Child cries or listens, or his eyes take on an intent expression.
	End of 2nd month	Examiner rings bells as above.	Child's eyes move slowly from side to side in search of sound.
	3 months	Mother asked whether child responds to music such as radio or songs. Examiner/mother may sing to child.	Child listens to music.
	4 months	Examiner rings bell as above.	Child makes small searching movements of head and eyes.
	5 months		Turns head deliberately to bell.
		Examiner activates c-note tuning fork by pressing prongs together, then releasing suddenly. Fork is held a few inches from each ear.	Child exhibits listening reaction or physical activity decreases.
		Mother asked whether child coos or ceases crying in response to music.	Coos or stops crying on hearing music.
		Mother/examiner vocally reassures crying infant.	Child ceases crying upon hearing mother's voice.
		Child is observed while several adults converse or as examiner speaks.	Child turns head to person speaking.
	7 months	Examiner calls softly to the child during the testing.	Child should look or turn head to examiner when called.
	8 months	Child is observed when adults or older children are talking.	Child turns head from one person to another, occasionally attempting to join in conversation.
	9 months	Examiner holds watch near child's right ear while steadying his/her head with the left hand. Say to the child, 'Listen, tick-tick'. Repeat on the other side.	Child must exhibit a quiet listening expression.
	11 months	Examiner/mother sings to child or mother questioned regarding child's reaction to music.	Child must exhibit vocal responses to music, singing or radio.

Test	Developmental Level	Item/Procedure	Response
Sequenced Inventory of Communication Development (SICD)	4 months	Examiner asks parent whether child responds to different sounds around the home: 'What does (baby) do if the phone rings or you turn on the vacuum cleaner?'	Parent describes a response to two sounds.
	8 months	Examiner says, 'Hi, there,' to child when he/she is not looking at the examiner	Child looks up or smiles.
		While child plays with a quiet toy, the examiner moves to a position behind him/her first to the right, then to the left. Examiner crinkles cellophane once from the right, then to the left. Examiner shakes rattle once from the left and once from the right.	Child turns to locate the stimulus source.
	8-12 months	Child is placed on a table facing away from both parent and examiner so that his/her line of vision is 90° from each. Examiner says child's name using a normal conversational loudness level. Parent says child's name using the same approach.	Child turns to localize each speaker.
	12 months	Examiner, from 3 feet, and at 90° from the child's line of vision, says, 'Look here'.	Child turns to locate the stimulus.
	16 months	Examiner questions parent about child's responses to environmental sounds: phone rings, plane overhead, refrigerator door opening and closing. Repeat with a container of rice and then with one of the pebbles or beans.	Child responds differently to sounds: goes to kitchen in response to refrigerator door, looks up for airplane.
	24 months	Examiner activates then allows child to explore a bell, a rattle, and cellophane. From behind a shield, examiner represents a sound from first the bell, then the rattle, and finally the cellophane. Objects must not be aligned in their order of presentation.	Child discriminates each noisemaker by looking at, touching, or pointing to each after hearing its sound.
	48 months	Examiner activates, then allows child to manipulate three bells, each of a different intensity: soft, medium and loud. From behind a shield, examiner	Child indicates by pointing to, touching, or giving the bell he/she heard after each presentation.

Table 13.3 continued

Test	Developmental Level	Item/Response	Response
		presents a sound from first the soft bell, then the loud bell, and then the medium bell.	
Haeusserman	24 months +	Examiner gently rings a small hand bell under the table as the child manipulates other testing materials.	Child stops activity and/or looks for sound source.
		As child manipulates table bell, examiner steps behind and shakes a container of sand in back of child's head, 10-12 inches away.	Child pauses and listens and may turn to look for sound source.
		As the child engages in manipulating a small handled bell, activate a metal cricket under the table.	Child indicates that he hears the cricket.
		Repeat the cricket sound as the child manipulates the table bell with a push button.	
		After sounding the cricket and toy, offer both the cricket and handbell to the child and ask him to select the one he/she think made the noise.	Child selects cricket.
		Examiner hands child two handbells, one of which has the clapper removed.	Child discards bell without clapper or manipulates only intact bell.
		Examiner hands child sound block with pebbles and sound block with rice and invites him/her to play with them.	Child may ignore medium-sound block but plays only with the louder sound block. He/she may shake the medium-sound block and exhibit a puzzled expression that he expected to hear the same noise from both blocks.
		As the child engages in play with testing material, the examiner activates a music box with a crank handle under the table.	Child looks for music box.
		The examiner then shows the music box to the child and goes through the circular turning motions but does not turn the crank.	Child indicates that he/she does not hear the music.
	42 months +	Examiner presents child with three sound blocks, one with sand, one with rice, and one with pebbles. Examiner allows child to manipulate each sound block. Using a duplicate set	Child matches each sound block correctly.

Test	Developmental Level	Item/Procedure	Response
		of sound blocks, the examiner picks up and shakes the loudest sound block and asks child to find the one among his/her set that sounds the same. Repeat with softest sound block, and middle-sound block in that sequence, having the child select his/her sound block that sounds same.	
	54 months +	The examiner demonstrates grading the sound blocks from softest to loudest. Ask the child to grade his/her set of sound blocks in the same way.	Child seriates his/her sound block from softest to loudest.
		The examiner provides the child with soft quiet toy or paper and crayon and then steps behind the child and stirs spoon inside cup, opens a box of crackers, or drops a wooden cube on the floor.	Child turns to search for sound source.
		Examiner may also sit in front of child and fling a wooden cube under the table on to the floor.	Child's pupils dilate.
		Examiner slides finger over the teeth of a comb behind the child's head.	Child searches for the comb or turns to see what produced the sound.
Psycho-educational Assessment of the Pre-school child	Pre-school	Examiner produces a sequence of claps at the rate of two per second. Child should replicate pattern: 1. one clap, 2. two claps, 3. one clap–pause–two claps 4. one clap–pause–one clap 5. two claps–pause–two claps.	

Skills Assessed. Visual, auditory, tactile and sensori-motor processes; sensori-motor cognitive skills such as object permanence and behaviours relating to objects, and pre-operational cognitive skills. Discrimination, association, inductive, deductive and quantitative reasoning, seriation, spatial relationships and motor-planning abilities are also tapped.

Standardization. Norm referenced.

Visually impaired, deaf-multi-handicapped and deaf–blind children included in standardization sample.

Validity and Reliability.   Data reported in manual.

Usefulness With Visually Impaired. The DASI has instructions for administration to the totally blind and the non-verbal child. Some items that are usually non-verbal are administered verbally. The DASI allows the observation of the student's fine motor and communication skills. The manual provides sequentially designed instructional strategies for each concept screened. The appendix contains an analysis of each assessment item by concept and/or process.

- *The Miller Assessment of Preschoolers (MAP)*

The MAP (Miller 1982) is a 27-item screening tool developed for use by teachers and clinical personnel to identify children in need of further evaluation.

Developmental Range.   Two years, nine months to five years, eight months.

Skills Assessed.   Sensory and motor abilities, memory, sequencing comprehension, association verbal expression, visualization, performance of mental manipulations and the interpretation of visual–spatial information. These skills are divided into five performance indexes: foundations, co-ordination, verbal, non-verbal, and complex behaviours.

Standardization.   Norm referenced.
Visually impaired students were not included in the standardization sample.

Validity and Reliability. The MAP has proven to be a highly theoretically and statistically sound instrument, both valid and reliable.

Usefulness With Visually Impaired.   The 'Foundations' index of the MAP is very relevant to assessment of a student with visual impairment as this section addresses the sense of position and movement, the sense of touch and basic movement components. Of special diagnostic value are the following seven items: General Information, Follow Direction, Stereognosis, Hand–nose, Finger Localization, Stepping and Object Memory.
    Although the administration of these items will require adaptation, only the General Information and Following Direction items depend on comprehension of verbal or signed-directions and some form of verbal or gestural response is needed to perform the General Information item. These items yield critical information about the student's tactile-kinaesthetic senses, his awareness of his relationship to space and gravity and his knowledge of objects and situational problem-solving.
    An estimated developmental range may be obtained for each item.

Individual profiles for recording clinical observations of the student's performance and for recording behaviour state during the assessment accompany the screening form.

- *The Uzgiris–Hunt Ordinal Scales of Psychological Development (U–H)*

The U–H scales (Uzgiris and Hunt 1975) are an ordinal set of Piagetian sensori-motor scales developed to assess a student's placement in a hierarchy of conceptual development.

Developmental Range.   Two months to 24 months.

Skills Assessed.   Uses seven sets of independent scales: Visual Pursuit and Permanence of Objects, Means–Ends Relationships, Vocal Imitation, Gestural Imitation, Construction of Objects in Space, Causality, and Behaviours Relating to Objects.

Standardization.   Ordinal sequences of behaviour.
  Visually and hearing impaired students were not included in the standardization sample, only normal infants.

Validity and Reliability.   Reported in manual.

Usefulness With Visually Impaired.   Perhaps the most desirable aspect of the U–H scales is their focus on concept development and the variety of materials which can be collected, adapted or constructed for eliciting targeted behaviours. The ingenuity of the evaluator is the most variable factor in the administration of the scales. A thorough understanding of the developmental pattern of sensorily impaired students is required for using the U–H scales with this population in order to obtain optimal performance levels.
  The Object Permanence scale can be adapted by referring to guidelines on the blind child's approach to objects as supplied by Fraiberg (1977) and revised by Langley (see Table 13.4). This scale offers valuable information on the student's ability to organize, scan and explore his environment.
  The Behaviours Relating to Objects, the Vocal and Gestural Imitation, and the Causality scales provide excellent means for assessing the multi-handicapped student's interactions with and ability to acquire information from people, objects and his environment. These three scales are highly predictive of a student's communication abilities (Dunst 1981; Brown and Langley 1984). Use of these scales will help determine where in the communication process the multi-handicapped student has significant deficits. They will differentiate the student who exhibits only echolalia and the student who possesses a true communication system, whether verbal or non-verbal. Additionally, these scales can be used to determine a student's readiness for natural gestures or formal sign training. The Means–Ends

Table 13.4: The Developmental Progression of Pursuit and Permanence of Objects in the Blind Infant: Touch Versus Sound

Chronological age	Touch cue	Sound cue
6-7 months	When a toy is removed from the child's hands, the action of the hands briefly continues. A toy touched to the hand activates a grasping response.	The sound of a toy elicits alertness but no orientation of the head to the sound source. A sound elicits no motion of the infant's hands.
7-8 months	When a toy is removed from the child's grasp, rudimentary behaviour occasionally occurs. The hand moves randomly across the place where contact was lost. The search is brief and unsystematic. A chance encounter with the toy elicits grasping behaviour.	If a toy is removed from a child's grasp prior to the activation of its sound, searching movements will not occur when the sound is turned on, but the hand will open and close. Isolated instances of head turning towards the sound can now be observed. There is no use of sound to track or locate a toy.
8-11 months	Frequent intentional reaching occurs in the locale where the infant lost contact with the toy.	If the toy makes sounds, the infant can occasionally find its location through its sound cue. The fingers move to the sound cue alone. No searching is observed.
11-13months	Search patterns now take into account the place where the lost object had been tactually experienced.	The infant reaches directly to the sound cue alone. The infant pursues an out-of-reach object on the basis of the sound cue alone.

Source: adapted from Fraiberg (1977).

scale will suggest the student's readiness for participation in self-care skills and his ability to act purposively on his environment.

The Construction of Objects in Space scale yields critical evidence of the earliest understanding and development of concepts related to orientation and mobility. This scale assesses such skills as knowing the functional end or side of an object, having an appreciation for gravity, and being able to circumvent obstacles in the environment in order to obtain a toy or reach a desired locale. It is a valuable scale when sign language may be the mode of communication, as it will be imperative to know how the student organizes movements in space and movements related to his own body and posture.

- *The Reynell–Zinkin Scales*

These scales (Reynell 1979) were designed specifically to 'enable professional people concerned with young visually handicapped children to have some guidelines for assessment and developmental advice' (manual, p. 11).

Developmental Range. Two months through five years.

Skills Assessed. Five primary domains are tapped: social adaptation, sensori-motor understanding, exploration of environment, response to sound and verbal comprehension, and expressive language. An additional subscale of communication is provided for assessing the communicative mode of students who are hearing impaired, deaf–blind, cerebral palsied, or have severe verbal language handicaps.

Standardization. Norm referenced.
   The Reynell–Zinkin Scales were standardized on blind and partially sighted children as well as visually impaired multi-handicapped children.

Validity and Reliability. Data are not reported.

Usefulness With Visually Impaired. The Reynell–Zinkin Scales have been a most welcomed addition to the field of assessment. The items are practical and realistic, and clearly delineate between students who are visually impaired and those visually impaired students with additional handicapping conditions. The scales are one of the few resources that assess skills related to orientation and mobility training. The flexibility of the scales permits the evaluator to modify the items as dictated by the student's impairments and still obtain valuable developmental data. Because the age scores were derived from the performance of a wide variety of visually handicapped children, the scores appear to be inflated when compared with scores obtained on other developmental scales. However, having used these scales for two years in conjunction with other assessment tools, the author has found that the scales yield performance profiles that parallel those obtained with other scales. In particular, the author has found the Reynell–Zinkin Scales to correlate with the Maxfield–Buchholz, the Developmental Activities Screening Inventory, and the Griffiths Mental Development Scales (Griffiths 1954).

• *The Griffiths Mental Development Scales*

A set of comprehensive developmental scales (Griffiths 1954, 1970) designed with handicapped as well as normal children in mind.

Developmental Range. Birth to eight years.

Skills Assessed. The Griffiths is divided into five subscales: Locomotor, Personal–Social, Hearing and Speech, Hand and Eye, and Performance.

Standardization. Norm referenced.
   Visually and hearing impaired children were included in the standardization sample as well as children of other natures of handicaps and normal children.

Validity and Reliability.   Data are reported in the manual.

Usefulness With Visually Impaired.   The flexibility of administration and the practicality of the items makes the Griffiths a useful instrument for assessing the needs of the visually impaired. The manual (Griffiths 1954, p. 108) profiles the performance of a deaf and a blind baby. The profile is quite valuable for assisting in the decision as to whether a visually impaired or a hearing impaired student's development is similar to that of other visually or hearing impaired students or is indicative of additional handicaps. The Personal–Social scale employs items related to the development of orientation and mobility skills. Items from the first two years of the scales are minimally dependent on vision with the exception of those within the Eye and Hand Scale. A separate developmental level may be assigned to each scale, thus the Eye and Hand scale can be used as an indicator of the degree of visual impairment and a guide for intervention needs. Scores obtained on the other scales may then reflect a more functional estimate of the visually impaired child's true abilities.

When using the scales with partially sighted children, the evaluator should be cognizant that the picture cards from the Hearing and Speech scale are difficult perceptually for the child due to the poor figure–ground contrast and the abstractness of the designs. When possible, the student should be taken to a concrete representative of the picture. An alternative method, and perhaps more meaningful for a multi-handicapped visually impaired child, is to describe the picture in terms of function. While the response to this adaptation requires a higher level of skill than the original item, it will provide an estimate of the student's classification and functional language abilities.

The Haeussermann Scale of Developmental Potential of Preschool Children

The Haeussermann (1958) is a clinical process for evaluation of adaptive capacity in handicapped children. The Haeussermann is directed toward determining 'whether a student can function in all areas related to learning and to developing and what level he has reached in each area' (manual, p. 61).

Developmental Levels.   Two through six years with directions for assessing lower functioning children.

Skills Assessed.   Sensory processes, fine motor, receptive and expressive communication abilities. Motor planning, concept of self and self-help functions are explored through a structured interview and observation process. Perceptual abilities, the ability to abstract above the level of identity, the ability to arrive at a solution by process of elimination, spatial reconstruction of configuration done mentally, ability to count, the ability to shift from previous mind set, and rate of learning are among other skills and processes assessed.

Standardization. The Haeussermann is a clinical process and does not provide standardization data. Items are norm-referenced.

Twenty-five years of experience with handicapped children including visually and hearing impaired, severely mentally handicapped, and severely physically involved children.

Usefulness With Visually Impaired. While Haeussermann does not specifically address the totally blind child, her manual provides excellent ideas for adapting items and for probing concepts that have direct application for a visually impaired multi-handicapped child and for a non-verbal child. The manual specifies the concepts tapped by each item and suggests numerous innovative ways of eliciting the concept from the child. The tactile, auditory and visual motor screening items are particularly beneficial.

- *The Callier–Azusa Scales*

The Callier–Azusa (Stillman 1978) is a set of structured behaviour checklists designed for assessment of deaf–blind children.

Developmental Range. Birth to 108 months.

Skills Assessed. The Callier–Azusa is composed of five subscales: Socialization, Daily Living Skills, Motor Development, Perceptual Abilities, and Language Development.

Standardization. Norm referenced.

The scales were developed by staff of the Callier Center who had two or more years' experience with deaf–blind children. Stillman (1978, p. 4) reported 'items included (in the scale) would describe normal developmental milestones observable among deaf–blind children'. The scales have been used with deaf–blind children, but not standardized on a deaf–blind population.

Validity and Reliability. None reported as, to date, no standardization has been attempted.

Usefulness With Visually and Hearing Impaired. Although these scales are advocated for use with deaf–blind children, unlike the Reynell–Zinkin Scales, they provide no developmental patterns of these children nor have age scores been adjusted as a result of a deaf–blind population's performance on these scales. Although purported to be sequentially and developmentally based, children exhibit extreme scatter on these scales.

The Perceptual Abilities subscale, in particular reflects a lack of research-based sequentially ordered items. The tactile development section does not consider the evolution of early protopathic or epicritic skills. Examples of expected behaviours are provided for some of the eliciting items but inconsistently reflect either behaviours expected from a normal system or the Callier staff's activities with deaf–blind children. The Motor Development subscales are very well constructed and are the most useful scales.

While individual items and subscales will provide a resource of behaviours to draw upon in an assessment, Stillman (1978) advises that the scales 'must be administered by individuals who are thoroughly familiar with the child's behaviour' and the 'child be observed for at least two weeks' (manual, p. 4). The Callier–Azusa Scales are currently in revision to update and expand their relevance to deaf–blind and multi-handicapped students; see Chapter 15, this volume.

● *The Vulpe Assessment Battery*

The Vulpe (1977) is a 'unified approach to developmental assessment, performance analysis and program planning for atypically developing children' (manual, p. 49).

Developmental Range.   Birth through five years.

Skills Assessed.   The Vulpe is a very comprehensive tool which assesses not only child behaviours but also the state of the environment and care-givers as they relate to the child. Specific subscales include: Basic Senses and Functions, Gross and Fine Motor Skills, Expressive and Receptive Language Skills, Cognitive Processes and Specific Concepts, and Organizational Behaviours.

Standardization.   Norm referenced.
    Multi-handicapped children, including visually impaired.

Validity and Reliability.   Not a standardized test but a 'systematic overview of many aspects of the individual child's pattern of interacting with the world' (Manual, p. 4). Reliability data indicate that the Vulpe can be reliably administered by a variety of child-care professionals to children of different handicapping conditions.

Usefulness With Visually Impaired.   Because the Vulpe was specifically concerned with assessing a child's own specific abilities and nature of interference by the handicapping impairment, its format readily lends itself to a thorough assessment of a visually limited multi-handicapped child. The seven-step scoring procedure permits scoring of the quality of the response, suggests a level of behavioural integration, and facilitates the expression of subtle changes in the child's performance over time. Additionally, the scoring system enables modifications of item administration mode, environment, materials and child's physical status to be recorded quickly and easily.

Very appropriate for the visually impaired multi-handicapped student is the subscale Basic Senses and Functions. Designed to assess behaviours of the central nervous system considered essential to performing any activity: 'This section attempts to provide an organized means to assess the responses of various components of the central nervous system to stimuli, e.g., response of visual, auditory, olfactory, tactile, proprioceptive, kinesthetic and vestibular systems to stimuli' (manual, p. 25). Also included is the assessment of gross motor co-ordination, motor planning, strength, joint range of motion, balance, muscle tone, reflex testing, fine motor co-ordination, and breathing.

The Vulpe is valuable for the assessment of students who are severely impaired with a minimum of overt behaviour responses.

- *The Psychological Stimulus/Response Evaluation for Severely Multiply Handicapped Children (PSR)*

The PSR (Mullen, Danella and Myers 1977) was designed 'to minimize the physical aspects of the tasks while tapping behaviour which demonstrates acquisition of concepts traditionally associated with levels of intellectual development' (p. 2).

Developmental Range. Birth to five years.

Skills Assessed. Three primary components are the Auditory Language scale, the Visual–Motor scale, and the Tactile Differentiation scale. The Auditory–Vocal and the Visual–Motor scales are each divided into four levels of performance.

Standardization. Norm referenced.

Not specific to visually impaired but was constructed for 'severely multiply handicapped children who cannot participate in standardized testing in one or more learning areas' (manual, p. 3).

Validity and Reliability. None reported. The PSR yields a functional age and was developed to provide an estimate of a student's optimal intake and processing channel and most efficient response mode.

Usefulness With Visually Impaired. The first levels of the Visual–Motor scales are excellent for screening the intactness of visual systems. The Auditory–Vocal scale is a sound resource for tapping the visually impaired student's functional hearing and receptive and expressive language ability. The student can respond with vocalizations, head, facial or body movements. Mullen *et al.* suggest that non-verbal children may use a communication board or sign language to receive credit since these modes produce the symbolic equivalent of the spoken word. Items from the Visual–Motor scale may be selected as the needs of the assessment process and visual abilities of the student dictate. Individual levels are assigned for each item. The PSR is best used as a supplement to more comprehensive assessment instruments.

- *The Early Intervention Developmental Profile (EIDP)*

The EIDP (Rogers and D'Eugenio 1977) is a comprehensive assessment for use by either an individual or a multi-disciplinary team for 'planning comprehensive developmental programs for children with all types of handi-caps who function below the 36-month level. It is intended to supplement … standard … evaluation data' (p. 2).

Developmental Range.   Birth to 36 months.

Skills Assessed.   The EIDP is comprised of six scales: Perceptual/Fine Motor, Social/Emotional, Self-Care (feeding, toileting, and dressing/hygiene) and Gross Motor Development.

Standardization.   Norm referenced.
   The manual states that standardization occurred with handicapped children. It is not known whether visually impaired children were included.

Validity and Reliability.   Reported in manual.

Usefulness with Visually Impaired.   The flexibility of administration, assessment setting, and materials enables the evaluator to use the EIDP with a variety of multi-handicapped students. Many of the cognitive items are Piagetian-based and many of the gross motor items are neuro-developmentally based so that components of movement rather than isolated skills are addressed. This approach is valuable when assessing students whose movements have been influenced by sensory impairment.
   The most valuable assets of the EIDP are the stimulation activities which are designed for every item assessed. The activities are complemented with suggestions for implementation with deaf, blind or motorically impaired students.

- *The Adaptive Performance Instrument (API)*

The API (Gentry 1980) evolved from the need for a comprehensive, alternative measurement system for assessing severely and multi-handi-capped students functioning developmentally below two years.

Developmental Range.   Birth to two years.

Skills Assessed.   The API is divided into three booklets which encompass eight separate curricular domains; Physical Intactness, Reflexes and Reactions, Gross Motor, Fine Motor, Self-care, Sensori-motor, Social, and Communication.

Standardization.   Norm referenced.
The API has been used with children who exhibit all natures of handicapping conditions.

Validity and Reliability.   None reported.

Usefulness With Visually Impaired.   The API is a cumbersome, detailed instrument that is best used within a multi-disciplinary framework. However, a wealth of information can be accrued by using it. It purports to assess skills which enable a child to function in the environment and many of the behaviours may be assessed by observation of the student in familiar and routine settings. The major advantages of the API over other instruments are the adaptations which accompany a majority of the items; these, however, are not always appropriate nor detailed enough to assist the evaluator naïve to a specific handicapping condition.

- *The Merrill Palmer Tests of Mental Abilities*

The Merrill Palmer (Stutsman 1931) is a scale of perceptual-motor and language items designed to tap cognitive abilities of young children.

Developmental Range.   Eighteen months through six years.

Skills Assessed.   Sensori-motor problem-solving skills, long and short-term memory, goal directedness, visual-motor integration, gross and fine motor skills, receptive and expressive language abilities, visual sequential skills, seriation and spatial relationships, body image and inductive and deductive reasoning.

Standardization.   Norm referenced.
No sensorily impaired students were included in the standardization sample.

Validity and Reliability.   Reported in manual.

Usefulness With Visually Impaired.   The Merrill Palmer has long been a choice for assessment with multi-handicapped students because of the variety of materials and flexibility in administration and scoring systems. There are quite a number of items that can be administered to a blind child and the majority of the items can be administered non-verbally. The manipulative nature of most items makes this an enjoyable test for students. Adjustments in scoring can be made for items that are refused, omitted or failed because of language difficulties. Drawbacks to the Merrill Palmer are the outdated norms and the time factor of any of the items. However, the Merrill Palmer yields valuable diagnostic data regarding learning style and modality preference as well as being indicative of pre-vocational potential and readiness.

Use of Assessment Scales for Infants and Children With Adolescent and Young Adult Handicapped People

The experiential ranges and cognitive scatter typically seen in older multi-handicapped youth dictate that developmental scales and assessment instruments intended for younger children be used with this group. The compromise to use developmental scales that measure early evolving skills unfortunately often leads to programming that focuses on attainment of infant and pre-school abilities. However, cognizance of the relationship of sensori-motor and pre-operational abilities to the development of self-care, motor planning, communication and social skills leads to chronologically appropriate instructional goals and methodologies (McLean, Snyder–McLean, Rowland and Jacobs 1981).

Selection of instrumentation for the older student must consider the aetiology, onset and extent of sensory impairments. Often older students have developed a functional language and communication system prior to the onset of a significant hearing or vision loss. Knowledge of the types of experiences the student had prior to the sensory loss will affect interpretation of the student's performance and, subsequently, the design of instructional priorities.

Evoking behaviours directly relevant to functional life, work and leisure skills is of foremost importance in the assessment of older students. Regardless of which instruments are administered, the evaluator must be able to collect data on the student's knowledge of objects and of how he uses objects as tools to accomplish a desired result. These two skills are basic to the development of self-care behaviours. Langley (1980a) found that some level of left-to-right movement orientation, discrimination, one-to-one correspondence, sequential, spatial and motor planning abilities was critical to the development of sheltered workshop-type behaviours (i.e. matching, sorting, packaging). Observations of the conditions in which the student is happiest, the types of media he most often relates to, and activities he is most likely to initiate, either spontaneously or selected in a forced choice situation, will indicate some notion of a leisure and work orientation towards which the student should be directed. Ecological assessments and observations (Carlson, Scott and Eklund 1980; Smith 1980) add valuable supplementary information to the assessment of the older student for whom many tasks found in infant and pre-school scales are inappropriate.

When it is anticipated that the student may function in some type of sheltered work environment, an ecological assessment will help the evaluator gather beneficial data against which to assess the student. Observations of several vocational settings can determine the nature of skills and expectations that will be demanded of the student. The evaluator, then, can arrange similar tasks within the assessment to look at the student's potential to develop expected behaviours. Mithaug, Hagmeier and Haring (1977) have constructed a thorough checklist of behaviours severely handicapped clients should exhibit for entrance into a sheltered workshop. Langley (1980a) described a hierarchy of pre-vocational abilities and tasks exemplary of each hierarchical phase that evolved from her work with older severely handicapped visually impaired students. An excellent resource for observing and analysing a student's performance in work experience is the *San Francisco Vocational Competency Scale* (Levine and Elzey 1968).

A Systematic Approach to Vocational Education (Wadler 1983) is a curriculum developed for moderately and severely handicapped students at the Florida School for Deaf and Blind. It is divided into four areas that may serve as an adjunct to assessment. The curriculum has been used success-fully with deaf–blind multi-handicapped students.

Becker, Schur and Paoletti-Schelp (1983) published a criterion and norm-referenced instrument designed to assess life skills of deaf–blind students ten years of age and older: *The Basic Life Skills Screening Inventory* (BLSSI). The BLSSI assesses physical functioning, personal management, home management, community living, language, work habits and behaviours, responsibility/social maturity, maladaptive behaviour, and an actual work sample (nut and bolt assembly and/or ballpoint pen assembly). Each assessment item is divided into three priority levels: priority 1, beginning formal vocational and life skills training; priority 2, skills required for sheltered workshop and supervised living; priority 3, skills for competitive employment and independent living.

Other instruments that offer insight into pre-vocational, vocational, social, and adaptive behaviours of multi-handicapped students, and practical and age-appropriate teaching suggestions are described below.

- *The Lakeland Village Adaptive Behavior Grid*

The Grid (1976) is a performance-based checklist of adaptive behaviour designed for assessing skills, training needs and progress of institutional clients.

Developmental Range.   Birth through 16 years.

Skills Assessed.   The Grid consists of ten skill clusters: eating, toileting; dressing; health and grooming; communicating; mobility and dexterity; vocation and recreation; socialization; orientation; behaviour control.

Standardization.   Norm referenced.
The Grid was standardized on an institutional population of mentally handicapped clients whose average developmental level was approximately four years. It is not known whether sensorily impaired clients were included in the standardization sample.

Validity and Reliability.   Reported in manual.

Usefulness With Visually Impaired.   The Grid's primary advantages over other scales of adaptive behaviour are:

1.   items in all clusters extend down to birth;
2.   individual developmental levels can be assigned to each cluster;
3.   items can be scored through interview of care-givers or direct observation.

The clusters of orientation, vocation and recreation are particularly useful for determining potential for vocational development. The items on the Grid focus on behaviours necessary for social interaction and independence and thus are concerned with how the student functions in the environment regardless of sensory impairment. The weakest cluster is that of communication although it addresses the use of gestures and signs.

- *The Maxfield–Buchholz Scale of Social Maturity for Preschool Blind Children*

This scale (Maxfield and Buchholz 1957) is an adaptation of the Vineland Social Maturity Scale.

Developmental Range.   Birth through five years.

Skills Assessed.   Seven categories of social development are assessed: General Items of Personal–Social Growth, Dressing, Eating, Communication, Locomotion, Socialization and Occupation.

Standardization.   Norm referenced.
Based on the performance profiles of legally blind and partially seeing children.

Validity and Reliability.   None reported.

Usefulness With Visually Impaired. Most appropriately used with students who have vision as one, if not the primary, handicapping condition. The evaluator can compare visually impaired children with other visually impaired children to determine whether social development is evolving at a rate expected for his age. When used with older students, an estimate of his functioning level in adaptive behaviour skills may be obtained. The authors caution: 'It is important to keep in mind that this is not a test of intelligence. Its level of expected performance is based on what blind children are actually found to do at different age levels. Capacity to do is not measured except indirectly' (manual, p. 11).

The scale may be used with deaf–blind if vision is significantly affected. As the scale is developed to be an interview scale administered to a primary care-giver, scores obtained often tend to be inflated. A more accurate reflection of the student's abilities may be obtained through direct observation of the student. When used in conjunction with the Reynell–Zinkin Scales, a global view of the most consistent behaviours within the student's repertoire is achieved.

- *The Reading–Free Vocational Interest Inventory*

The Inventory (Becker 1975) is a non-reading picture vocational preference test for use with older, mentally handicapped students. 'The Inventory was devised to provide systematic information on the interest patterns of mentally retarded males and females engaged in occupations at the unskilled and semi-skilled levels' (manual, p. 1).

Developmental Range. Suggested for educable mentally handicapped students at the high school level, grades nine through twelve.

Skills Assessed. The Inventory has both a male and a female form. Female interest areas include 'laundry service', 'light industrial' and 'personal service', while male areas include 'automotive', 'building trades' and 'animal care'.

Standardization. Separate norms for public (state) school and for institutions.

Used with public (state) and institutional populations of educable mentally handicapped students. It is not known whether students with sensory deficits were included in the sample.

Validity and Reliability. Reported in manual.

Usefulness With Visually and Hearing Impaired. The student points to one of three pictures which represent the type of work he would enjoy. If the student is partially sighted the evaluator can verbally describe the pictures to augment the student's perceptions. If totally blind, the student can respond verbally to the choices. Although a few jobs could be performed by blind students, the majority of the jobs could be executed by partially sighted students. One strong asset of this scale is its potential to distinguish between preferences for mechanical vs. people-orientated vocations.

Subtests from previously mentioned comprehensive measures can be used to provide additional data on adaptive behaviour. The Personal–Social scale from the Griffiths, the Social Adaptation and Exploration of the Environment scales from the Reynell–Zinkin, and selected subscales from the EMR and TMR Performance Profiles are particularly useful for observations of the older student's ability to function in daily life activities.

Assessment of Language and Communication

While the focus of this chapter is the psychological assessment of visually impaired populations, understanding the relationships among social, cognitive and linguistic processes is mandatory. The performance of visually impaired populations is significantly affected by severe language and communication deficits. It is not unusual for multi-handicapped students to have a fairly large vocabulary of words or signs but still not be able to initiate or maintain an exchange in a communicative interaction. Muma (1978) explained that form is secondary to function and that only after a student has established a purpose for communication should one be concerned with the efficiency of the student's ability to encode his message. To appreciate the significance of Muma's statement, one only has to observe an echolalic blind child who expresses, out of context, previous dormitory incidents in complex syntactical constructions but who never spontaneously or appropriately communicates hunger, pain or a desire for social interaction. Echolalic and 'verbalism' (Harley 1963) tendencies have frequently been associated with visually impaired children but hearing impaired multi-handicapped students exhibit the same characteristics when learning sign language (Langley 1984). Multi-handicapped students seem to acquire the basic problem-solving processes necessary to learn and store labels but lack the interpersonal social–causal relationships critical for initiating a communicative interaction (Dunst 1981; Brown and Langley 1984). While a formal speech/language/communication assessment is the role of the speech pathologist, the psychologist and teacher must address issues related to the development of functional communicative abilities. Such issues are concerned with determining whether the student can or has established meaningful relationships with people at some level, whether he understands his potential to direct others to do things for him, whether he truly appreciates the functional uses of common objects, and whether he can use those objects to attract an adult or a peer's attention or to use people to help him identify and use novel objects in the way they are intended to be acted upon. These concerns can be woven into the assessment process as the child is engaged in formal and informal tasks of social development, independence and cognitive development. Communication patterns of visually impaired (Fraiberg 1977; Warren 1977) and hearing-impaired (Stuckless and Birch 1966; Meadow 1968 and Wilbur 1979) have been well documented and should be used as references against which to index a sensorily impaired (Fraiberg 1977; Warren 1977) and hearing-impaired (Stuckless adapted to a verbal or a sign mode (Davis 1977) but a few scales deserve special attention as they have been designed specifically for more severely impaired students. Consultation with a speech pathologist as to a student's communicative performance should be an active and essential responsibility.

- *The Receptive Expressive Language Assessment for the Visually Impaired (RELA)*

The RELA (Anderson 1977), constructed for visually impaired infants and pre-primary children, evolved from the need for a measurement that did not rely on 'responses and reactions to visual clues and materials' (manual, preface).

Developmental Range.   Birth through six years.

Skills Assessed.   Auditory awareness; imitation; vocalization; vocabulary, receptively and expressively; knowledge of object use; concept of body image, numbers, environmental sounds, size, position, texture and length; direction following; verbal reasoning; short-term memory; past and future tense, and pluralization.

Standardization.   Norm referenced.
    Intended for use with severely visually impaired and blind children.

Validity and Reliability.   No information is reported.

Usefulness With Visually Impaired.   The RELA is very useful when one is confronted with a totally blind child. While a set of materials has been produced for use with the scale, the materials can be easily assembled from household objects or the local hardware store. The most valuable components are items that address the use, association and function of objects in the child's environment. Of concern is the omission of structured opportunities to assess how the student communicates interpersonally or directs the actions of others. As this is a major gap in the language development of many visually impaired and particularly multihandicapped students, it is crucial to have some information about this aspect. The RELA is best used to supplement other information.

- *The Gestural Assessment of Thought and Expression (GATE)*

The GATE (Langley 1984) was designed to assess a student's cognitive and social readiness for, and development of, a gestural mode of communication.

Developmental Range.   Birth through three years.

Skills Assessed.   Seven components of non-verbal communication are assessed: turn-taking, signalling, object permanence, social–causality, imitation, behaviours relating to objects, and sign behaviour.

Standardization.   Norm referenced.
   Normal hearing infants and pre-schoolers, deaf–blind, multi-sensorily disabled, and severely mentally handicapped students were included in the standardization sample.

Validity and Reliability.   Reported in manual.

Usefulness With Visually Impaired.   The GATE was designed for use with the multi-sensorily disabled and other multi-handicapped children, for recording the most rudimentary to the most sophisticated gestural mode of communication. Where necessary, adaptations are provided for the totally blind child. The GATE is administered by directly eliciting target behaviours and by observing the student in familiar environments over a period no longer than five days. The performance profile is used for selecting instructional objectives and activities that accompany the manual.

- *The Uzgiris–Hunt Scales*

Three scales of the U–H Scales (Uzgiris and Hunt 1975) are particularly relevant for the assessment of pragmatic communicative abilities: Causality, Behaviours Relating to Objects, and Imitation (see earlier description of Uzgiris–Hunt Scales).

- *The Generic Skills Assessment Inventory*

The Generic Inventory (McLean, Snyder-McLean, Rowland and Jacobs 1981) is a prescriptive assessment tool whose content reflects a model of language, communication and related skills that is hierarchical and generic in nature.

Developmental Range.   Birth through 24 months.

Skills Assessed.   The Generic Inventory is divided into People skills and Object skills assessed across four levels of performance on five scales: Object Relationships, Representation, Dyadic Interaction, Expressive Communication and Comprehension and Imitation.

Standardization. Norm referenced.

The Generic Inventory was developed for non-verbal and language impaired severely handicapped students. It is not known whether students with specific sensory impairments were included in the norming sample.

Validity and Reliability. Not reported.

Usefulness With Visually Impaired. The Generic Inventory is an excellent tool to be used by an interdisciplinary team. It allows great flexibility in administration as the authors recognized that structured testing procedures are the least effective with severely handicapped. Scoring can accommodate individual differences of students. Specific age scores are not obtained, but levels of competency in the five areas can be pinpointed.

Translation of Assessment Data Into Intervention Priorities

Perhaps the most difficult component of any assessment is deciding what the data mean and what to do with them. Typically, a student is tested primarily for making school placement decisions, a score or performance level is assigned, and the report filed away. What and how to teach, however, should be the direct outcomes from an assessment. Specifically, the following information should be addressed in the results and interpretations section of an assessment report:

1. Delineation of ranges of performance in all areas assessed.
2. Performance strengths and deficits and hypothesis as to why the student performed as he did and why there may be gaps in skills, and discrepancies in performance of similar skills.
3. Specification of the student's learning style, primary learning modality, conditions under which he learned optimally, and learning rate.
4. Suggestions as to situations, materials, contexts and time frames which will elicit optimum performance.
5. Suggestions as to types of students with whom he should learn and interact.
6. Types of related personnel and services required to optimize developmental potential (resource vision or hearing teacher, occupational or physical therapist, direct speech and language services, specialized equipment and transportation).
7. Suggested intervention priorities, goals and objectives.

Armed with this data, a teacher should easily be able to design an individual teaching plan and the assessment becomes an ongoing process rather than an end result tucked away in a drawer.

Summary

A process-orientated multivariant assessment is a systematic approach to synthesizing how and why a multi-sensorily disabled student behaves as he does. Such an approach permits an eclectic data base obtained from structured and unstructured observations and a variety of assessment methodologies. The key to a process-orientated assessment is awareness of the implications of sensory impairments on development, of appropriate assessment instrumentation, and of how and when to apply it. The process yields information about a student that will be immediately relevant to enhancing developmental progress and it ensures that no student is 'untestable'.

References

Adelson, E. and Fraiberg, S. (1974) 'Gross motor development in infants blind from birth', *Child Development, 45*, 114-26

Anderson, G.M. (1977) *Receptive expressive emergent language assessment for the visually impaired 0-6*, Ingham Intermediate School District, Mason, Michigan

Barraga, N.C. and Morris, J. (1978) *Program to develop efficiency in visual functioning*, American Printing House for the Blind, Louisville, Ky

Becker, H., Schur, G and Paoletti-Schelp, M. (1983) *The Basic Life Skills Screening Inventory: An instrument to assess vocational readiness in the Deaf-blind developmentally disabled*, South Central Regional Deaf-Blind Center, Dallas, Texas

Becker, R.L. (1975) *A.A.M.D.—Becker Reading—Free Vocational Interest Inventory*, American Association on Mental Deficiency, Washington DC

Bower, T.G.R. (1977) *Development in Infancy*, Freeman, San Francisco, Col.

Brown, C. and Langley, M.B. (1984) 'The diagnostic—prescriptive model for training interdisciplinary personnel working with profoundly handicapped learners', Project, Bureau of Education for Exceptional Students, Tallahassee, Florida

Budoff, M. (1973) *Learning potential and educability among educable mentally retarded* (Progress report, Grant OEG-0-8-08056-4597 from National Institute of Education, NEW), Research Institute for Educational Problems, Cambridge, MA

Burlingham, D. (1965) 'Some problems of ego development in blind children', *Psychoanalytic Study of the Child, 20*, 194-208

Carlson, C.I., Scott, M. and Eklund, S.J. (1980) 'Ecological theory and method for behavioural assessment', *School Psychology Review, IX*, 75-82

Danella, E.A. (1973) 'Tactile preference in multiply handicapped children', *The American Journal of Occupational Therapy, 27*, 457-63

Davis, J.M. (1977) *Reliability of hearing-impaired childrens responses to oral and total presentations of the Test of Auditory of Language*

DuBose, R.F., Langley, M.B. and Stagg, V. (1977) 'Assessing severely handicapped children', *Focus on Exceptional Children, 9*, 1-15

Dunst, C.J. (1981) *Infant Learning: A Cognitive-linguistic Approach*, Teaching Resources Division of Developmental Learning Materials, Allen, Texas

Faye, E. (1970) *Low Vision*, Charles C. Thomas, Springfield, Ill.

Fewell, R.R. and Langley, M.B. *The developmental activities screening inventory, II.* Austin, Texas: Pro-Ed Corporation, 1984

——, —— and Roll, A. (1982) 'Informant versus direct screening: A preliminary comparative study', *Diagnostique, 7*, 163-7

Fraiberg, S. (1977) *Insights from the Blind*, Basic Books, New York

Freedman, D.G. (1964) 'Smiling in blind infants and the issue of innate vs acquired', *Journal of Child Psychology and Psychiatry*, 5, 171-84

Fuerstein, R. (1970) 'A dynamic approach to the causation, prevention and alleviation of retarded performance' in H.C. Haywood (ed.), *Social Cultural Aspects of Mental Retardation*, Appleton Century Crofts, New York

Gentry, D. (ed.) (1980) *The Adaptive Performance Inventory*, University of Idaho, Moscow, Idaho

Griffiths, R. (1954) *The Abilities of Babies*, Association for Research in Infant & Child Development, Great Britain

—— (1970) *The Abilities of Young Children*. Child Development Research Centre, London

Haeussermann, E. (1958) *Developmental Potential for Preschool Children*, Grune and Stratton, New York

Harley, R.K. (1963) *Verbalism among Blind Children*, Research Series, No. 10, American Foundation for the Blind

Hart, V. (1978) 'Motor development in blind children' in M.E. Mulholland and M.Z. Wurster (eds.), *Help me become everything I can be*, Proceedings of the North American Conference on Visually Handicapped Infants and Preschool Children, American Foundation for the Blind, Minneapolis, MN.

Hill, E.E., Rosen, S., Correa, V.I. and Langley, M.B. (1984) 'Pre-school Orientation and Mobility: An expanded definition', *Education of the Visually Handicapped, 16*(2), 58-72

Kukla, D. and Connolly, T. (1978) *Assessment of Auditory Functioning of Deaf–blind/Multihandicapped Children*, South Central Regional Center for Services to Deaf–blind Children, Dallas, TX.

Langley, M.B. (1980a) *Assessment of multihandicapped visually impaired learners*, Stoelting Co, Chicago, Ill.

—— (1980b) *Functional Vision Inventory for the Multiple and Severely Handicapped*, Stoelting Co., Chicago, Ill.

—— (1984) 'The gestural approach to thought and expression: An index to nonverbal communicative behaviors', mimeographed, Nina Harris Exceptional Education Center, St Petersburg, Fl.

—— and Brown, C. (1983) 'A diagnostic–prescriptive program for profoundly mentally handicapped learners: A model for training interdisciplinary personnel', *Counterpoint*, May/June, 3

Levine, S. and Elzey, F.K. (1968) *San Francisco Vocational Competency Scale*, The Psychological Corporation, New York

Lidz, C.S. (1983) 'Dynamic assessment and the preschool child', *Journal of Psychoeducational Assessment*, 1, 59-72

McLean, J., Snyder-McLean, L., Rowland, C. and Jacobs, (1981) *Process-oriented Educational Programs for the Severely/Profoundly Handicapped Adolescent*, Bureau of Child Research, University of Kansas, Parsons Research Center, Parsons, Ks.

Maxfield, K.E. and Buchholz, S.B. (1957) *A Social Maturity Scale for Blind Preschool Children*, American Foundation for the Blind, New York

Meadow, K. (1968) 'Early manual communication in relation to the deaf child's intellectual, social and communicative functioning', *American Annals of the Deaf, 113*, 29-41

Mori, A.A. and Olive, J.E. (1978) 'The blind and visually handicapped mentally retarded: Suggestions for intervention in infancy', *Journal of Visual Impairment and Blindness, 72*, 273-9

Miller, L. (1982) *The Miller Assessment of Preschoolers*, KID Foundation, Colorado

Miller, L.R. (1977) 'Abilities structure of congenitally blind persons: A factor analysis', *Journal of Visual Impairment & Blindness, 71*, 145-53

Mithaug, D.E., Hagmeier, E. and Haring, N. (1977) 'The relationship between training activities and job placement in vocational education of the severely and profoundly handicapped', *American Association for the Education of the Severely/Profoundly Handicapped, 2*, 37-49

Mullen, E.M., Danella, E. and Myers, M. (1977) *Psychological S-R Evaluation for severely multiple handicapped children*, Meeting Street School, East Providence, R.I.

Muma, J.R. (1978) *Language Handbook: Concepts Assessment, Intervention*, Prentice-Hall, Inc., Englewood Cliffs, NJ

Northern, J.L. and Downs, M.T. (1978) *Hearing in Children* (2nd ed.), Williams and Wilkins, Baltimore, Md.

Ohwaki, S. and Stayton, S. (1976) 'Preference by the retarded for vibratory and visual stimulation as a function of mental age and psychotic reaction', *Journal of Abnormal Psychology, 85*, 576-82

Reynell, J. (1979) *The Reynell–Zinkin Scales: Developmental scales for young visually handicapped children — Part 1: Mental development*, NFER, Slough

Rogers, S.J. and D'Eugenio, D.B. (1977) *Developmental Programming for Infants and Young Children: Assessment and Application*, University of Michigan Press, Ann Arbor, Michigan

Sanford, A.R. (1975) *Learning Accomplishment Profile-Diagnostic edition*, Kaplan Press, Winston-Salem, N.C.

Schucman, H. (1957) 'A study in the learning ability of the severely retarded: a method for obtaining a quantitative index of the educability for severely mentally retarded children', unpublished dissertation, New York University

Scott, E.P., Jan, J.E. and Freeman, R.D. (1977) *Can't Your Child See?* University Park Press, Baltimore, Md.

Sheridan, M.D. (1973) *Children's Developmental Progress from Birth to Five Years: The STYCAR Sequences*, NFER, Slough

Simmeonson, R.J., Huntington, G.S. and Parse, S.A. (1980) 'Assessment of children with severe handicaps: Multiple problems — multi-variate goals', *Journal of the Association for the Severely Handicapped, 5*, 55-72

Smith, C.R. (1980) 'Assessment alternatives: Non-standardized procedure', *School Psychology Review, IX*, 46-57

Stephens, W.B., Fitzgerald, J., Hitt, J. and Grube, C. (1980) *Student activity guide: A Piagetian perspective*, Stoelting Co., Chicago, Ill.

Stillman, R. (1978) *Assessment of Deaf--Blind Children: The Callier–Azusa Scale*, Council for Exceptional Children, Reston, Va.

—— *The Callier-Azusa Assessment Tool*, Revised. Dallas, Texas: Callier Center for Speech and Hearing, in preparation.

Stuckless, E. and Birch, J. (1966) 'The influence of early manual communication on the linguistic development of deaf children', *American Annals of the Deaf, 111*, 542-604

Stutsman, R. (1931) *Merrill Palmer Scale of Mental Tests*, Stoelting Co., Chicago, Ill.

Sullivan, P.M. and Vernon, M. (1979) 'Psychological assessment of hearing impaired children', *School Psychology Digest, 8*, 271-90

The Lakeland Village Adaptive Behavior Grid (1976), Lakeland Village, Medical Lake Washington

Uzgiris, I.C. and Hunt, J. McV. (1975) *Assessment in Infancy: Ordinal Scales of Psychological Development*, University of Illinois Press, Urbana, Ill.

Vander Kolk, C.J. (1977) 'Intelligence testing for visually impaired persons', *Journal of Visual Impairment & Blindness, 71*, 158-63

Vernon, M. (1967) 'A guide for the psychological evaluation of deaf and severely hard of hearing adults', *The Deaf American, 19*, 9

—— and Green, D. (1980) 'A guide to the psychological assessment of deaf-blind adults', *Journal of Visual Impairment and Blindness, 74*, 229-31

Vulpe, S.G. (1977) *Vulpe Assessment Battery*, National Institute on Mental Retardation, Toronto, Ontario, Canada

Wadler, F. (1983) *Systematic approach to vocational education*, Florida School for the Deaf and Blind, St Augustine, Fl.

Warren, D.H. (1976a) 'Blindness and early development: Issues in research methodology', *The New Outlook for the Blind, 70*, 53-60

—— (1976b) 'Blindness and early development: what is known and what needs to be studied', *The New Outlook for the Blind, 70*, 5-16

—— (1977) *Blindness and Early Childhood Development*, American Foundation for the Blind, New York

—— (1978) 'Childhood visual impairment: Sources and uses of knowledge', *Journal of Visual Impairment and Blindness, 72*, 404-11.

Wilbur, R.B. (1979) *American Sign Language and Sign Systems*, University Park Press, Baltimore, Md.

14 PSYCHOLOGICAL ASSESSMENT OF THE HEARING IMPAIRED, ADDITIONALLY IMPAIRED AND MULTI-HANDICAPPED DEAF

David E. Bond

Introduction

Survey reports on the prevalence of hearing-impaired people who are inappropriately placed in facilities for the mentally handicapped (Tempowski, Felstead and Simon 1974; Kropka 1979; Kropka and Williams 1980) and reports of clinical experience with inappropriately assessed and placed hearing impaired (Vernon and Brown 1964; Vernon 1967a; Bond 1979, 1981) appear to suggest that misdiagnosis and inadequate assessment techniques continue to occur in intervention with the hearing impaired. In clinical and field experience with the hearing impaired, particularly those hearing persons who have additional impairments or handicaps (e.g. handicap arising through physical, visual, cultural and environmental impairments), unsuitable placement and intervention frequently arises through inadequate psychometric assessment techniques, and assumptions which are not relevant to hearing impairment. Uninformed or inappropriate recommendations and advice may result in placement of hearing-impaired people in environments where the hearing-impaired person's needs and ability are unique and cannot be adequately met. Inappropriate placement may endanger the behaviour, cognitive performance, mental health and development of the hearing-impaired person.

Reasons for unsuitable assessment may be understood in terms of inadequacies in training, experience, knowledge or in relation to logistic problems of inadequate provision of psychologists, facilities, non-availability of consultant services or personnel. However valid these reasons may be, the needs of the client group must be paramount in psychological diagnosis, assessment, intervention and advice. The psychologist needs to be more than a 'tester' when working with any client group, particularly those whose needs and abilities are as heterogeneous and as complex as the needs and abilities of those who are hearing impaired (see Levine 1981). Consequently it is appropriate to outline general principles which psychologists should take into consideration when working with the hearing impaired, including work with clients from both the overall population of the hearing impaired, and from those who have additional impairments or handicaps.

297

PRINCIPLES IN PSYCHOLOGICAL INTERVENTION WITH THE HEARING-IMPAIRED CLIENT

1. Psychological and other tests, observational, behavioural, and systems analysis, information gathering and other techniques are among the repertoire of procedures which psychologists should use systematically and objectively to investigate the client's needs and abilities, and the environment in which the client functions. This systematic and objective investigation should lead to identification and diagnosis of problems, abilities and needs; formulation and testing of hypotheses relating to potential cause and extent of difficulties and abilities; and the formulation of possible solutions, treatment or other intervention procedures to meet the needs of the client or the client group.

2. Psychological tests involving the use of verbal language, including written language, or which are based on norms solely derived with hearing populations, are not usually valid in use with the hearing impaired, as verbally based tests usually measure linguistic limitations arising from hearing impairment and not the measure for which the test was originally designed (Vernon 1969; Levine 1981). Some tests which appear non-verbal may still penalize the hearing impaired, as skills in verbal reasoning may be necessary to perform the non-verbal function, e.g. visual analogous reasoning, sequencing of picture stories (see Myklebust 1964).

3. Even when a client has only a mild hearing loss, or when the hearing-impaired client's speech appears intelligible and linguistic structures appear intact, it would appear crucial that non-verbal measures standardized on, and appropriate to, the hearing impaired are used. Slight fluctuating or mild hearing impairment may significantly distort verbal understanding and reception (Hamilton and Owrid 1974; Webster, Saunders and Bamford 1984) and consequently significantly depress function on verbal tests, in comparison with function on non-verbal tests.

4. Psychologists and other 'assessors' or 'interveners' should recognize:

    (i) The hearing-impaired population is essentially heterogeneous with a wide diversity of needs, ability, additional impairments, and handicaps. Consequently there may be needs, abilities or difficulties which do not necessarily arise through hearing impairment and which may be found in other groups in the 'hearing' population (Bond 1979; 1981).

    (ii) Within the population of the hearing impaired there are groups who have common needs and may have an above-average incidence of additional difficulties. Where the aetiology of hearing impairment involves trauma factors such as Rubella, anoxia, meningitis, etc., the possibility of the client having additional impairments increases significantly (Vernon 1967b, 1969; Van Dijk 1982; Bond 1982,

1984). In addition some groups who show other primary handicaps or impairments, such as Down's syndrome clients, may show a significantly higher prevalence of hearing impairment (Lloyd 1970; Balkany 1980; Bond 1982). Psychological assessment and intervention with clients who have one or more additional impairments may necessitate creativity and imagination in psychological assessment in order to achieve measures which are valid in relation to the clients' abilities and functions. Assessment and intervention which fails to take into consideration the aetiology and additional impairments which a hearing-impaired client may have is at best naïve and may be totally irrelevant and damaging to the client and his needs.

5. The results of psychological, educational or any other tests, and method of analysis, should be checked and validated against other and local criteria wherever possible. It is useful to use at least two measures of general ability when assessing a hearing-impaired client — at least one test should measure function on untimed or 'power' tasks with the other measuring function on timed or 'speed' tasks. It is possible for the hearing-impaired client to function poorly on normatively standardized measures or on one particular type of test task (e.g. speed tasks) and yet to function at a significantly different level in relation to different tests (e.g. power tasks) or in a different environment.

6. Tests used by psychologists or individuals who are inexperienced in working with the hearing impaired tend to be subject to appreciably greater error than tests used by those who are experienced and familiar with the hearing impaired (Vernon 1967a). It would appear important that psychologists have at least consultative availability of psychologists who have experience and training in working with the hearing impaired.

7. Results from group assessment of the hearing impaired should be regarded with caution; at best, group testing should only be regarded as a screening technique (Vernon 1969).

PURPOSES OF ASSESSMENT OF THE HEARING IMPAIRED

Reasons for referral of hearing-impaired clients for psychological assessment are as varied as the reasons for referral of hearing clients. As with the hearing client referred for assessment or treatment, analysis of the reasons or motivation for referral, initial analysis of background to referral, and the circumstances in which the referral was made may lead appropriately to a completely different type of assessment and intervention than that expected by the referring agency. Again the primary aim of the psychologist must be to assess, diagnose and advise on the client's needs. Cases referred to the writer with requests for 'individual psychological assessment', 'behavioural assessment' and 'behaviour modification advice' have on occasions (following assessment including behavioural and systems analysis) led to advice/recommendations to modify or alter management, staffing, systems, communication, curriculum and organization with a much more positive overall and long-term effect than simple individual assessment and treatment would have achieved.

Psychological assessment may well take different forms according to the reasons for assessment. In general there would appear to be six main reasons for psychological assessment which have been identified by various writers (Vernon 1969; Levine 1981; Vernon and Alles 1982). The following list is based on the above works and on clinical and applied experience:

1. survey information to identify groups with common needs — to assist in initial establishment or organization of provision to meet basic common needs;
2. aids in planning future facilities, treatment, rehabilitation, education, curriculum, staff provision and training;
3. placement i.e. in facilities, environments, groups to meet common or special needs such as communication, behavioural, educational or other needs;
4. diagnosis of specific learning problems, psycho-neurological disorders, behavioural, emotional, intellectual problems;
5. prediction of future performance and curricular or behavioural and other management needs; guide to intervention strategies such as counselling and guidance, vocational training;
6. assessment of change over time, to evaluate both learning skills, motivation and capacity of the individual, and the effects and effectiveness of intervention, environments, management, programmes and procedures.

The reasons for psychological assessment and intervention are obviously inter-related. Thus the psychologist who has clients referred primarily for assessment may well be in a position over time to identify groups with common treatment needs or to comment on the relative effectiveness or otherwise of different placements, treatment programmes, or intervention techniques in relation to specific individual difficulties and needs. To be effective in assessment the psychologist working with the hearing impaired should be aware of factors related to hearing impairment and familiar with factors which affect the hearing impaired.

HEARING IMPAIRMENT AND ADDITIONAL IMPAIRMENTS OR MULTIPLE HANDICAPS

Identification and classification of individuals in terms of additional impairments or multiple handicaps often appear to reflect more the nature and state of the total environment, than the degree or nature of the impairment; i.e. in an environment of manually communicating hearing-impaired persons, the non-manually communicating, hearing, talking person might be considered impaired or handicapped.

The communication philosophy and practice would appear to be a significant factor in determining classification; in many cases, non-oral/aural hearing-impaired clients may be classified as multi-handicapped in view of their communication difficulties in aural/oral communication (non-signing) systems. These clients may be inappropriately assigned to facilities for the language-disordered, the intellectually handicapped or the psychiatrically ill. Many cases who have these apparent problems are inappropriately placed, yet when thoroughly assessed and placed in environments where peers and personnel communicate through a common sign language (including total communication in which sign, speech and amplification through hearing aids are used simultaneously), may function as a hearing-impaired person who needs total communication and who has no additional handicaps or impairments.

The writer finds it useful to use several groups in which hearing-impaired people with additional impairments have similar needs. These were originally derived from groups outlined by Murphy (1977) and adapted in subsequent papers by the writer (Bond 1979, 1982, 1984).

1. The hearing-impaired child who may have slight or significant additional impairments which do not significantly interfere with his function or success in his/her environment, e.g. in one case, a hearing-impaired girl (severely deaf with visual problems including congenital nystagmus and myopia) coped quite successfully, in a mainstream education programme — yet her combined hearing and visual impairments were substantial.
2. The child who is additionally impaired by exogenous factors such as late diagnosis, bilingual background, inappropriate expectations by those managing the child, inappropriate educational placement, and inappropriate methods of communication.
3. The child with a primary severe hearing loss who has hidden specific learning disabilities, including neuro-muscular and/or aphasoid behaviours as described by Vernon (1967b), Murphy (1977), Bond (1979, 1982, 1984), van Uden (1980, 1981).
4. The child with severe multiple handicaps which adversely affect learning, such as physical, visual, physiological, emotional, behavioural, intellectual, and which are likely to necessitate shelter or care throughout the individual's life.

Groups 1 and 2: Minor Additional Impairments

The psychologist who is aware of special assessment requirements, needs of, and provision for the hearing impaired, and who carries out a systematic, thorough and objective investigation, should be able to identify the major abilities, difficulties and needs of the first two groups.

Group 3: Hidden Learning Difficulties

As Murphy (1977) indicated, the group which is the easiest to overlook contains those who have hidden learning impairments. In cases of hidden impairments additional handicaps may result through inappropriate intervention and placement, particularly placement in environments where the individual is unable to communicate and experiences a high level of failure and/or rejection.

The writer has previously outlined features of behaviour commonly found, in clinical and applied experience, in hearing-impaired clients who have hidden learning impairments (Bond 1979, 1982, 1984). These difficulties tend to occur in various combinations of some or all of the following areas:

Perceptual, Memory Processing, Cognitive

1. Visual spatial, perception, planning and organization: e.g. Copying drawings-designs, copying patterns, jigsaw assembly tasks, complex block assembly tasks.
2. Imitation, e.g. of movement, rhythmical patterns.
3. Short-term visual memory for spatial information such as memory of position, size, number, shape, designs.
4. Short-term visual memory for sequences of information such as memory for digits, words, pictures, colours, bead patterns, designs, patterns of movement.
5. Visual learning and hand–eye co-ordination, e.g. repetitive copying tasks.
6. Visual analogous and associative reasoning tasks.
7. Sequencing visual information as in size shape, number, pictorial sequences, etc.

Neuro-muscular, Behavioural, Emotional

1. Visual attention span, poor concentration, variable motivation, easily distracted. Limited span for receptive communication or information.
2. Attention-seeking, attention demanding, possibly manipulative in attempts to evoke or provoke adverse reactive behaviour from others. May require less sleep than peers.

3. Difficulties in interpersonal relationships.
4. Impulsive with no or little obvious control over self, possibly over-reactive; low tolerance of stress or frustration.
5. Muscular rigidity, tension.
6. Involuntary motor behaviour, e.g. tremors, jerks, twitches.
7. Clumsiness; early developmental history of falling, being bruised, dropping objects, etc.
8. Anxiety, nervous tics, particularly when doing e.g. schoolwork, pencil and paper work, reading, maths.
9. Poor or inadequate self-concept, lacking in confidence, possibly withdrawn, and may become easily depressed.

Educational

1. Failure and frustration in some approaches to communication, e.g. aural/oral communication problems.
2. Underachievement in written work, reading and number in comparison with totally communicated knowledge (i.e. through signs supported simultaneously with speech, hearing aids, etc.).
3. Reports of occasional flashes of apparent brilliance at a much higher level than originally supposed.
4. Practical and communication skills significantly in advance of academic attainments in comparison with hearing-impaired peers of similar ability.

General

1. Aetiology involving trauma or insult in early development, e.g. aetiologies of Rubella, rhesus, anoxia, low birthweight, meningitis.
2. Educational or other records which may describe the client, as e.g., naughty, lazy, a trouble-maker.
3. Problems with symbolic communication compared with iconic or ideographic; problems with fingerspelling as opposed to signing.

It must be noted that some hearing-impaired clients may display some of the above features when there is no relationship of their behaviour to hidden learning impairments. From general clinical experience the writer would suggest short-term memory problems and neuro-muscular difficulties, with combinations of some or all of the remaining problems, tend to be associated with the more significantly additionally impaired client with hidden learning difficulty.

Information from psycho-neurological assessment, behaviour observation and behaviour analysis may assist in identification, verification, intervention and placement with clients who have hidden learning difficulties.

Group 4: Severe Multiple Handicaps

Like the hearing-impaired client who has hidden impairments, the multi-handicapped client requires provision and aids inclusive of, and beyond those which are normally required to meet the complex needs of the hearing impaired. Appropriate communication with both peers and supervising adults, and placement in environments in which there is a careful structure of activities, positive management techniques, and ample opportunity for success, appear key factors in appropriate placement and management of the multi-handicapped hearing-impaired client.

In the following sections of this chapter, the writer has attempted to provide general guidelines of areas which would appear worthy of investigation when assessing hearing-impaired clients with additional impairments.

INDIVIDUAL ASSESSMENT

A number of writers (Levine 1960, 1981; Vernon 1969; Bond 1979; Vernon and Alles 1982; Quigley and Kretschmer 1982; Galbraith 1984) have suggested factors for psychologists to consider in assessment and intervention with hearing-impaired clients. These primary areas for consideration are adapted from the above works and include:

1. Aetiology or cause of hearing impairment. The aetiology may provide clues to the site and nature of the hearing loss (see Tucker and Nolan, Chapter 11, this volume) and to a variety of additional impairments and consequent needs (Vernon 1969; Bond 1982; 1984); e.g. Rubella syndrome may result in additional impairments involving vision, heart, lungs, skeletal structure, liver, testes, growth, endocrine system, hormonal balance, diabetes, cerebral/cognitive damage, specific learning difficulties (see van Dijk 1982; Murdoch 1984).
2. Time of onset, nature, degree and extent of hearing loss. Presence of secondary overlaying hearing impairment; e.g. conductive hearing impairment overlay to a sensori-neural hearing loss (see Tucker and Nolan, Chapter 11; Webster, *et al.*, 1984). Pre-lingual hearing impairment obviously has different effects on the development of speech, language and communication than a hearing loss which occurs after language has developed. Fluctuating, conductive and other hearing losses may adversely affect communication and may at the same time affect general health, mental health, etc. (see Webster *et al.*, 1984).
3. Presence of familial hearing impairment and mode(s) of communication within the home and at school or other placement.
4. Preferred communication mode and mode of interaction with the out-

side world, i.e. is communication through auditory/articulatory skills (aural/oral) or through visual/spatial (sign, gesture, etc.)?

5. Presence of additional impairments, deprivation of experience; e.g. a visual or physical handicap in addition to hearing impairment may adversely affect the validity of non-verbal test results even when the test is designed and standardized for use with the hearing impaired.

6. Communication skills and ability of the assessor and/or the effect of interpreter presence on the dynamics of assessment; i.e. wherever possible the assessor should be able to relate to, and communicate with, the hearing-impaired client in the client's primary mode of communication. If communication is not possible owing to the client relying totally on e.g., the native sign language or total communication (e.g. signed English) an interpreter (preferably the main worker with the client such as teacher, care staff, etc.) can be very helpful. However, as in any other case, consideration must be given to any adverse or positive effects which the presence of the interpreter may have on the interview.

7. The site of assessment may have a significant effect on the client's behaviour. Assessment of the emotionally disturbed, behaviourally difficult or apprehensive client in an unfamiliar environment may tell us very little about the client's behaviour other than how he functions in an unusual environment. Wherever possible, particularly when assessing the multi-handicapped deaf (including the multi-sensorily impaired), the writer prefers to assess in environments familiar to the client and to observe clients during this assessment in a variety of activities and places. In the case of a school-based client this may involve observation and assessment working 1:1 with teacher, small group, free-time activities, mealtime, outdoors, with familiar and unfamiliar adults.

MODELS OF ASSESSMENT

The broad framework of assessment which the writer prefers to use in psychological assessment of the hearing impaired is the model outlined by Hammer (1977). This model assumes three stages: the normative stage, the within-group stage and the ipsative stage.

The Normative Stage

In this stage it is assumed that:

1. there is a range of function relative to chronological and maturational/developmental attainments;
2. true function fits into this normative range;
3. there are some tests which can tell us where a client falls into these

normative ranges, as compared with peers of the same age or maturational level (Hammer 1977).

The baselines and reference points provided in normative measures may be invaluable in assistance with placement, management and intervention, but educational decisions based solely on 'normative scores', IQs, standard scores, etc., from normatively standardized tests must remain open to serious question (see Anastasi 1968). The population on which most measures are standardized tends to be different from the hearing-impaired population, particularly those who have additional impairments or handicaps (Bond 1979). In addition, the typical standardized instrument with a limited number of items is unable to evaluate the myriad behaviours which comprise intelligent functioning (Neyhus 1978).

The Within-group Stage

In this stage it is assumed that it is possible to compare clients with each other and to tell how the client varies from, or is similar to, other clients with the same handicap or impairment; i.e. there are tests which are standardized for the assessment of the hearing impaired and thus one is able to compare the function of a hearing-impaired client on these tests with the performance of other hearing-impaired subjects. Obviously this stage of assessment has significant advantages in assessing for placement within the population of the hearing impaired.

The Ipsative Stage

This stage probably offers the most value for evaluation of programmes, placement, intervention effectiveness, individual motivation, learning abilities and capacity. In this stage the client's current performance is compared against earlier performances over a period of time.

Assessment within these stages may be affected by the nature and degree of the individual's impairments. In some cases additional impairments may be such that it is not possible or valid to use either normative or within-group standardized measures. In other cases it may be more appropriate to use combinations of subtests, rating scales and other investigation techniques to investigate the needs of the client.

AREAS FOR ASSESSMENT AND REPORT

What information should be included in a psychological assessment of a hearing-impaired client? To some extent, assessment and subsequent reporting will be tailored to the reasons for referral, considerations in relation to the people who referred the client, and for whom the report may be intended. However, as indicated elsewhere in this chapter, the psychologist must be prepared to assess systematically and objectively all aspects of a client's needs. Vernon (1969), Levine (1981), Vernon and Ottinger (1981), Vernon and Alles (1982) and others have suggested various important aspects which should be investigated and reported on in a psychological assessment of the needs of the hearing impaired. The following sections are adapted from their work, and from clinical and applied experience in professional work with the hearing impaired. The areas are mainly relevant to assessment for diagnosis, placement, prediction and evaluation of intervention, although other aspects of assessment often arise through investigation of the following areas.

Background Information

This should provide an outline which includes reasons for referral, relevant educational, family and case history, previous psychological involvement, aetiology, indication of hearing levels, use of residual hearing, indication of visual impairments (including colour vision), indication of other impairments or medical condition(s) particularly those which may affect performance during assessment or which may affect needs, and any other relevant information.

Non-verbal Cognitive Function and Psycho-neurological Status

Overall Level of Function (Abilities) on Non-verbal Tests

Preferably two or more tests should be used and, as indicated earlier in this chapter, it may be important to comment on function on both timed or speed tests and on untimed or power tests. There are a number of standardized non-verbal tests which may be suitable in the assessment of the hearing-impaired person's level of function. These tests include:

1. Wechsler Scales of Intelligence Performance Tests (Wechsler 1955, 1967, 1976): Wechsler Adult Intelligence Scale (WAIS age 16+ years), Wechsler Intelligence Scale for Children — Revised (WISC-R age 6-16 years), Wechsler Pre-school and Primary Scale of Intelligence (WPPSI age 4½-6 years). There is a standardization for the Hearing Impaired for the WISC-R (Anderson and Sisco 1976).
2. Hiskey Nebraska Test of Learning Aptitude (Deaf and Hearing norms, age range 3-18 years) (Hiskey 1966).
3. Leiter International Performance Scale — Revised (age range 2-18 years), (Leiter 1948, 1969).

4. Raven's Standard Progressive Matrices (Raven 1965).
5. Arthur Point Scale of Performance Tests — Revised II (age range 5-15 years) (Arthur 1947).
6. Snijders-Oomen Non-verbal Intelligence Scales (age range 3-16 years) (1959).
7. Columbia Mental Maturity Scale (Burgemeister, Blum and Lorge 1972).
8. Goodenough–Harris Drawing Test (Harris 1963).
9. Merrill Palmer Performance tests.

It remains necessary for the psychologist to consider results from any of the tests with caution. A test is basically a method of systematically and object-ively structuring an interview or a range of tasks to enable the tester to obtain a maximum amount of 'objective' information about the client's behaviours in the minimum possible time. On some of these tests there are difficulties in presentation, explanation, over-emphasis on speed of com-pletion, large differences in standard or derived age score resulting from relatively minimal difference in raw score (i.e. a raw score variation of 1 may be scored as a learning age difference of up to three years on some tests), and small apparatus which may cause difficulties in manipulation for even mildly physically impaired clients. Experience of the psychologist working with the hearing impaired is an important factor in the administration of most tests, particularly in establishing rapport, relation-ships and communication. The psychologist may also need to evaluate subjectively the fact validity of the test or subtests and to use only those subtests which do not appear to test the extent of the effects of hearing impairment or the effects of other impairments when the aim of assessment is to assess ability, e.g. a non-verbal test involving use of fine motor skills indicates the fine manipulation-motoric level at which a physically impaired hearing person is able to function and is not an indication of his ability.

Developmental Tests

Normatively based developmental rating scales and tests, particularly when used in conjunction with other normative tests, can be useful in assisting in the assessment of the multi-handicapped, additionally impaired, culturally/ experientially impaired, low-functioning, young hearing-impaired person. As with other apparently non-verbal measures, the psychologist should examine task requirements to assess face validity of the measure as an indicator of ability rather than a measure of the handicap.

Tests, or developmental screening inventories, which may provide useful information to get an indication of overall ability include:

1. Vineland Social Maturity Scale (Doll 1953);

2. Normal Developmental Scales (Moonblatt, Decker and Franklin 1971);
3. Developmental Screening Inventories (Gesell 1954; Knoblock and Pasamanick 1974);
4. STYCAR Developmental Scales (Sheridan 1975);
5. Griffiths Mental Development Scales (Griffiths 1970);
6. Portage Guide to Early Education (Weber, Jesien, Shearer, Bluma, Hilliard, Shearer, Schortinghuis and Boyd, 1975).

Obviously constraints on interpretation of standarized tests should also be applied to the above measures. As behaviour or attainments vary, the writer usually finds it most useful to interpret results in terms of a basal age baseline (in which all tasks presented at that level were passed) with subsequent indications of the percentage pass at each age level until a ceiling is achieved (e.g. basal level = 24 months; 60 per cent items at 30 months level; 20 per cent at 33 months; 10 per cent at 36 months; 0 per cent at 39-42 months). This can be effected for an overall indication of ability and at a diagnostic level in relation to comparison of specific developmental skills as in the following areas:

reflexes and reactions;
adaptation;
gross motor — locomotion;
fine motor — prehension and manipulation, hand-eye co-ordination;
performance — practical skills and reasoning;
personal — social emotional development (excluding verbal-communication items);
self-help skills (e.g. self-care, sleeping, eating, occupation).

Psycho-neurological Assessment

Owing to the high incidence of psycho-neurological disorders in hearing-impaired clients (Vernon 1969; Murphy 1977; Bond 1979; Vernon and Ottinger 1981), it appears important that the hearing-impaired client's psycho-neurological function is investigated. This involves comparison of function in a range of activities, identification of areas of specific strength and weakness, and identification of targets for training/remedial programming. Skill areas which should be evaluated include:

1. Matching tasks
   (i) three-dimensional matching (e.g. everyday objects through to abstract in size, shape, colour, weight);
   (ii) two-dimensional matching (pictures, designs, patterns, shapes, numbers, letters, words) — (from simple to complex); two-dimensional copying tasks — (from simple to complex);

     (iii) two dimensions (plans) to three-dimensional construction tasks (e.g. block construction);
     (iv) three-dimensional construction tasks;
     (v) simple imitation tasks.

2. Memory tasks: short-term visual memory
     (i) visual–spatial recall for objects, patterns, designs;
     (ii) visual recall for items/objects, numbers, pictures, letters, words;
     (iii) visual recall for sequences in rhythm, actions, movement;
     (iv) objects, numbers, pictures, drawing designs from memory (from simple to complex).

3. Processing tasks
     (i) sequencing visual information (shape, size, height);
     (ii) sequencing pictorial information (e.g. in order of occurrence);
     (iii) analogous or associative matching and reasoning tasks;
     (iv) imitation, sequencing and recall of gesture.

4. Fine-motor and hand–eye co-ordination tasks
Where performance on a task or a set of tasks shows approximately one or more standard deviations of variation from function on other tasks, it is probable that the variation could be significant as an indicator of a specific difficulty. The usual areas of difficulty involve poor performance on tasks involving memory (particularly sequence), processing information and fine-motor and hand–eye co-ordination tasks.

Psycho-neurological Tests.   Tests which can provide useful information in psycho-neurological diagnostic assessment include:

1. Information from the various psychological tests of ability as outlined earlier in this section, and their various subtests.
2. Graham–Kendall Memory for Designs Test (Graham and Kendall 1960).
3. Bender Visual Motor Gestalt Test (Bender 1938).
4. Benton Visual Retention Test (Benton 1974).
5. Imitation of gesture tests (Berges and Lézine 1965).
6. Finger movement, imitation and rhythm tests (van Uden 1980, also cited in van Dijk 1982).
7. Developmental tests of visual perception (Frostig 1963).
8. Bruininks–Oseretsky Test of Motor Proficiency (Bruininks 1978)
9. Illinois Test of Psycho-Linguistic Abilities (non-verbal tasks) (Kirk, McCarthy and Kirk 1968).

Once an area of apparent difficulty has been identified, the psychologist should systematically verify and define the specific area of difficulty through use of alternative measures and investigation of function on co-related tasks. As with non-verbal tests of ability, it remains necessary for psychologists to consider the results from tests with caution, as both validity and reliability may be suspect. However, in the hands of a competent and experienced clinician, useful information may be obtained from the above and other tests.

Communication and Language Skills

Assessment in this area should include an evaluation of the client's mode(s) of communication and the relative effectiveness in both receptive and expressive modes. The evaluation should preferably be carried out by observation in more than one environment and where possible and relevant should also include a systematic comparison of the different modes of communication. In evaluating communication the writer prefers to use the following structure depending on the client's needs and environment:

1. Observations: classroom, working in a group, individually with a familiar adult, interacting with peers in class or home, interacting with peers — including (if available) hearing peers. Children or peers can provide invaluable information as they are usually less likely to have rigid ideas about any communication mode and consequently tend to use the most effective means of communication with a hearing-impaired person.

2. Formal evaluation of optimum communication: comparative examination on tests (usually normatively standardized) using more than one communication mode: e.g. aural/speech reading compared with finger spelling compared with total communication (signed English). Preferably tests should have parallel forms or parallel alternatives, but this is not always feasible. Tests and assessment techniques which the writer prefers to use include, e.g., Peabody Picture Vocabulary Test (Dunn 1959); British Picture Vocabulary Scale (Dunn, Dunn, Whetton and Pintilie 1982); Tests of Receptive and Expressive Language Ability (Bunch 1981); Reynell Developmental Language Scales (Revised) (Reynell 1977); Normative Developmental Scales as noted above.

3. Informal assessments using optimum mode of communication: actions, etc., description of pictures, following simple instructions, answering questions, conversation with peers. Schemes such as the Derbyshire Language Scheme (Masidlover and Knowles 1982) or LARSP (Crystal, Fletcher and Garman 1976), may assist in more formal evaluation of language structures, and assist in establishment of target and treatment areas for communication.

Verbal Educational Attainment

Assessment can include number knowledge, application of number to solve simple problems, word recognition and reading skills, written language and, using the main communication system used by the client, verbal information processing, language, general knowledge, verbal skills and reasoning, social comprehension.

Tests of verbal educational attainments must be chosen carefully in relation to the needs and abilities of the client. There is a wide range of normatively standardized measures which might provide useful systematic information in initial placement of a client or in decisions about, or evaluation of, placement of a hearing-impaired client in a class with hearing pupils of similar age abilities and functional skills. However, for most hearing-impaired clients, particularly those who have additional impairments or handicaps, criterion-referenced verbal-educational assessment based on structured developmental curriculum should provide useful guidance for those involved in intervention (curriculum- and criterion-referenced assessment are discussed in Chapter 17).

Behaviour and Adjustment

Patterns of behaviour and adjustment are probably the most important area for the hearing-impaired client. Most stereotypes relating to hearing impairment appear to focus around behaviour. The hearing impaired are said by some (who appear to fail to appreciate the heterogeneous nature of the population of the hearing impaired) to be rigid, inflexible, over-reactive and impulsive, physical and egocentric.

Academic excellence and aural/oral competence are not necessarily passports to successful function in the community. There are many hearing impaired who have limited aural/oral communication skills who are able to cope at least adequately and often successfully in the hearing world, including many who have additional impairments or handicaps.

Investigations of the hearing-impaired client's behaviour or adjustment through projective techniques, written questionnaires and personality tests are at best dubious, even when the examiner is a fluent user of manual communication. The client may have difficulty understanding questions, forms or language and, as Vernon (1967a, 1969) indicated, there is some question as to whether the norms for personality structure of hearing people are appropriate for the hearing impaired. Hearing impairment, especially pre-lingual hearing impairment, appears to alter the individual's perceptions of his environment, in some cases to that of a iconic, visual-spatial and visual movement world, giving a different organizational perspective from the normally hearing person (see Vernon 1967a). In professional experience with a wide range of hearing-impaired clients, the writer has found observations, behavioural investigations and self-reports most useful in identifying problems and treating the hearing impaired. Where possible, behaviour should be observed in a variety of environments and contexts during the process of assessment. In addition observations of parents or other professionals should provide useful indications about behaviour.

Observable Behaviour

Assessment should note behaviours which are likely to affect the individual's response in interaction with others. The structure which the writer finds useful includes:

1. Work Habits
   (i)   attention to task and on-task behaviour;
   (ii)   constructive perseverance on tasks;
   (iii) motivation;
   (iv)   flexibility of approach;
   (v)   ability to learn from demonstration;
   (vi)   ability to learn from trial and error responses.
2. Work skills
   (i)   manual dexterity and mechanical skills;
   (ii)   organization of response;
   (iii) speed and accuracy;
   (iv)   neatness.
3. Personal
   (i)   honesty and truthfulness;
   (ii)   temperament;
   (iii) self-confidence — relations to self;
   (iv)   anxiety;
   (v)   emotional reactions;
   (vi)   leadership;
   (vii) attitude to correction;
   (viii) attitude to others peers and supervision helpers.

(For a useful checklist relating to abnormal behaviours see Vernon 1969.)

Very careful observation of overall behaviour, enquiry about behaviour on structured guidance checklists such as the above, and noting discrepancies in behaviour, may assist the psychologist to identify (or to train others to identify) areas of difficulty in function; for example, a small number of hearing-impaired clients who were reported to have normal visual acuity have on occasions shown difficulty in perception of forms, or outlines where there were little or no other cues (i.e. lines, colours etc.), jumpy nervous behaviour particularly when moving objects or people approached from the sides, excessive head movement when following objects across the visual field and delayed awareness of objects moving from the periphery of the visual field. Further investigation revealed limited peripheral visual field, and subsequent medical investigation resulted in diagnosis of Usher's syndrome in a large number of these cases. Usher's syndrome is a genetic condition which links hearing impairment and a progressive deterioration of the retina through retinitis pigmentosa (see English 1978).

Behaviour Rating Scales

Behaviour rating scales are a useful method of structuring informants' observations about a hearing-impaired client's behaviour. Some scales, such as the Bristol Social Adjustment Guides (Stott 1974) are standardized to identify 'hearing' maladaptive behaviours. Caution in interpretation is, therefore, necessary when scales such as this are used with hearing-impaired clients. Other useful scales include the Meadow-Kendall Social Emotional Inventory for Deaf Students (Meadow-Kendall, Karchmer, Peterson and Rudner 1980), The Behaviour Rating Scale, Controlled Observation Sheets (Ives 1979), checklists for symptoms of mental illness (Vernon 1969).

Systematic Applied Behaviour Analysis

Behaviour analysis offers some of the most useful techniques in investigation of the additionally impaired or multi-handicapped hearing-impaired person's behavioural or other problems (see Gagne 1965; Vance Hall 1971; and Ferster and Culbertson 1982). Behaviour analysis offers systematic methods of:

1. identifying a problem and precisely describing the problem;
2. specifying the nature, degree and extent of the problem; when it occurs, at what times and for how long;
3. identifying factors which may be contributing to the problem, such as inappropriate reinforcers, curricular and organizational problems, hormonal and metabolic disorders, etc., and consequently
4. identifying methods of treating, or areas for intervening in problems, to arrive at a solution;
5. monitoring the effectiveness of treatment.

Cases which demonstrate the value of systematic behaviour analysis include:

1. An intelligent adolescent who had a very severe hereditary (familial genetic) hearing impairment. She displayed excessive uncontrolled emotions, mood changes, precipitative action, aggression, etc. When all the case history details were brought together (teacher's records, court, police and social worker records), the behavioural outbursts had occurred over a three-to-four-year period, at approximately

monthly intervals and difficulties usually lasted approximately 1 to 1½ weeks. After a considerable and rather unfortunate delay, further medical investigations revealed a hormonal imbalance and premenstrual tension syndrome was diagnosed. The client was subsequently offered an effective simple medical treatment (Bond 1979; 1982).

2. In an experimental programme a number of multi-handicapped hearing-impaired clients whose behaviours included apparent neuro-muscular disorders, high level of impulsive, behaviour, poor on-task and attention-to-task behaviour, poor sleep were selected for study. Treatment through removal of, e.g. white sugar, cow's milk, food additives, etc., from their diet was arranged. Target behaviours were monitored noting increases in attention span, on task behaviour, decreases in impulsive behaviours (e.g. destruction, temper tantrums). Approximately 30 per cent of the cases showed behavioural improvement which correlated closely with the absence of certain foodstuffs from diet.

The writer usually asks referring agencies (teacher, parents, etc.) to carry out an analysis of the intended client's behaviour in the case of behavioural problems after carefully detailing the requirements of the analysis. In many cases the referring agency has been able to identify and subsequently treat the cause of the problem as a result of the analysis. In other cases the deviant behaviour extinguishes as the client's appropriate behaviours are monitored and thus reinforced at the same time as the deviant responses.

Aptitudes and Interests

Indication of aptitudes and interests can be useful in assisting with vocational/recreational training and experience. In the past the writer used pictorial enquiries (self-made and commercially produced) to investigate interest. However, more reliable and valid results can usually be obtained directly from discussion with the client and discussion with supervising adults and parents.

Results

Results should be summarized, conclusions derived and subsequently followed with a statement of needs, accompanied by plans for current and future intervention.

SUMMARY

Assessment is not an activity which is the exclusive territory of psychologists. Thorough assessment is highly dependent on comprehensive interdisciplinary teamwork.

From the psychologist, the hearing impaired deserve no less than the hearing. Clinical and applied experience would appear to suggest that some hearing-impaired clients are adversely affected as a result of misguided assessments and interventions. The hearing impaired deserve systematic objective investigation, appropriate provision for needs and intervention to help them to realize their abilities. Careful systematic assessment is essential. This should either be carried out by psychologists who are aware of the complexities and needs of the hearing impaired, or by psychologists who have consultative availability of psychologists who have experience, training and competence in working with the hearing impaired.

References

Anastasi, A. (1968) *Psychological Testing* (3rd edn.), MacMillan, New York
Anderson and Sisco (1976) *Standardisation of the WISC-R Performance Scale for Deaf Children*, Gaulladet
Arthur, G. (1947) *A Point Scale of Performance Tests*, The Psychological Corporation, New York
Balkany, T.J. (1980) 'Otologic Aspects of Downs Syndrome', *Seminars in Speech, Language and Hearing, 1* (1)
Bate, M., Smith, M. and James, J. (undated) *Review of Tests and Assessment in Early Education (3-5 years)*, NFER–Nelson, Windsor
Bender, L. (1938) *A Visual Motor Gestalt Test and its Clinical Use*, American Orthopsychiatric Association, New York
Benton, A.L. (1974) *Revised Visual Retention Test* (4th edn.), The Psychological Corporation, New York
Bergès, J. and Lézine, I. (1965) *The Imitation of Gestures*, trans. A.H. Parmalee, Clinics in Developmental Medicine Series, Spastics Society and William Heineman, London
Bond, D.E. (1979) 'Aspects of Psycho-Educational Assessment of Hearing Impaired Children with Additional Handicaps', *Journal British Association. Teachers of the Deaf, 3* (3), 76-9
—— (1981) 'Aspects of Behaviour and Management of Adolescents who are Hearing Impaired', *Journal British Association. Teachers of the Deaf, 5*(2), 41-8
—— (1982) 'Management of Hearing Impaired Children who have Additional Learning and Behavioural Difficulties', Paper presented to Heads of Services and Schools Hearing Impaired Conference, University of Manchester
—— (1984) 'Hearing Impaired Children: Some aspects of additional impairment and multiple handicaps' in D.E. Bond and R. Reid (eds.) Special Edition on Hearing Impairment, *Journal of the Association of Educational Psychologists, 6*(5), 50-61
Bruininks, R.H. (1978) *Bruininks–Oseretsky Test of Motor Proficiency*, American Guidance Service, Minnesota
Bunch, G. (1981) *Tests of Receptive and Expressive Language Ability*, G.B. Services, Toronto
Burgemeister, B., Blum, L. and Lorge, I. (1972) *Columbia Mental Maturity Scale*, Harcourt Brace Jovanovich Inc., New York
Crystall, D., Fletcher, P. and Garman, M. (1976) *The Grammatical Analysis of Language*

Disability: a Procedure for Assessment and Remediation, Studies in Language Disability and Rehabilitation, Edward Arnold, London

Doll, E.A. (1953) *Measurement of Social Competence*, American Guidance Service Inc.

Dunn, L.M. (1959) *Peabody Picture Vocabulary Test*, American Guidance Service, Minnesota

Dunn, L., Dunn, L.M., Whetton, C. and Pintilie, D. (1982) *British Picture Vocabulary Scale*. NFER–Nelson, Windsor

English, J. (ed.) (1978) 'Ushers Syndrome. The Personal Social and Emotional Implications', Monograph. *American Annals of the Deaf, 123*(3)

Ferster, C.B. and Culbertson, S.A. (1982) *Behaviour Principles*. Prentice Hall, New Jersey

Frostig, M. (1966) *Developmental Test of Visual Perception*, Consulting Psychologists Press, Palo Alto, California

Gagne, R.M. (1965) *The Conditions of Learning*, Holt, Rinehart and Winston Inc., New York

Galbraith, D. (1984) 'The Psychological Assessment of Deaf Children' in D.E. Bond and R. Reid (ed.) Special Edition on Hearing Impairment, *Journal of the Association of Educational Psychologists, 6*(5), 19-27

Gesell, A. (1954) *The first five years of life*, Methuen and Co., London

Graham, F.K. and Kendall, B.S. (1960) *Memory for Designs Test* Southern University Press, Monograph 2-VII

Griffiths, R. (1970) *The Abilities of Young Children*, Young and Son, Somerset, England

Hamilton, P. and Owrid, L. (1974) 'Comparisons of hearing impairment and socio-cultural disadvantages in relation to verbal retardation', *British Journal of Audiology, 8*, 27-32

Hammer, E.K. (1977) 'Appraisal: A process for identification of problems and potentials of the severely handicapped', Paper presented at the National Topical Conference of Appraisal of the Severely Handicapped, Washington DC

Harris, D. (1963) *The Goodenough Harris Drawing Test*, Harcourt, Brace and World, New York

Hiskey, M. (1966) *Hiskey Nebraska Test of Learning Aptitude*, Amon College Press, Nebraska

Ives, L.A. (1979) 'Some Aspects of Social Emotional Development in Hearing Impaired Children (Behaviour Observation Sheets)', Occasional Paper, Royal Schools for the Deaf, Manchester

Kirk, S.A., McCarthy, J.A. and Kirk, W.D. (1968) *Illinois Test of Psycho-linguistic Abilities*, University of Illinois Press, Urbana

Knoblock, H. and Pasamanick, B. (1974) *Gesell and Amatruda's Developmental Diagnosis* (3rd ed.) Harper and Row, New York

Kropka, B.I. (1979) 'A study of the deaf and partially hearing population in the mental handicap hospitals of Devon', A report to the Royal National Institute for the Deaf, London

—— and Williams, C. (1980) 'The Deaf and Partially Hearing in Mental Handicap Hospitals. The disadvantaged Minority?', *British Journal of Mental Subnormality, 26*, 89-93

Leiter, R.G. (1969) *The Leiter International Performance Scale*, Stoelting Co., Chicago

Levine, E.S. (1981) *The Ecology of Early Deafness*, Columbia University Press, New York

Lloyd, L.L. (1970) 'Audiologic Aspects of Mental Retardation' in N.R. Ellis (ed.) *International Review of Research in Mental Retardation, 4*, Academic Press, New York, pp. 311-74

Masidlover, M. and Knowles, W. (1982) *The Derbyshire Language Scheme*, Derbyshire County Council

Meadow-Kendall, K.P., Karchmer, M.A., Peterson, L.M. and Rudner, L. (1980) *The Meadow-Kendall Social--Emotional Inventory for Deaf Children*, Gaulladet College, Pre-College Programs, Washington, DC

Moonblatt, L. and Decker, N. (1971) *Normal Developmental Scales* (ed. B. Franklin), Multi-handicapped Deaf–Blind Program, Dept. of Special Education, San Francisco State College

Murdoch, H. (1984) 'Maternal Rubella: The Implications' in D.E. Bond, and R. Reid (eds.) Special Edition on Hearing Impairment, *Journal of the Association of Educational Psychologists, 6*(5), 3-6

Murphy, L.J. (1977) 'The Multi-Handicapped Deaf Child' in *Proceedings. N.Z. Conference of Teachers of the Deaf*, Kelston, NZ

Myklebust, H.R. (1964) *The Psychology of Deafness* (2nd Edn.), Grune and Stratton, New York

Neyhus, A.L. (1978) 'Assessment for Individualised Educational Programming', *Volta Review, 80*, pp. 286-95

Quigley, S.P. and Kretschmer, R.E. (1982) *The Education of Deaf Children: Issues Theories and Practice*, Arnold, London

Raven, J.C. (1965) *The Progressive Matrices Scales*, H.K. Lewis, London

Reynell, J. (1977) *Reynell Developmental Language Scales*, NFER, Slough

Sheridan, M.C. (1975) 'The Stycar Language Test', *Developmental Medicine Child Neurology, 17*, 164

Snijders, J. Th. and Snijders-Oomen, N. (1970) *Non-verbal Tests for Deaf and Hearing Subjects* (4th edn.), Groningen

Stott, D.E. (1974) *Bristol Social Adjustment Guides*, Hodder and Stoughton, London

Tempowski, I., Felstead, H. and Simon, G. (1974) 'Deafness and the mentally retarded', *Apex 2*, 4-5

Vance Hall, R., Panyan, M.C., Wheeler, A.H. and Fox, W.L. (1971) *Managing behaviour 1-5*, Hand H Enterprises Inc., Kansas

van Dijk, J. (1982) *Rubella Handicapped Children*, Swets and Zeitlinger, BV, Lisse

van Uden, A. (1980) 'Finger movement, imitation and rhythm Tests', personal communication

—— (1981) 'Early Diagnosis of those Multiple Handicaps in Pre-lingually Profoundly Deaf Children which Endanger an Education According to the Purely Oral Way', *Teacher of the Deaf, 5*(4)

Vernon, M. (1967a) 'A Guide for the Psychological Evaluation of Deaf and Severely Hard of Hearing Adults', *The Deaf American, 19*(9)

—— (1967b) *Multiply Handicapped Deaf Children: The Causes, Manifestations and Significances of the Problem*, NAD, Maryland

—— (1969) 'Techniques for Screening Mental Illness among Deaf Clients', *Journal of Rehabilitation of the Deaf*, pp. 23-26

—— and Alles, B. (1982) 'Psychological Evaluation of Multi-handicapped Deaf and Hard of Hearing Youth', *Directions, 3*(2), 2-18

—— and Brown, D.W. (1964) 'A guide to psychological Tests and testing procedures in the evaluation of deaf and hard of hearing children', *Journal of Speech and Hearing Disorders, 29*, 414-23

—— and Ottinger, P. (1981) 'Psychological Evaluation of the Deaf and Hard of Hearing' in Stein, Mindel and Jabaley (eds)., *Deafness and Mental Health*. Grune and Stratton, New York, pp. 49-64

Weber, S.J., Jesien, G.S., Shearer, D., Bluma, S., Hilliard, J.M., Shearer, M., Shortinghuis, N.E. and Boyd, M.S. (1975) *The Portage Guide to Home Teaching*, Co-operative Educational Service Agency, Wisconsin, also NFER—Nelson, Windsor

Webster, A., Saunders, E. and Bamford, J.M. (1984) 'Fluctuating conductive Hearing Impairment' in D.E. Bond and R. Reid (eds.), Special Edition on Hearing Impairment, *Journal of the Association of Educational Psychologists, 6*(5), 6-19

Wechsler, D. (1955) *Wechsler Adult Intelligence Scale*, Psychological Corporation, New York

—— (1967) *Wechsler Pre-school and Primary Scale of Intelligence*, Psychological Corporation, New York

—— (1976) *Wechsler Intelligence Scale for Children — Revised* Psychological Corporation, New York

15 DEVELOPMENTAL ASSESSMENT OF COMMUNICATIVE ABILITIES IN THE DEAF–BLIND

Robert D. Stillman and Christy W. Battle

Introduction

Recent advances in understanding both normal and atypical human development owe much to the application of developmental assessment procedures and observational protocols to study behaviour in both structured and naturalistic settings. In the area of communicative development, the application of assessment techniques to normally developing and communicatively impaired populations has helped to begin the process of unravelling the complex and inter-related cognitive, social and linguistic factors which underlie early communicative competence (e.g. Corrigan 1979; Nicolich 1981; Wetherby and Gaines 1982; Sigman and Ungerer 1984; Wetherby and Prutting 1984). The following describes our efforts to design developmental assessment procedures and observational protocols incorporating the cognitive, social and linguistic domains which appear relevant to the development of communicative competence, and to assess the social–interactive context in which communicative exchanges occur. The assessment methods to be described were designed for use primarily in educational settings and to be applicable for deaf–blind and multi-handicapped individuals regardless of the severity of their impairments or their chronological age.

Developmental Assessment

Implicit in the construction of developmental assessment instruments is the assumption of the orderly, hierarchical nature of development within each assessment domain (Uzgiris and Hunt, 1975; Hunt 1976). A catalogue or checklist of abilities or behaviours observed in normally developing children as a function of age does not constitute a developmental assessment scale unless there is the assumption that each ability or behaviour on the scale is a prerequisite for the appearance of succeeding abilities or behaviours. Implicit also in developmental-assessment instruments is the assumption that, while the developmental sequence within domains is invariant, the rate at which new abilities emerge, and the manner in which they are revealed in behaviour, are affected by both experiential and biological factors. Thus, in the design of developmental assessment procedures applicable for deaf–blind and multi-handicapped individuals, it is assumed that the emergence of abilities follows the same sequential and hierarchical pattern observed in normally developing children. It is not assumed, nor is

319

there compelling evidence, for a unique course of development among deaf–blind and multi-handicapped individuals. However, the appearance of successively more complex levels of abilities within developmental domains may be delayed or even unattainable as a consequence of experiential and biological factors. Furthermore, the observable behaviours indicative of the presence of specific abilities and the diversity of behaviours generated by the ability reflect the individual's experiences and the nature of his impairments. The assessed behaviours, therefore, may differ considerably in quality and quantity from those typically observed among normally developing individuals.

The selection of items and examples in a developmental assessment scale is guided by the author's conception of underlying developmental processes, and how these processes are revealed in behaviour. Behaviours described in a developmental assessment scale are, therefore, probes selected because of the likelihood that their presence suggests the status of the underlying processes the scale purports to measure. Thus, the sequence of behavioural items on a scale is a reflection of, but is not synonymous with, the underlying developmental processes. In order to interpret assessment results in terms of developmental status, rather than in terms of the presence or absence of specific behaviours, the user must be thoroughly familiar with the particular conception of development which served as the framework for the scale's construction.

Day (1983) has provided a comprehensive review and critique of developmental assessment scales currently used to assess the cognitive, social and communicative abilities of deaf–blind individuals. Among the scales reviewed are those designed especially for use with deaf–blind, and others which may be applicable provided suitable modifications are made such as changing or eliminating items requiring intact auditory, visual or motor abilities. However, none of the assessment scales reviewed appears to have achieved general acceptance.

The Callier-Azusa Scale

One of the developmental assessment scales designed specifically for use with the deaf–blind is the Callier-Azusa Scale, Edition G (Stillman, 1978). This scale approaches the assessment of communicative abilities, as do most scales, through the separate assessment of expressive and receptive communication, cognitive abilities and social skills. However, since the publication of the Callier-Azusa Scale-G, there have been significant advances in understanding the inter-relationships between social, cognitive and communicative development and in identifying those aspects of cognitive development and social experience which appear to predict later communicative development (e.g. Bates 1979; Schaffer 1979; Wolf and Gardner 1981). These studies, in conjunction with our own research on communicative development in the deaf–blind (Battle 1981; Stillman, Aylmer and Vandivort 1983; Stillman and Battle, 1984), have led to a major revision and reorganization of the Callier-Azusa Scale. The following discussion focuses on the revised Callier-Azusa Scale, Edition H (Stillman and Battle 1983).

The Callier-Azusa Scale-H is an assessment scale designed to offer the educator and clinician a comprehensive, developmentally-based framework for viewing the communicative abilities of deaf–blind and multi-handicapped individuals. The Callier-Azusa-H is composed of a hierarchical progression of items within four developmental domains: *Representational and Symbolic Abilities, Receptive Communication, Intentional Communication* and *Reciprocity*. Its purpose is to provide the educator and clinician with assessment information relevant to planning individualized, communication-based intervention programmes; to provide a means for documenting developmental change in both communicative competence and the cognitive and social abilities related to communicative development; and to elucidate patterns of development across cognitive, social and linguistic domains which may prove useful both in understanding the behaviours of deaf–blind and multi-handicapped individuals, and in fostering the design of more effective assessment procedures and intervention techniques. While description of the entire scale is beyond the scope of this chapter, it is hoped that the following discussion of its contents and administration will help to clarify some of the problems and issues in assessment of deaf–blind and multi-handicapped individuals, and assist the educator and clinician better to assess and understand the communicative abilities and communicative behaviours of deaf–blind and multi-handicapped individuals.

Population

The target population for whom the Callier-Azusa-H was designed is the deaf–blind. It is important to note that deaf–blindness rarely means total loss of vision and hearing. Recent surveys indicate that 65-70 per cent of the deaf–blind have usable vision, and 30-5 per cent have sufficient residual hearing to benefit from amplification (Stein, Palmer and Weinberg 1982; Curtis and Donlon 1983). Most deaf–blind individuals, however, are pre-verbal and exhibit pronounced developmental delays in addition to their combined auditory and visual impairments. Neuro-motor dysfunctions, autism and other neurological and physical abnormalities are also common among this population. In general, these impairments are congenital or result from trauma or disease in early development. Although the assessment scale was designed for application with the deaf–blind, the items and examples are appropriate for use with other sensorily impaired, multi-handicapped individuals, especially those functioning at lower developmental levels.

Assessment Procedures

Assessments using the Callier-Azusa Scale are derived from observations of the individual's behaviour in familiar environments, especially the classroom. There are no formal testing procedures because lower functioning deaf–blind individuals generally perform poorly in formal testing (Day 1983). However, the absence of formal testing procedures means that the context in which assessments take place may affect assessment results. Because the Callier-Azusa Scale-H focuses on communication, context means not only the physical setting, but also the interactive style of the adult partner, and the demands and constraints of the activity in which the child is assessed. Thus, the adult partner's skill in eliciting, sustaining, initiating and responding in interactions, and in devising activities likely to lead to the optimal demonstration of a child's communicative ability, will influence the child's performance and, thus, the assessment results. To assure accurate assessments it is, therefore, essential that adequate opportunity be provided to observe the individual in a variety of relevant physical and interpersonal contexts. An observation period of two weeks is suggested. The extended assessment period also reduces the possibility of inaccurate assessments resulting from the often substantial day-to-day variations in behaviour exhibited by deaf–blind and multi-handicapped individuals.

It is recommended, also, that several observers familiar with the child participate jointly in the assessment. In this way, observers with differing professional perspectives and differing interactive styles can pool their knowledge and learn from each other's experiences and interpretations of the behaviours observed.

Assessments based on the observation of naturally occurring behaviour always require judgements and decisions. In deciding whether an individual possesses a certain ability, one should ascertain whether the ability is demonstrated in a variety of different behaviours, whether it is consistently observed, whether it is observed in the absence of prompting and manipulation, and whether the ability is observed in a variety of relevant contexts. Application of these assessment criteria is critical because of the frequent occurrence among deaf–blind individuals of isolated or 'splinter' skills which usually appear following training to perform specific behaviours or when obtaining food, physical stimulation or extrinsic reinforcement is the goal of the behaviour observed (Stillman and Battle 1984). 'Splinter' skills, however, are rarely a true indicator of the child's level of ability since they do not predict the child's performance beyond a restricted context (i.e. situations in which need gratification or extrinsic reinforcement are available). Because the purpose of developmental assessment is to deduce an individual's abilities through the observation of behaviour rather than to document the presence of specific behaviours, the distinction between communicative abilities and communicative behaviours is critical. Communicative abilities are intrinsic cognitive–social–

communicative competencies and are revealed in a variety of behaviours. Specific communicative behaviours, however, may be either an expression of cognitive–social–communicative abilities or the demonstration of sensitivity to reinforcement contingencies. In the latter case, the ability revealed is the ability to perform a designated action in order to obtain reinforcement. Within the Callier-Azusa-H, assessment items were designed to make the distinction between communicative abilities and communicative behaviours explicit.

The following summarizes the content, particularly at the lower developmental levels, of the four scales included in the Callier-Azusa Scale-H. These summaries are intended to familiarize the reader with the developmental domains included in the assessment scale, and to describe how the abilities assessed may be manifested in the behaviour of deaf–blind and multi-handicapped individuals.

Representational and Symbolic Abilities

Representational ability is the ability to form and retrieve mental images or schemas which stand for objects, people and events. The child who is able to represent experience mentally is, thereby, enabled to communicate experience to others by means of a symbolic vehicle. A symbolic vehicle is anything used to make reference to experience including words, drawings or the imitated actions of objects and people manifested in the child's gestures and play. The development, use and refinement of symbolic vehicles culminates in the use of language symbols to convey thoughts to others.

The Representational and Symbolic Abilities scale assesses aspects of development which indicate progress towards representational abilities, and aspects of representational development related to the use of symbolic vehicles (Piaget 1962; Werner and Kaplan 1963; Bates 1979; Nicolich 1981). Pre-representational and representational abilities are assessed through observation of the development of anticipation, imitation, gestures, language and symbolic play.

The development of representational ability is an outcome of the process of distancing or differentiation between self and the external world. Initially, the child does not separate himself and the external world. From the child's perspective, objects, people and events are fused with his own actions and sensations. What the child recognizes are his own familiar sensations and the contexts in which they occur, not people, objects and events. It is through the process of distancing or differentiation that the child comes to appreciate the existence of a world distinct from his own actions and sensations, and is, thereby, enabled to form mental representations which stand for the objects, people and events he has observed.

The child's differentiation of self from the external world is a gradual process which can be observed in his decreasing reliance on immediate and familiar contexts to anticipate external events, his increasing ability to understand the correspondence between his own actions and those he observes, and his increasing ability to depict through imitation the observed actions of people and objects. The increasing focus on the external world, rather than on his own actions and sensations, also allows the child to anticipate events which he has not experienced and to imitate actions he has not previously performed. The following describes the assessment of pre-representational anticipation and imitation abilities.

The sequence of items assessing anticipation begins with the child's ability to anticipate familiar events in the context of whole body cues. For example, the child becomes excited, or smiles when held in position associated with a familiar game, or for the chronologically older child, begins rocking when seated in a familiar rocking chair. At the next level, the child anticipates familiar events without the necessity for extensive physical cues. For example, the child smiles or vocalizes when given a familiar toy.

The child then begins to anticipate an activity when in the place where the activity regularly occurs or when given an object or signal associated with the activity. For example, the child goes directly to the trampoline when he enters the gym, begins pulling down his pants when he enters the bathroom, goes to the table when given a plate, begins a 'pat-a-cake' game when the adult holds out her hands, or picks up his cup when the adult signs or says 'drink'. Finally, the child anticipates an event from observation of activities which typically precede the event. For example, the child goes to the door when the adult puts on her coat, goes to the sand table when the adult takes out a toy typically played with at the sand table, or recognizes that a cooking activity is about to start when given any object typically associated with the activity.

The earliest stages of imitation are observed when the child occasionally repeats a behaviour which was imitated by the adult; for example, when the child is waving his arms, the adult waves, and the child notices and begins waving again. The child may also inconsistently perform a familiar action in imitation of an adult action such as slapping the table or vocalizing even if he was not engaged in the behaviour when the adult performed it. At the next level, the child consistently imitates a few familiar movements and/or sounds produced by the adult. However, these imitations occur only while the adult is performing the action. For example, when the adult begins to crawl, the child crawls with her, or when the adult rolls a toy car back and forth, the child copies the action with his own car. At the next level, the child imitates a broad range of actions and successfully imitates actions that are similar to, but not identical with, his own familiar actions. For example, the child who imitates clapping can also imitate a similar movement such as rubbing the hands together, even though he has not previously been observed to perform that movement.

The emergence of the pointing gesture indicates the onset of representational abilities. The pointing gesture, used to make reference to something in the external world, is a clear indicator that the child is able to turn his focus away from himself and towards the world outside. It is also the child's first use of a symbolic vehicle, an action used to make reference to something. Although totally blind children may not point to things at a distance, they may point to make reference to face and body parts, or reach to touch objects to make reference to them, rather than to explore or manipulate.

The following summarizes the processes of differentiation which underlie the continuing development of representational abilities and the progression of items in the higher levels of the scale.

First, there is a decreasing reliance on contextual cues to retrieve mental representations and to produce symbolic vehicles. As a result, the child gradually becomes able to produce symbolic vehicles outside of the context in which they were learned. For example, the child who learns to understand and use the pushing gesture, sign or spoken word in relation to pushing his chair to the table becomes able to understand and use the same symbolic vehicle at other times, in reference to other acts of pushing. The context of a present model also becomes less important in the child's imitation, and the child may imitate an observed sequence of actions some time after the event occurred. For example, the child who has observed an adult wiping the sink may attempt the same action the next day without again observing the adult's action. In symbolic play, the child first pretends to eat only at mealtime. As the context becomes less necessary in eliciting play behaviour, the child pretends to eat outside mealtimes.

Second, there is an increasing differentiation of the child from the form of the symbolic vehicle. Initially, the forms of the symbolic vehicles the child understands and uses are his own actions. For example, the child indicates 'throwing' with his own throwing motion. The symbolic vehicle is, therefore, idiosyncratic and cannot be unambiguously understood by those unfamiliar with the child's interests and experiences. The child's throwing gesture, for example, might be interpreted as, and for some children might mean, put, give or discard. As the child differentiates himself from the symbolic vehicle, he begins to understand and use symbolic vehicles which are formed not of his typical actions, but of sounds or manual signs. For example, he uses the word 'throw' formed of sounds or the abbreviated motion of the manual sign for 'throw' to refer to throwing. As a result, the child's expressions can be more readily understood by others.

Third, there is an increasing differentiation between the child and the meaning of the symbolic vehicle. At first, the child only understands and uses symbolic vehicles which refer to his own actions. For example, he understands and uses the throwing gesture, spoken word or sign only to describe his act of throwing. But with increasing differentiation, he becomes able to understand and use symbolic vehicles to refer to the actions of others; for example, to describe another person's act of throwing or to request that another person throw. In symbolic play, the child initially depicts his own activities; for example, his sleeping, his eating, his dressing and his washing. He then becomes able to pretend at the behaviour of others; for example, sweeping, going to work, dusting or driving a car.

Fourth, there is increasing differentiation between the symbolic vehicle and that which it represents. Initially, the child only understands and uses symbolic vehicles which are perceptually similar to that which they represent. For example, the throwing gesture looks like the motion of throwing, the sound 'meow' sounds like the cat's cry, or 'tick-tock' sounds like the clock. With increasing differentiation the child becomes able to understand and use symbolic vehicles which are not perceptually similar to the thing represented; for example, signed or spoken words for 'throw', 'cat', or 'clock'. In play, the child initially pretends to eat only using the usual utensils. With increasing differentiation, the child pretends to eat using a stick for a fork, a block for a bowl and a chair for a table. The child also becomes able to pretend to be other people and things such as an aeroplane.

Receptive Communication

The Receptive Communication scale assesses the ability to respond to the communicative expressions of others. The assessment of receptive abilities focuses not only on the form and content of expressions to which the child responds, but also the contexts in which the expressions are understood. Specifically, the scale assesses receptive abilities as they develop from understanding communications related to the child's present needs and actions to understanding communications concerning topics unrelated to the child's immediate concerns; from understanding familiar communications about familiar events to understanding novel communications about novel events; and from understanding only with the assistance of contextual cues to understanding independent of contextual cues. Throughout, the child's ability to understand increasingly complex and abstract communicative forms is assessed. The Receptive Communication scale is primarily of our own design and is based on our observations of how deaf–blind and multi-handicapped individuals respond to the directed social–communicative actions of adult partners.

The processes of differentiation, described in the discussion of the Representational and Symbolic Abilities scale, provides the framework for items on the Receptive Communication scale. The gradual differentiation of self from the external world allows the child to begin to understand and interpret the communications of others rather than simply to respond to familiar stimuli with particular actions. It also frees the child from reliance on context to interpret communications. Differentiation between self and the form of the symbolic vehicle results in a shift from understanding only gestures which mimic the child's own actions to understanding more abstract symbolic vehicles which refer to the child's actions, such as conventional gestures, spoken words or manual signs. Differentiation between self and the meaning of the symbolic vehicle results in a shift in the child's understanding of communication from assuming that communications refer only to himself and his actions, to understanding that communications can refer to the actions and characteristics of objects and others. Differentiation between the symbolic vehicle and that which it represents results in the child's increasing ability to understand symbolic vehicles which are less depictive of what they represent and more arbitrary in form.

At the earliest level, receptive ability is assessed by observing the child's responses to social acts intended to elicit attention or to modify ongoing behaviours. For example, the child quietens or attends to gentle physical stimulation, attends to interesting visual or auditory events produced by the adult, and can be comforted when distressed. At the next level, the child responds to familiar contextual cues such as position, movement or a particular object or person by anticipating events associated with that particular context. For example, the child becomes excited, tenses or smiles when held or placed in a position associated with a familiar 'game'; begins to participate in a familiar movement, such as rocking when the adult begins to rock the child; becomes excited when presented with a familiar toy; or becomes excited upon seeing, hearing or touching a familiar person.

At the next level, the child recognizes that one action signals the occurrence of another action in the context of familiar interactive 'games'. For example, in a 'tickling game' which includes a fixed sequence of adult actions culminating in tickling, after a number of repetitions of the sequence, the child anticipates being tickled from the adult's actions which always precede tickling. At this level, the child also responds to adult attempts to direct attention to objects or events in the immediate environment. For example, the child looks at or sits in a chair when the adult taps or shakes the chair, or the child looks at or picks up an object when the adult moves or shakes it.

At the next level, responses are observed to signals intended by the adult to be communicative and to elicit from the child a particular behaviour. The child's response to these signals reflects associations learned between the signal, the context in which the signal is observed, and the behaviour expected in response to the signal. Items on the scale assess the forms of communicative signals to which the child responds including demonstrations, gestures and offered objects. For example, the child picks up a lunch tray following the adult, pats the adult's hands when the adult holds out her hands to initiate a 'pat-a-cake' game, or goes to the lunch table when given a plate. In each case, the response reflects a learned behaviour to a signal occurring within a familiar context.

The child may respond also to a few spoken words or manual signs presented in familiar contexts. For example, the child may respond to the spoken word or manual sign for 'sit' when standing next to a chair. Language symbols, however, at this level, are responded to as context-bound signals for actions. Thus, the word 'sit' presented when no chair is available is unlikely to indicate to the child to sit on the floor, unless this specific association was taught.

Further progress in receptive ability occurs when the child demonstrates greater understanding of the communicative expression itself with less reliance on context and learned associations. Items at this level assess the ability to distinguish between signals in ambiguous contexts. For example, the child consistently responds correctly to gestures to 'pick up' and 'push' an object on the table when either action is appropriate in the context. Other items at this level assess the ability to copy demonstrations which differ slightly from those the child has copied previously. For example, without specific training, the child who copies carrying a chair to the table, copies pushing the chair.

At the next level, the scale assesses the beginning of understanding that clearly depictive communicative expressions represent familiar actions, objects and activities. For example, without training, the child responds to stirring or scooping gestures made over a bowl by stirring or scooping its contents. The child also understands that any object used in an activity can represent the activity. For example, without training, the child goes to the bath area when given his towel, soap, flannel or bath toy. Drawings depicting familiar objects and which are the same size and colour as the object are also understood to represent the object. For example, without training, when the child is shown a drawing of a spoon, he picks a real spoon from among several objects. The child also responds to pointing gestures when the adult's hand and the object of reference can be seen simultaneously. For example, the child follows the adult's point to a toy and looks at it, picks it up or activates it.

Further understanding of the representational nature of communicative expressions is evident when gestures which demonstrate a requested action are understood in new, but appropriate contexts. For example, the child who understands that a pushing gesture made next to a chair means to push the chair, understands that the same motion made next to the door means to close the door. Gestures which depict one aspect of an activity are understood to mean the whole activity rather than only one component. For example, a sweeping gesture is understood to mean start a clean-up activity rather than just to sweep. The child also understands routine requests communicated through drawing, when the drawing clearly depicts the requested action. A few spoken words or manual signs are understood in the context of familiar activities. For example, when the adult signs or says 'ball', the child gets the ball which is in view on a shelf; or when the adult signs or says 'give', the child gives the adult the object he is holding.

Over the next few levels, the child gradually begins to respond to familiar gestures and verbalizations outside their usual contexts, and to understand new gestures and verbalizations independent of context. The child also gradually expands his receptive vocabulary beyond names for present people and objects to include names for absent people and objects, words for new actions, and words which refer to past, present and future.

Intentional Communication

The Intentional Communication scale was designed to focus the assessment of expressive communicative abilities on the level of intentionality of the child's expressions. Within each level of intentionality, the scale assesses the purposes the communications serve and the forms they take. The sequence of items in the scale was derived from a variety of sources (Piaget 1962; Werner and Kaplan 1963; Dore 1977; Clark 1978; Bates 1979; Newson 1979; Prutting 1979; Schaffer 1979) and our own experiences with deaf–blind and multi-handicapped individuals.

At the early levels of development, the child does not communicate intentionally. Rather, the child performs actions in response to internal states and to sensations resulting from environmental stimuli. These actions are communicative only in the sense that they can be interpreted and responded to by the partner as indicators of the child's needs and desires. Until the child has differentiated self from the external world, he cannot communicate intentionally because he is unaware of the independent existence of others beyond his own actions and sensations. The child's focus on himself, his actions and his sensations means also that those actions which have a communicative effect can relate only to himself and will appear only in familiar contexts. It is only when the child has differentiated himself from people, objects and events that intentional communication, communications about the external world, and communications outside familiar contexts are possible.

In identifying early communicative expressions, we have followed Spitz's definition: 'any perceivable change of behaviour, be it intentional or not, directed or not, with the help of which one or several persons can influence the perceptions, the feelings, the thoughts, or the actions of one or several persons, be that influence intended or not ...' (1965, p. 128) and Clark's definition: 'whatever it is that enables the activities of individuals to be co-ordinated with one another ...' (1978, p. 257). Thus, the earliest communicative expressions are actions emitted in response to internal states and which serve to assure the meeting of basic adaptive needs. In assessing communicative abilities at this level, one looks for behaviours which elicit contact from others, keep others in close proximity, and terminate interpersonal contact. Behaviours which may serve these purposes include crying, generalized excitement, looking towards, reaching towards, clinging, squirming, looking away and, in some individuals, self-abuse. Whether the behaviours observed are communicative, and the specific communicative purposes exhibited, however, can be established only with reference to the context in which they occur and the effect of the partner's attempts to respond to the perceived purpose of the expression.

At the next level, one examines the child's ability to participate in, sustain and modulate interactive activities. Initially, one looks for the presence of actions which serve to maintain contact with others for social rather than need satisfaction purposes. Example behaviours include social smiling, vocalizing in the presence of the partner and reaching towards and grasping at the partner.

At the next level, one looks for the presence of actions which indicate participation in interactive 'games'. For example, in games where the adult and child bounce, rock or jump together, when the adult pauses, the child makes some movement, touches the adult, or vocalizes. The particular action may vary from pause to pause, but the actions are perceived and responded to by the partner as a request to continue the activity. Initially, these expressions are unintentional actions which occur during pauses in interactive games. However, through repeated experience, in interactive games, these unintentional actions evolve into intentional actions: actions performed deliberately with the anticipation of a specific effect. The action is now performed in order to achieve a certain immediate goal. However, the actions are not intentionally communicative because the focus is an immediate one, to bring about a change in his own sensations rather than to convey information to others about his desires. Consistent use of such signals are observed first in a few activities and then in many activities having a start/pause/restart structure. The form of the signals also becomes specific to the particular activity; for example, bobbing the head to signal to continue bouncing, making a jump to restart jumping with the teacher or clapping to continue a clapping activity. These signals are generated spontaneously by the child, but occur only in the context of ongoing interactive games.

Signals to terminate activities also appear; for example, removing the partner's hands, withdrawing hands, pushing the partner away, or moving away. In some instances, termination signals may take the form of emotional protests such as angry vocalizations, agitation and, in some cases, self-abuse. Termination signals may be observed, in addition, to refuse to participate when the adult attempts to initiate an activity or to protest the termination of an activity the child wishes to continue. Termination and protest signals are included in the assessment because they represent both a legitimate purpose of communication and an important means by which the child utilizes his actions to manage the social and physical environment.

At the next level, the child uses intentional actions to signal the adult to initiate specific activities or to request specific objects and actions. The signals now appear outside the context of ongoing interactions. The focus of the expressions, however, remains on the goal (the object, the adult's body part which performs the action, or the place where the desired activity typically occurs) and often appears to be an inseparable component of a goal-directed action sequence. For example, the child holds out his hands to initiate a patting game, goes to the sink or water fountain and waits for the teacher to turn on the water, or pushes the adult into a chair to initiate a game typically played in the chair. Use of the adult's hands as a tool to obtain or activate objects, or to solve minor problems, is also commonly observed. For example, the child may put the teacher's hand on a milk carton to have it opened, on a door knob to have the door opened, on his pants to have them pulled up, or on a toy to have it activated. In these examples, the child's focus of attention is on the hands which perform the action, rather than on enlisting the adult's assistance. If the adult's hands are not readily available, the child will seek them out, become distressed or discontinue the activity rather than request the adult's assistance through an alternative expression.

Trained signals including trained gestures, manual signs and vocalizations used to initiate activities are also intentional actions. For example, following training in which the teacher forms the child's hands into the manual signs for 'drink' and then gives the child a drink, the child uses the 'drink' sign to request a drink. Communicative expressions learned in this manner and spontaneously used generally serve to request food, drink, physical stimulation or objects for stimulation.

The spontaneous sequencing of signals is observed as the child develops an understanding of the effects of his signals. For example, the child may push the teacher's leg to sit, then pat the teacher's hand to initiate a clapping game usually played while sitting. The individual's signals may have been trained, but the sequence of signals was not. Signals to refuse, protest or terminate take the form of specific intentional actions such as trained 'finished' signs, signals redirecting the teacher to another activity, or picking up an object or performing a behaviour associated with the end of the activity. These signals are consistently used in place of emotional reactions.

The child, at this level, is thoroughly aware that his actions can bring about anticipated effects, and he uses these actions to control the environment. For many deaf–blind and multi-handicapped individuals, the use of an increasingly broad repertoire of signals and their application in a variety of contexts appears to be the highest level achieved in the development of intentional communication.

Further progress towards the development of true intentional communication is observed when the focus of the child's communicative actions shifts from the goal, to gaining the partner's attention in order to communicate. For example, the child may elicit the adult's attention to an object by showing it, request objects by making reaching motions towards the object even when the object is within reach, and varying the form of the communicative expression until success is achieved in gaining the adult's attention. The child's actions indicate an understanding of the role of the partner in achieving communicative goals, and communicative expressions are directed to the partner rather than to the goal or the body part of the partner which helps to achieve the goal. Communicative purposes other than requests, terminations and protests also emerge. For example, the child begins to point out things in the environment for the purpose of sharing knowledge rather than to request specific actions. A few spontaneously occurring gestures also emerge. Some of these are abbreviated forms of earlier goal-directed actions; for example, pushing motions to request that the adult move or sit rather than actually pushing the adult. Other gestures emerge from imitation of observed actions such as waving the hands back and forth in order to get the partner to shake her head.

At the highest level assessed, the child creates and uses a variety of idiosyncratic gestures for communicative purposes. Conventional gestural forms and language symbols then emerge to become the primary means of communication.

Reciprocity

The Reciprocity scale assesses the child's developing ability to participate in reciprocal communicative exchanges, and to understand the patterns and conventions of social conversation. It has been our observation that many deaf–blind and multi-handicapped individuals use their communicative abilities primarily to respond to adult demands or to initiate specific requests, but not to engage in or maintain social interactions. The atypical appearance of the communicative behaviour among many severely handicapped individuals may be related to their lack of understanding or experience in using their communicative abilities for conversational purposes. The assessment of reciprocity is included as a separate scale to focus attention on those aspects of communicative abilities which relate to conversational skills. Because conversation requires both expressive and receptive abilities, some items from the Intentional Communication and Receptive Communication scales which relate to the development of conversational abilities are included in the Reciprocity scale.

The Reciprocity scale is divided into three broad levels each of which includes several sequential steps. The earliest level assesses the child's repertoire of actions which serve to initiate, sustain and terminate social exchanges. This early level is distinguished from subsequent levels in that the child emits these behaviours unintentionally and without awareness of their affect on the partner. It is the partner's response, sensitivity to the child's actions, and ability to interpose actions in the regular pauses in ongoing activities that make it appear that the child is participating in a conversational exchange.

At the next level, the scale assesses the child's use of intentional actions to initiate, sustain, terminate and to protest at the termination of an exchange. The child's focus, however, remains on his actions and their effects, rather than on the establishment and maintenance of an exchange with a partner. At this level, the child also becomes more adept at eliciting the adult's attention and responding to the adult's attempts to gain the child's attention. An expanded repertoire of social conventional gestures accompanying exchanges are also observed.

At the highest level, the scale assesses the child's use of intentionally communicative behaviours to participate in conversation. The child's focus is on the partner and the exchange, rather than on his actions and their effects. It is at this point that the child can lead and pace communicative exchanges on a variety of topics and eventually incorporate gesture and words (oral or manual) into conversational exchanges.

Summary

In the construction of items and examples for scales of normal development, it is generally assumed that there is a chronological age-related correspondence between physical and mental development, that sensory and motor abilities are intact, and that there is a core of early experiences common to all children. The validity of these assumptions, however, cannot be assured among the deaf—blind. For example, among deaf—blind children, physical maturation often exceeds cognitive development. Thus, the deaf—blind child's abilities may be expressed through behaviours of which the normally developing child, at the same cognitive level, is incapable. Furthermore, specific sensory and motor impairments frequently restrict or alter the ways in which cognitive and communicative abilities are expressed. Finally, the early experiences and opportunities for the deaf—blind child to interact with the social and material environment generally differ considerably from his normally developing counterpart. Some of the differences in experiences directly result from the presence of severe impairments (e.g. decreased or distorted sensory input, lack of mobility, decreased social contact). Others, however, relate to the educational interventions to which deaf—blind children are exposed. For example, normally developing children rarely encounter the type of skill training prevalent in educational programmes for low-functioning, deaf—blind individuals. Instead, 'early intervention' for the normally developing child features responsiveness to the child's needs and desires, involvement in reciprocal interactions, and organization of the child's environment for the purpose of encouraging self-directed and self-paced exploration and learning. These differences in early and ongoing experiences mean that the deaf—blind individual's behaviours, more so than his normally developing peer, will reflect adult-imposed skills, often maintained by extrinsic reinforcement, rather than the individual's intrinsically generated and self-supported abilities.

In designing the Callier-Azusa Scale-H, we have attempted to make developmental assessment applicable to the deaf—blind by relating behaviours commonly observed among deaf—blind individuals to the developmental levels they indicate. At the same time, we have attempted to construct items and item sequences which reflect underlying developmental processes common to all individuals. Through relating observed behaviours among the deaf—blind to normal developmental processes, we hope to refocus assessment on developmental processes rather than behaviour, and, thereby, promote the design of individualized intervention procedures aimed at facilitating development, rather than the establishment, modification or elimination of behaviours.

References

Bates, E. (1979) *The Emergence of Symbols*, Academic Press, New York

Battle, C.W. (1981) 'Teacher Responsiveness to the Communicative Expressions of Their Severely Handicapped Students' unpublished master's thesis, University of Texas at Dallas

Clark, R. (1978) 'The Transition from Action to Gesture' in A. Lock (ed.), *Action, Gesture and Symbol*, Academic Press, New York

Corrigan, R. (1979) 'Cognitive Correlates of Language: Differential Criteria Yield Differential Results', *Child Development, 50*, 617-31

Curtis, W. and Donlon, E. (1983) 'A Ten-Year Follow-up Study of Deaf-Blind Children', *Exceptional Children, 50*, 449-55

Day, P.S. (1983) 'Assessment of Deaf—Blind Children' in S. Ray and M.J. O'Neill (eds.), *Low-Incidence Children: A Guide to Psycho-educational Assessment*, Natchitoches, Louisiana

Dore, J. (1977) '"Oh Them Sheriff": A Pragmatic Analysis of Children's Responses to Questions' in S. Ervin-Tripp and C. Mitchell-Kernan (eds.), *Child Discourse*, Academic Press, New York

Hunt, J. (1976) 'The Utility of Ordinal Scales Inspired by Piaget's Observations', *Merrill-Palmer Quarterly, 22*, 31-45

Newson, J. (1979) 'Intentional Behavior in the Young Infant' in D. Shaffer and J. Dunn (eds.), *The First Year of Life*, John Wiley and Sons, London

Nicolich, L.M. (1981) 'Toward Symbolic Functioning: Structure of Early Pretend Games and Potential Parallels with Language', *Child Development, 52*, 785-97

Piaget, J. (1962) *Play, Dreams and Imitation in Childhood*, W.W. Norton, New York

Prutting, C. (1979) 'Process, 'pra/, ses n: The Action of Moving Forward Progressively From One Point To Another On the Way To Completion', *Journal of Speech and Hearing Disorders, 44*, 3-30

Schaffer, H.R. (1979) 'Acquiring the Concept of Dialogue' in M. Bornstein and W. Kessen (eds.), *Psychological Development from Infancy: Image to Intention*, Lawrence Erlbaum Associates, Hillsdale

Sigman, M. and Ungerer, J. (1984) 'Cognitive and Language Skills in Autistic, Mentally Retarded and Normal Children', *Developmental Psychology, 20*, 293-302

Spitz, R. (1965) *The First Year of Life: A Psychological Study of Normal and Deviant Development of Object Relations*, International Universities Press, New York

Stein, L., Palmer, P. and Weinberg, B. (1982) 'Characteristics of a Young Deaf—Blind Population', *American Annals of the Deaf, 127*, 828-37

Stillman, R. (1978) *The Callier Azusa Scale-G*, University of Texas at Dallas

——, Aylmer, J. and Vandivort, J. (1983) 'The Functions of Signalling Behaviors in Profoundly-Impaired, Deaf—Blind Children and Adolescents', Paper presented at the Annual Meeting of the American Association on Mental Deficiency, Dallas, Texas

—— and Battle, C. (1983) *Callier-Azusa Scale-H: Cognition and Communication*, University of Texas at Dallas

—— and —— (1984) 'Developing Prelanguage Communication in the Severely Handicapped: An Interpretation of Van Dijk Methods', *Seminars in Speech and Language, 5*, 159-70

Uzgiris, I. and Hunt, J. (1975) *Assessment in Infancy: Ordinal Scales of Psychological Development*, University of Illinois Press, Urbana

Werner, H. and Kaplan, B. (1963) *Symbol Formation*, John Wiley and Sons, New York

Wetherby, A.M. and Gaines, B.H. (1982) 'Cognition and Language Development in Autism', *Journal of Speech and Hearing Disorders, 47,* 63-70
—— and Prutting, C.A. (1984) 'Profiles of Communicative and Cognitive Social Abilities in Autistic Children', *Journal of Speech and Hearing Research, 27,* 364-77
Wolf, D. and Gardner, H. (1981) 'On the Structure of Early Symbolization' in R.L. Schiefelbusch and D.D. Bricker (eds.), *Early Language: Acquisition and Intervention,* University Park Press, Baltimore

PART SIX

CURRICULUM PLANNING AND TRAINING METHODS

16 APPROACHES TO TEACHING PEOPLE WITH VISUAL AND MENTAL HANDICAPS

Anthony B. Best

Introduction

In this chapter we shall start by examining the special needs created by blindness or severe visual impairment and then relate these to mentally/ visually handicapped people. This is followed by a discussion on specialist teaching approaches appropriate for this population and, finally, some examples are given of teaching activities and resources which have been used successfully with the mentally/visually handicapped.

IMPLICATIONS OF VISUAL IMPAIRMENT

Severe visual impairment restricts the quality and quantity of experiences available. From a very early age a visually handicapped person is limited in what he can experience of the world. Firstly, his direct access to information is restricted. He cannot see objects around him such as chairs, books, ornaments, trees. Unless he is able to touch these objects, or examine them closely, he may not be aware of their existence. As a result of this, the child may grow up aware of what, for example, a chair is, but unaware of the variety of objects what can come into this category. His concept will extend to those chairs of which he has personal experience and, over several years, this may be only a handful. This inability to see objects also means that they are not available to act as a stimulus to action. The young child will learn to crawl partly because he sees objects he wants to crawl towards; we may think of getting a drink because we see an attractive jug of juice on the table. These stimulus objects serve to give us new ideas and sustain our interest in our surroundings, but are not available to a blind person. A third effect of this difficulty is that the visually handicapped child is unable to monitor the effect of his own actions. This can apply to a wide range of activities from seeing what happens as he moves muscles and limbs (and so developing a clear body image) to watching the reactions of other people to his actions.

Secondly, a visually handicapped person has difficulty in incidental learning. The sighted use this medium extensively (particularly children) for copying actions, play, social behaviour or work skills. Even simple skills, such as sitting up straight, using a knife, or, at a later age, kissing a friend, are largely acquired through noticing others and attempting to model their behaviour. We develop our idea of concepts — such as pouring and the properties of liquids — through incidentally noticing an activity going on around us; children develop their first reading skills through noticing brand names hundreds of times during their first three to four years; we can learn about size and shape by noticing a newspaper being unfolded and folded up. All of these important formative experiences are unavailable to visually handicapped people.

Thirdly, visual handicap can limit the quality of information available. A clear example of this is meeting a person. Compare the sound of the voice with the experience of seeing the person and his clothes, size, shape, facial expressions, eye movements, stance and so on. It is quite possible that a simple wooden chair would be more interesting to a mentally/visually handicapped child than would be a person with a dull voice and whom he was not allowed to touch! To return to a previous example, the concept of a chair may be built up through tactually experiencing chairs but the impressions which make up that concept — perhaps of texture, temperature, details of shape — will be less precise and detailed than those available to a sighted person. Lowenfeld (1974) has provided an illustration of how those factors may affect a daily activity. Both the quantity and quality of information, then, is limited and this has several implications. Visually handicapped children tend to show a developmental lag in the first few years of their lives. Although this lag is not inevitable and it has been shown that appropriate remedial training can compensate for many of the difficulties (e.g. Norris, Spaulding and Brodie 1957; Fraiberg 1977), it is commonly found in children and can be significant by the age of nine months. A large number of researchers have identified this lag (e.g. Gomulicki 1961; Piaget 1970: Tobin 1972; Gottesman 1976) and have found that, in some areas of development, a lag of 18 months at the age of six would be typical for a congenitally blind child who has no additional handicaps. The child who is not held back as much as this is likely to be very bright and to have received expert guidance and stimulation from a very early age. These conditions are, of course, the opposite of those likely to be found in the mentally handicapped population with which we are primarily concerned. Reynell and Zinkin (1979) investigated the development of over 100 visually handicapped children and some of their findings are shown in graph form in Figures 16.1 and 16.2. Performance relates to items on their developmental scales but the graphs themselves show clearly the gap which can emerge between visually handicapped children and the sighted. It is important to note several specific areas where a lag may be found as these relate directly to teaching areas requiring special attention.

Motor Development

Motor development is often severely affected by visual handicap. The motivation to move may be lacking, or maybe the example from others of

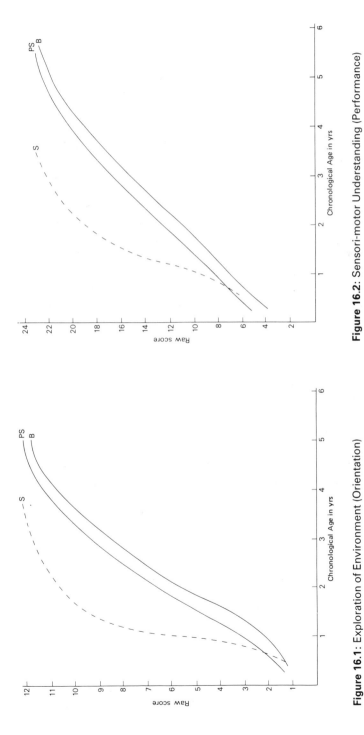

Figure 16.1: Exploration of Environment (Orientation)

Figure 16.2: Sensori-motor Understanding (Performance)

Source: J. Reynell, 'Developmental Patterns of Visually Handicapped Children' in *Child: Care, Health and Development*, vol. 4, pp. 291-303 (Blackwell Scientific Publications Ltd., 1978)

what can be achieved through body movement. The lack of visual information also means it is more hazardous to attempt to crawl and walk across a floor. Not only are the motor skills, such as walking, bending, reaching, not practised, but blind people face a difficulty in developing the orientation skills necessary for movement. These skills include the ability to perceive the relationship between objects in a room, the shape of the surroundings, distance and direction from the person to fixed objects, the interpretation of sounds, air currents and temperatures. These are all abilities that blind people can acquire with the help of special training but which are much more difficult to develop without some specialist help or if the visually handicapped person has difficulty integrating a number of pieces of information. Detailed discussion of this area is given by Hart and Blasch in Welsh and Blasch (1980).

The encouragement of movement is often a difficult area for parents who fear the accidents that may result from children becoming too confident. Other care-givers may also be hesitant about this, particularly if the blind person is amongst other people who could be knocked over by the blind person or would become aggressive if bumped into. Underachievement may, therefore, result from this secondary handicap rather than because of the visual impairment itself.

Language Development

Another major area of concern is language development. The problem does not seem to be innately linked with visual handicap but rather is more likely to be attributable to experiential poverty. If care-givers are not aware of the importance of talking to, stimulating and playing with children and of giving them concrete first-hand experiences, then the child may grow up with incomplete or inaccurate concepts. The attachment of meaning to words is another aspect of interest. Many researchers and practitioners have pointed out that blind children will have difficulty in understanding words unless they have first-hand experience of the object, action or attribute represented by the word. Even if they are able to use the word appropriately, they may not attach the same meaning to it as would a sighted child, as their experiences are likely to be different from those of fully sighted children. In extreme cases children may display 'verbalisms' — the use of words without any real understanding of their meaning — and careful questioning is necessary to check if this is happening. Some mentally/visually handicapped people talk a lot but may include nonsense words and phrases or repeat familiar colloquial expressions amongst their utterances. These are indications of the possible lack of real understanding of many of the words that are being used. Language development has been discussed in some detail by a number of writers such as Fraiberg (1977), Warren (1977) and Urwin (1978). Mills (1983), in the preface to a book on language development in the blind child, states: 'it would seem that blindness alone is not sufficient to produce deviant language acquisition. When blindness comes together with other handicaps of whatever kind, the chances of language disorders are increased.'

Cognitive Development

The developmental lag in cognitive development is the area which has received most attention from researchers as it is central to the emergence of an understanding of the world. The findings of researchers has been summarized by Warren (1977) and he identifies three main reasons which are suggested as being responsible for this lag. These reasons are:

1. cumulative lag;
2. restricted experiences;
3. less sophisticated discriminatory ability.

Piaget (in a lecture given in 1970, quoted in Gottesman (1976)) supported the idea of a cumulative lag when he stated:

> Blind infants have the great disadvantage of not being able to make the same coordinations in space that normal children are capable of during the first year or two, so that the development of sensory-motor intelligence and the coordination of actions at this level are seriously impeded in blind children. For this reason, we find there are even greater delays in their development at the level of representational thinking and that language is not sufficient to compensate for the deficiency in the coordination of actions. The delay is made up ultimately, of course, but it is significant and much more considerable than the delay in the development of logic in deaf and dumb children.

The idea of restricted experiences is based on the reduced number of experiences available to the visually handicapped child. In particular, sighted children gain a great deal of information from incidental learning. Much of this is not available to the visually handicapped child. They do not see liquid being poured from a tall jug into a wide bowl or a piece of paper crumpled up into a small ball. Tobin (1972) made this point when he stated:

> How far this developmental lag is attributable to restrictions in the extent and quality of the visually handicapped child's learning experiences and interactions with his environment is difficult to assess. It may be that visual impairment reduces the number of those entirely fortuitous experiences in which, for the sighted child, the inadequacy of

his existing schemata is borne in upon him. A comparison of the home and other pre-school backgrounds of, for example, conserving and non-conserving blind 6-year olds, would be one indirect way of testing the hypothesis that differences are traceable to the nature and complexity of the stimulation received. An alternative, and more direct, method of investigating this hypothesis would be through experimental comparison of different kinds and intensities of training along the lines of those used by Smedslund (e.g. 1961). The importance of the school in making good these deficits (if these are, in fact, the cause of the observed wide disparities in performance) would seem to need little underlining. (p. 97.)

In addition to this lack of quantity of experiences, Gomulicki (1961) suggested that the lack of the integrative functions of vision means that less sense can be made of any information which the child can experience. Therefore, the experiences are restricted as the visually handicapped person often has difficulty in perceiving the relationship between objects or actions. They do not know who has opened the door, they cannot tell which vehicle is making a particular noise. Gottesmann's point (1976) — that the visually handicapped use a less sophisticated discriminatory ability — ties in with this, but his emphasis is on the quality of the information. He feels that there must be a lack of precision in the information coming to a visually handicapped child and indeed, if one compares, say, listening to water being poured to actually seeing it, this point seems most reasonable. In the early stages of conservation, the child will be heavily dependent on this sensory input and it is at this level that a delay is often observed. Gottesman summarizes this by saying:

Because of the lack of appropriate experiences for conserving, the blind subjects at the six and seven year age level lagged behind the performance of both sighted groups. But at the eight to eleven year age level, the blind group performed as well as the other groups. This phenomenon could be due to the fact that the tasks at the older age levels required an increased reliance on integrative processes of cognitive functioning, rather than a reliance on the less sophisticated sensory discriminatory abilities. More information is conveyed through the visual perceptual processes than through the tactual processes at an earlier stage, therefore, the blind children perform less accurately than the sighted ones at that age level. At a later stage, both perceptual modalities relay a sufficient amount of information required by the subject to make appropriate conservation responses. (p. 99.)

Touch

The blind person will use touch as an important way of gleaning information. But touch, and, to a lesser extent, hearing, differ from vision in being 'linear' and sequential. They do not give a complete image of an object or room in one glance as does vision. Separate impressions must be built up and fitted together to give an appreciation of the whole, and it seems reasonable to assume that this requires good short-term-memory concentration and reasoning to interpret contextual clues. When the blind person is searching for detail, the perceptual 'window' available through touch is little more than the size of one finger tip and so the identification of unfamiliar objects can present a considerable challenge to even non-additionally handicapped blind people. An important part in the deductive process of recognizing an object is the identification of critical features, and experienced staff can help considerably by directing the blind person's attention to those features which will carry most information for them (a point that will be explored fully later in this chapter).

A second aspect of the use of touch is the length of time required to explore an object in this sequential manner, through initial explorations, adding information from sound or smell, re-checking. Even finding out about a simple object such as a chair requires an initial contact, perhaps on the chair back, then a hand movement down the back to confirm identification, then a sweep across the seat to check on objects which might have been left there. This will take very much longer than the simple glance which is over in less than a second. A more difficult task — such as finding a sock amongst the bedclothes — may take much longer, and an advanced skill — such as locating a paragraph heading in a braille book — may require the finger to touch over and read hundreds of words before meeting the required heading.

Residual Vision

For the partially sighted, an area of special interest is the development of residual vision. Different eye defects have very different effects on vision, but several workers with children (e.g. Barraga 1970; Chapman and Tobin 1979; Langley 1980) have devised programmes that develop the use of residual vision through carefully sequenced activities. These activities strengthen areas such as fixation, tracking, scan and search procedures, recognition of critical features, and appreciation of perspective. Many mentally/visually handicapped people seem to make little use of the incomplete and unreliable images supplied through their residual vision. Their vision may vary under different lighting conditions causing confusion in their minds as to what is around them; they may have blurred images of distant objects which, confusingly, seem to change shape and become clearer at a closer distance; they may have a narrow field of vision which gives perfectly clear central vision but which results in the person bumping into objects on the floor or knocking over objects with their hands if the objects are not within their narrow area of clear vision. An additional factor which may limit the use of residual vision is the understanding and expectations of the staff. They may not appreciate the selective nature of some eye defects or misinterpret a report which indicates that a client is 'blind or nearly so', and so make few demands on him to use any of the residual vision which is present. Little, if any, research work has been carried out to show if systematic training does make a significant difference to their use of residual vision. However, in the absence of research findings on this population, the evidence from non-additionally handicapped children, and the impressions of experienced workers with mentally/visually handicapped people would seem to provide clear justification for the inclusion of this type of training in a curriculum for the mentally/visually handicapped.

On several occasions, reference has been made to the effect of specialist intervention. A secondary handicap is often created by the lack of a true understanding by care-givers of the effects of visual impairment. This phenomenon is not exclusive to visual handicap, as has been discussed by writers such as Fraser (1980), but the emotional overtones associated with blindness, the low incidence of visual impairment and the complex nature of its effects all make it likely that parents, teachers, therapists and care-workers will have unrealistic or low expectations of what a visually handicapped person can achieve.

Implications for the Mentally Handicapped Person

All of these effects and implications have direct relevance to the mentally/visually handicapped person. The presence of mental handicap is particularly important as many of the difficulties created by visual impairment can be most easily overcome by using contextual clues and inference to supplement the meagre first-hand experiences. Yet these two techniques require reasoning and attending skills which may not be well developed in mentally handicapped people. There is so little redundancy in the information usually available to a visually handicapped person that every clue must be attended to in order to make sense of a situation. The mentally/visually handicapped person, for example, may hear a food trolley passing and smell the food, but may not be attending when a member of staff, above the general hubbub of noise, says that everyone must wait in their seats. The mentally/visually handicapped person may start moving towards the food and then become confused when admonished and sent back. The more severely handicapped person, particularly if there is an additional hearing impairment, may grow to dislike contact with staff if initial approaches have been sudden, such as a spoon in the mouth, a hand under the shoulder or a cold plastic shape thrust into the hand. Other clients will have the sight of someone approaching, perhaps eye-contact, then the sight of the object and a friendly facial expression, each of which will help him to anticipate the contact. The mentally/visually handicapped are particularly disadvantaged in not being able to control their own environment, not being able to impose a structure on daily activities, having difficulty in initiating contact. This can lead to poor self-image in those able to differentiate themselves from their surroundings and depending on a simple fixed daily routine. A number of writers have discussed this as a tendency in blind adults (Cutsforth 1951; Cholden 1958; Zahl 1962) and others have suggested that this might be particularly true of the mentally/visually handicapped or the deaf−blind (Brown 1983; Brock 1984).

Summary

So far in this chapter we have identified some of the important effects of severe visual impairment. These can be summarized as follows:

 direct access to information is restricted;
 incidental learning is restricted;
 the quality of information available is poor;
 touch becomes an important channel for information;
 useful but incomplete or unreliable visual images may be available.

The implications of these effects are that:

 learning takes longer;
 there may be a developmental lag in children;
 mobility may be severely restricted;
 language development may be delayed;
 the meaning attached to words may be altered;
 more time must be available for exploration by touch;
 little use may be made of residual vision;
 care-givers may have low expectations.

SPECIAL CURRICULUM AREAS

A discussion of curriculum should begin with a decision on the theoretical model of curriculum design which will be used.

There have been many discussions on this topic in relation to mentally handicapped people (for example, Penfold 1980; Kiernan 1981; Brown 1983), and it is impossible to select a model that will be acceptable to all practitioners. A developmental objectives-based model seems to be most widely advocated and, as it is an appropriate framework when examining the special needs of the visually handicapped, will be used here. The component processes of the approach — defining objectives, analysing tasks, selecting reinforcers — will apply regardless of the handicaps of our client. One area contained in a training programme is likely to be that of self-care skills such as feeding and dressing.

The sequence of acquisition of these skills is unlikely to be greatly affected by the presence of visual impairment, although the length of time taken between 'steps' and the training techniques will be affected. Training programmes for mentally handicapped people, such as those provided by Portage (Bluma and Shearer 1976) or Balthazar (1981), give appropriate developmental lists of skills as do assessment tools such as the PAC (Gunzberg 1976). Simon (1981) has also provided guidance in this area for those working specifically with mentally/visually handicapped people.

Preparatory skills such as grasping, reaching, discrimination, matching and sorting will need to be acquired, as they will by a sighted child, and in some areas identical objects can be used (for example, sorting beads, plates, forks and spoons, clothes, and soap). The earlier skill areas may need some modification. Reaching is one such area. In the non-handicapped infant, reaching usually follows visual tracking and would emerge at about four months. Reaching to sound, its equivalent skill in the visually handicapped, appears much later and so might not be established before tactile discriminatory skills emerge. Sorting and matching will be by texture and shape or sound. Discrimination by weight, smell, taste or temperature seems to be much more difficult, although this may be because of a relative lack of practice. Those with some residual vision will be able to use colour as a variable, but care will be needed in extending this to a combination of colour and shape. It may be that a client can see enough to discriminate clear colours, but not be able to cope visually with shapes. It may be that using vision and touch together presents a particularly complex task (note the difference between this activity and that of *confirming* a visual impression by tactual exploration).

Many fine motor skills are often seen as leading towards drawing and writing, but for the mentally/visually handicapped person this is often not the case. These activities are not available to the mentally/visually handicapped person and there are no substitutes for them. However, the fingers need to be taught to explore and to gain information in addition to the usual manipulative functions such as unscrewing, fitting together and twisting. These special skills may be acquired through practice and exposure, as much as through systematic instruction, although specific ideas for activities are given later.

The curriculum area of communication can also remain comparatively intact using models provided for the severely handicapped such as those by Popovich (1977) and by Crawford (1980). The communication subscales of the Reynell–Zinkin (1979) mental scales were designed specifically for use with the visually handicapped and include identical items to those found in scales for the sighted. The differences are in the examples provided in some of the items. For example, in matching objects and in following instructions, objects such as spoon, brush and cup are specified which are easy to discriminate tactually. Skills based on using 2-D and 3-D representations (e.g. matching pictures to objects, pointing to pictures on request) present particular difficulties. Pictures may not be clear enough to be seen, or be too abstract for the visually impaired person to recognize any similarity between the seen object and the representation. Often 3-D representations do not feel anything like the real object and so are rarely meaningful to a blind person. It is, therefore, usually practice to omit these sections from developmental curricula and establish a word (i.e. sign or verbal)/object understanding when prerequisite concept development skills have been developed.

Imitation skills are often included in early communication development and physical imitation may need special attention as severe visual impairment can make this difficult. McInnes and Treffry (1982) suggest a sequence of co-active and then re-active movements in the development of imitation and this model is appropriate for use with mentally/visually handicapped people. The first stage, co-active movement, will usually involve the child sitting on the floor between the legs of the adult. The two people move together, the child with his back to the adult. The adult will build on any movements the child can make and take him through simple movements such as bending, stretching, twisting. From this stage the adult begins to take turns with the child, allowing him to feel — and see — any movements she makes until, eventually, the child is ready for true imitation of gross and fine movements.

Two further curriculum areas need particular attention. These are mobility and the use of residual vision. Movement and mobility for the mentally/visually handicapped include many skills which do not usually need to be taught, or, at least, do not need to be considered as major teaching objectives when working with the sighted. Not only do the visually handicapped need activities which will help them become aware of and understand their environment (orientation); they may also need guidance in learning how to explore and move around safely (mobility). These special skills will build on a basis of gross motor skills such as are identified in a scale of normal development (see also Chapter 20, this volume).

The relevant subscale of the Reynell–Zinkin Scales illustrates well these special needs as it includes a number of items which would require very little effort on the part of the sighted such as 'exploration of furniture within reach', 'finding the door of a room'.

A curriculum in these areas should include consideration of the following:

understanding sounds	(same; different; directions; distance; identification; meaning)

identifying objects	(e.g. furniture; parts of a room — doors, corners, windows)
movements	(e.g. walking; running; jumping; climbing stairs; trampolining)
following routes	(e.g. using clues — foot, hand, sound; locating objects; travelling in contact with objects; free travel across open spaces)

This area is examined comprehensively by Welsh and Blasch (1980).

Many practitioners working with children have given attention to exercises and activities which may help to develop the use of residual vision. Some of these activities would be appropriate for use with adults who have poor vision. Work in this area varies from highly structured assessment and training packages, such as the Look and Think Procedures (Chapman and Tobin 1979) and the Diagnostic Assessment Procedure (Barraga and Morris 1980) to an informal approach in which staff develop the use of residual vision through encouragement and advice. In the latter approach, attention might be given to visual clarity with training involving the use of progressively less contrasting backgrounds to an object through head movements and experimentation with the distance at which objects are viewed; attention might be drawn to an object by making a sound with it, or making a vigorous movement until the client becomes used to locating and identifying the object without the help of additional clues. An example of the former approach is the Functional Vision Inventory (Langley 1980). This contains ideas for activities to encourage early visual skills such as fixation, tracking and changing focus and then moves on to the more complex skills such as discrimination, figure–ground recognition and per-spective. This publication also provides a most helpful general discussion of the development and use of residual vision, as does the very comprehensive textbook on low vision edited by Jose (1983).

Teaching Approaches

Many aspects of the teaching approach appropriate to the mentally/visually handicapped person will be identical to that used with the sighted; the analysis of tasks, selection of rewards, careful control of prompting, will all need consideration. In each, the presence of a visual handicap will affect decisions but the process will be unchanged.

For example, the analysis of the tasks of setting a table will contain the same items as for a sighted client, but may also include items such as 'locate edge of table', 'feel for edge of table mat', as these will be additional steps needed by a blind client. In selecting rewards, physical contact may be more appropriate and useful than it would be when working with sighted clients, and sound-making equipment may have an important place in the 'menu' of rewards. There are also some special principles which can be incorporated in a teaching approach.

Remove Distractions

Distractions may be in the room in which you are working or may be immediately around the task. Those at a distance may create interest which can distract the visually handicapped person from the task in front of him while those nearby may cause clutter amongst which it is difficult to focus attention on the objects associated with the task. These distractions may be of three types.

Visual Distractions. If the visually handicapped person has some residual vision, ensure that the background to the task itself and the surroundings are not distracting. A patterned wallpaper may make an object in the foreground difficult to see. Bright splashes of colour near the work area may be visually attractive but detract from the task. Objects on the table top not connected with the activity may cause confusion to those who seem them as imperfect images. Visual distractions can be overcome by careful positioning of the visually handicapped person and by the removal of any unnecessary objects near the task.

Tactile Distractions. For the totally blind person, tactile distractions may interfere with concentration. Small objects and features can cause this type of distraction. For example, small irregularities on the surface of a table or interesting texture on the side of chair. They may be the frayed ends of an apron or a piece of torn cardboard on a box. Careful observation will identify what might be interfering with concentration on the task being learnt.

Sound Distractions. We may be better able than a visually handicapped person to ignore sounds which are around us as we can more easily anticipate them and spot where they come from. Although it may be difficult to control the sounds that are going on in a room, it is important to remember that some may be a source of interest, confusion or curiosity for the visually handicapped person and this may interfere with his concentration on the training activity.

Check Table Height

If seated at a table, the person using touch will need to have his forearms and hands on the table-top in order to explore with his hands. If the table-top is too high, this will cause hunched shoulders or uncomfortably arched wrists. These are not major problems but it is better to avoid them if possible.

Keep Objects Within a Frame

If a frame is placed around a table, this will prevent objects from dropping off the table or moving out of arms' reach. A box with low sides or a tray with a straight lip could also help. If the visually handicapped person is working on the floor, then objects can be placed within a old tyre or inner tube.

Explore the Whole Area

Make sure the visually handicapped person knows what is in front of him by allowing him, or making him, explore all the area in front of him with his hands. If he does not do this, he may not realize that objects are on the table.

Explore Objects

If you are helping a visually handicapped person to explore objects, you must consider whether to place yourself behind the person to guide his hands, or opposite him where you can hold his hands but also watch his eyes to find out what he is looking at. Allow time to explore with the fingers and allow for repetition of movements as all the details may not be discovered in the first exploration.

Descriptions

Always check that the words you use are absolutely clear. Do not use expressions like 'this one' or 'over here' unless you can indicate exactly what you mean by making a sound or letting the blind person touch the object.

Replace Objects

If you move an object in the room or on the table-top, think carefully when you replace it. If you do not put it exactly where it was, you may be adding a difficulty for the visually handicapped person. You must decide whether you want to do this or whether it could distract him from the task he is attempting.

Activities

Specific ideas for activities are more difficult to ennumerate because of the wide range of performance levels included under the term 'mentally/ visually handicapped'. However, a few ideas are included here, taken from a number of sources, and further ideas can be found in the publications listed at the end of this chapter.

Fine Motor

It is important to develop finger movements and finger strength in the hands of young mentally/visually handicapped children as their fingers will be so important in gathering information. Young children also need practice in the co-ordinated use of both hands, a skill which seems to be particularly difficult for blind children. The following ideas give an indication of the type of activities which may be appropriate:

crumpling paper — greaseproof paper is pleasantly noisy;
pressing push buttons — can be wired to bells, buzzers and toys;
pulling paper off a roll;
squeezing water from a sponge;
pushing objects in clay;
grating carrot, apple;
opening purses;
unzipping a pencil case;
putting on and taking off clothes pegs from a box rim;
twisting a partially inflated cycle inner tube.

These activities can be used to develop basic finger skills such as the ability to locate, grasp, release, squeeze, pick up, pull, push, turn and press. Each can be used with the whole hand and with a finger and thumb.

Many centres collect together objects to make a 'Treasure Chest' or 'Feely Box'. This contains objects which can provide experiences in manipulation for the visually handicapped person. The following list is drawn largely from the ideas of Lilli Neilson, a Danish play therapist.

plastic plates (dinner, soup);
plastic cups and saucers;
milk mugs (plastic and stainless steel);
tooth mugs (plastic and stainless steel);
washing-up brushes (wood, plastic);
pan cleaners;
nail brushes, clothes brushes, hairbrushes;
shoe brushes;
toothbrushes;
tins with screw tops (different sizes);
tins with press-on lids (different sizes);
small packets of raisins;
clothes pegs (wooden and plastic);
combs;
spectacle cases;
soap box with soap;
purses with different kinds of fasteners;
handbags;
pencil cases;
plastic and metal tins with a round hole in the lid;
magnets;

torches;
lengths of rope, leather thong, string;
plastic tin containing buttons (with slit in top like a moneybox);
doorlock with key;
bags made of cloth, strong canvas, leather;
balls of all sizes and material;
musical boxes;
large bolts with wing nuts;
vacuum cleaner hose;
comb in case;
rattles (football fan type);
balloons (inflated or inflatable with mouthpiece);
electric light switches;
spoons, teaspoons, 3 teaspoons bound together;
egg beater;
a net bag containing balls;
cloth bag with zipper (containing paper);
bicycle pump;
bicycle inner tube;
kitchen timer;
rubber horn;
plastic tubing (for blowing into water);
old clock;
partly-blown-up balloon with rice or peas inside.

Many of the fine motor activities help the mentally/visually handicapped person build up more than manual dexterity. They will help to form concepts of objects and what they can do. The suggested materials include those with a flexible shape such as an inner tube as well as rigid shapes. At a more general level, they will help him to discover things and understand the difference between himself and the outside world. Without vision, this differentiation seems particularly difficult and, at a later stage of development, this differentiation can be extended into an awareness of object permanence — the concept of objects existing even though they cannot be felt.

The non-handicapped infant is likely to grasp objects and shake, bang or mouth them at around five to six months. He will start to examine, explore and learn simple actions to produce an effect at around eight to ten months. It is at this developmental stage, before the emergence of experimentation, comparison or ordering, that many of the suggested activities are aimed. For example:

Playing with a balloon: feeling it; patting it; pressing it against his cheek; letting the air out and blowing it up again; feeling vibrations while making a noise with lips against the balloon; tying the ends of a partially inflated long balloon together to make a 'bracelet'; hanging a balloon mobile over the child.

Playing with nesting cups: putting them inside one another; shaking one inside the other; covering one with a smaller one; finding one under another; picking objects out of a cup; finding them and throwing them in a bucket.

Playing with cardboard boxes: climbing in and out; being pulled about; being put on head; filling with objects; attaching rope and pulling towards child; cutting holes and putting arms through them.

Mobility

A second group of activities is directed towards developing mobility. Many ideas for appropriate activities are included in literature such as that by Tooze (1981), McInnes and Treffry (1982), Leary and Von Schneden (1982) and Presland (1982). The work of Bobath (1980) is particularly helpful for the early stages.

With the early movements of stretching and reaching, vibrators can often be used as a reward. A vibrating pad (such as those supplied in the UK by Vibro-Medico of Hadleigh, Essex) can be placed near the client and, on reaching out, he is rewarded with a few seconds' sensation. Alternatively, a small battery-operated massager can be used. Some therapists prefer to work on a wooden board so that the sounds made by the client and the apparatus provide useful feedback. When this board is supported an inch or so off the floor, the resonance and movement provide even more feedback.

The visually handicapped client is likely to be most confident moving near a firm surface such as the floor. Crawling and walking practice can be given through the use of a mobility circuit containing obstacles such as a mattress, tyres, cushions, bench, plank, carpet strip, barrel. The items can be selected to match the ability and confidence of the client and the circuit arranged so that they can reach the end, and a reward, with the minimum of help. Many activities can be created which involve following a short route made with strip of carpet, a length of rope or the backs of chairs. Again, the client needs some motivation for moving and so a reward should be given at the end of the route.

As confidence develops, movement should become firm, and can include bouncing activities on a small trampoline, inner tube, or soft-play environment. Again, it may be best to start with movements while sitting or lying before attempting to kneel or stand up. A barrel or large inflatable ball could also be used at this stage to encourage movement with the feet off the ground. The client can be swung, just off the floor, in a blanket, turned around while sitting on a tyre on castors, or, if weight permits, carried around on a staff member's back with feet just off the floor. He may be guided over uneven surfaces such as rocks, grass or sand. As confidence develops even further, the opportunity can be presented to walk up and down planks or a set of stairs, on and off chairs and along a series of blocks. The client should then be ready for free movement, walking or running across open spaces, perhaps following a sound, holding on to the end of a rope or even changing directions at the sound of a whistle.

CONCLUSION

In this chapter an attempt has been made to identify the special needs of mentally/visually handicapped people and to provide some examples of specific activities which can help to meet those needs. Attention has been drawn to curriculum areas which are important to include in an adequate compensatory training programme.

With an impairment to the distance co-ordinating sense of vision, there are severe restrictions to the quantity of the information available to a visually handicapped person. Understanding and learning can take longer and, in particular, there may be difficulties with mobility and language development. In addition to a full range of self-care, social skill and recreational activities, the mentally/visually handicapped person may need extra training in developing the use of touch, utilizing residual vision and acquiring movement and mobility skills.

While it has been possible to identify these needs and training areas with some confidence, there is, unfortunately, still only a restricted selection of literature available which suggests ideas for activities. Staff, therefore, need imagination and creativity in addition to the usual familiarity with behavioural approaches and a sense of humour.

References

Balthazar, E.E. (1981) *Scales of Adaptive Behaviour*, NFER, Slough
Barraga, N. (ed.) (1970) *Visual Efficiency Scale*, American Printing House for the Blind, Louisville, Kentucky
—— and Morris, J.E. (1980) *Diagnostic Assessment Procedure* American Printing House for the Blind, Louisville, Kentucky
Bluma, S. and Shearer, M. (1976) *Portage Guide to Early Education*, NFER, Slough
Bobath, R. (1980) *A Neurophysiological Basis for the Treatment of Cerebral Palsy*, Heinemann, London
Brock, M. (1984) *Christopher: A Silent Life*, Bedford Square Press, London
Brown, R. (1983) *Development of Programmes for Visually Impaired Mentally Handicapped Young People*, Wessex Studies in Special Education: 3
Chapman, E.K., Tobin, M.J. (1979) *Look and Think*, Schools Council, London
Cholden, L. (1958) *A Psychiatrist Works with Blindness*, American Foundation for the Blind, New York
Crawford, N.B. (1980) *Curriculum Planning for the ESN(S) Child*, British Institute of Mental Handicap, Kidderminster
Cutsforth, T.D. (1951) *The Blind in School and Society*, American Foundation for the Blind, New York
Fraiberg, S. (1977) *Insights from the Blind*, Souvenir Press, London
Fraser, B.C. (1980) 'The Meaning of Handicap in Children', *Child: Care, Health and*

Development, 6 (2), 83-91.

Gomulicki, B.R. (1961) *The Development of Perception and Learning in Blind Children*, Psychological Laboratory, University of Cambridge

Gottesman, M. (1976) 'Stage Development of Blind Children. A Piagetian View', *New Outlook for the Blind*, 70, 94-100

Gunzberg, H. (1976) *Progress Assessment Charts*, SEFA (Publications) Ltd, Stratford upon-Avon

Jose, R.T. (1983) *Understanding Low Vision*, American Foundation for the Blind, New York

Kiernan, C. (1981) *Analysis of Programmes for Teaching*, Globe Education, Basingstoke

Langley, M.B. (1980) *Assessment of Functional Vision*, Stoetling, Chicago

Leary, B. and Von Schneden, M. (1982) *'Simon Says' is not the Only Game*, American Foundation for the Blind, New York

Lowenfeld, B. (1974) *The Visually Handicapped Child in School*, Constable, London

McInnes, J. and Treffry, J. (1982) *Deaf–Blind Infants and Children*, Open University Press, Milton Keynes

Mills, A.E. (1983) *Language Acquisition in the Blind Child*, Croom Helm, London

Norris, M., Spaulding, P.J. and Brodie, F.H. (1957) *Blindness in Children*, University of Chicago Press

Penfold, J. (1980) 'Development of a Curriculum for Profoundly Handicapped Children', *Apex* 6 (3), 25-6

Piaget, J. (1970) *Genetic Epistemology*, Columbia University Press, New York

Popovich, D. (1977) *Prescriptive Behavioral Checklist for the Severely and Profoundly Retarded*, University Park Press, Baltimore

Presland, J. (1982) *Paths to Mobility*, British Institute of Mental Handicap, Kidderminster

Reynell, J. and Zinkin, P. (1979) *Developmental Scales for Young Visually Handicapped Children*, NFER, Slough

Simon, G.B. (1981) *Next Step on the Ladder*, British Institute of Mental Handicap, Kidderminster

Tobin, M.J. (1972) 'Conservation and Substance in the Blind and Partially Sighted', *British Journal of Educational Psychology*, 42, 192-7

Tooze, D. (1981) *Independence Training for Visually Handicapped Children*, Croom Helm, London

Urwin, C. (1978) 'Early Language Development in Blind Children', *British Psychological Society Occasional Papers*, 2 (2), 73-87

Warren, D.H. (1977) *Blindness and Early Childhood Development*, American Foundation for the Blind, New York

Welsh, R.L. and Blasch, B.B. (1980) *Foundations of Orientation and Mobility*, American Foundation for the Blind, New York

Zahl, P.K. (ed) (1962) *Blindness*, Hafner, New York

17 ORGANIZATION, MANAGEMENT AND CURRICULUM: SOME CONSIDERATIONS IN EDUCATIONAL PROVISION FOR THE MULTI-HANDICAPPED HEARING IMPAIRED

David E. Bond

Introduction

In this chapter the writer uses the terms hearing impaired and deafness to describe the whole range of hearing loss. It is also important to emphasize that most people with a hearing loss have residual hearing which should be stimulated and encouraged to the optimum to assist communication (see Bond 1983; Reed 1984; Tucker and Nolan 1984). Different degrees of hearing loss affect individuals differently; some with minimum losses may function as profoundly deaf, whilst others with profound hearing loss may function as having a minimum hearing loss. For the additionally impaired hearing impaired (AIHI) and multi-handicapped hearing impaired (MHHI) even very slight hearing loss or unilateral loss may have a severe to profound handicapping influence. The intellectually or mentally handicapped person, or person with specific learning difficulties who is hearing impaired (HI), may not develop techniques of looking for other visual cues, watching eye movements, facial expressions, body movements etc., or filling in the unheard gaps in communication through using contextual or other cues. Thus the AIHI or MHHI person can become significantly more handicapped by a hearing impairment which would not affect his 'normal' peers to the same degree and as a consequence the AIHI or MHHI may appear much more handicapped than they really are. Acoustically poor environments, poor lighting conditions, and generally difficult environmental conditions in which many HI, intellectually handicapped, or psychiatrically disturbed persons may work or reside (e.g. hospital environments with noisy wards) may also significantly exacerbate the problems created by HI and make persons with HI appear more handicapped than they are.

It is important to define the terms used in this chapter. AIHI are hearing-impaired persons who have additional impairments, but who are able to use residual skills and abilities to compensate sufficiently to enable them to function within open society as independent or potentially independent 'normal' hearing-impaired persons. The educational needs for this group may be within the range of integrated education or in special schools for the deaf (see later) depending on the severity of hearing impairment and other impairments and needs.

MHHI are hearing-impaired persons whose additional handicaps make, or appear to make, functioning as independent 'normal' hearing-impaired persons in open society impossible. The educational needs of this group are probably best met in special units or departments either within special schools for deaf or other areas of special education (see later) depending on the severity of hearing and other handicaps, and communicational, educational and other needs.

The label MHHI should not be considered synonymous with mental handicap. There tends to be a wide range of intellectual ability among many groups of MHHI individuals, although actual function may appear to be within the range of mental handicap. Consequently, when referring to the mentally handicapped, the writer prefers to use the terms intellectual or learning impairment as this would appear more consistent with the term hearing impairment, i.e. leaving an implication of an impaired faculty where there is useful residual capacity remaining.

In Education, problems in prescribing organization, management and curriculum for the AIHI and MHHI often appear to be exacerbated by the heterogeneous characteristics and needs of the population of the HI and which include failure of professionals to appreciate the effects and consequences of hearing loss, and rigid adherence to clinical definitions of impairment without recognizing the devastating additional difficulties caused by combinations of impairments. Clinical definitions based solely on information such as degree of hearing impairment (from pure-tone audiometry), the degree of visual, physical or other physiological handicap, criteria such as intelligence quotients, etc. would appear to have limited usefulness in describing the educational and management needs of the client. Cases which demonstrate this include the case described by the writer in Chapter 14, who, if classified on the severity of her hearing and visual problems, may well have been a candidate for facilities for the deaf–blind. As it was, she was able to function successfully in a mainstream class with a minimum of additional assistance. Other cases include intellectually or learning impaired, severely HI clients able to cope in aural environments in open society and employment.

For the hearing person in a normal environment, communication is an auditory, temporal, sequential, receptive and expressive experience. Communication is a flow of information which reinforces and assists in interpretation of the environment, actions and events. It may be direct or indirect, intentionally or accidentally overheard. For the hearing-impaired person auditory-aural communication may be distorted, unpleasant and difficult to cope with even when aided by hearing aids (Bond 1983).

Mode of communication may also become the criteria in classification of multi-handicap. At a simplistic level, communication problems of the hearing impaired may be reflected in:

articulation difficulties, if there is any intelligible articulation;
severely limited language: limited vocabulary; omissions of pivots, articles, prepositions; incorrect usage of tense, possessions, etc.;

temporal, sequential and structural difficulties in sentences;
inappropriate, irrelevant responses to questions;
physical responses in gesticulation
(see Conrad 1979; Quigley and Paul 1984).

Observation of hearing-impaired persons who have been inappropriately placed (e.g. in facilities for language-disordered, autistic, mentally handicapped), subsequent discussion with their 'supervisors', and survey and clinical information on the hearing impaired in mental handicap hospitals (e.g. Kropka and Williams 1980) appear to indicate that the communication difficulties experienced by the AIHI and MHHI often lead to inappropriate or exaggerated diagnosis of more limited intellectual ability than is the case, and behavioural–emotional-psychiatric difficulties.

Similar problems may occur for the HI, AIHI and MHHI whose main mode of learning and communication is visual–shape–spatial as opposed to auditory–articulatory encoding (see Conrad 1979). When placed in environments in which aural–oral mode of communication is practised rigidly (hopefully because of the needs of the majority of the clients in that environment), HI, AIHI and MHHI may all be classified as MHHI as a result of failure to progress with the aural–oral mode of communication. When, appropriately assessed, and placed in a total communication (TC), Signs–Supporting English (SSE) or Signed English (SE) environment, indications of additional impairments or handicaps either diminish or disappear.

Placement Problems

In addition to problems created by difficulties in clinical definitions of additional or multiple handicap and environmental factors and attitudes, problems may occur where recognition is given to one, some, or separate aspects of impairment and hearing impairment without adequate recognition of the effect of hearing impairment and its combined effect with other impairments on function (see Chapter 14).

As a result of priority listing of impairments without consideration of combined effects of sensory impairments, MHHI individuals may be placed in environments for the autistic, language disordered or mentally handicapped. Of cases seen by the writer who were inappropriately placed (most of these cases were visual–tactile encoders, learners and communicators), problems which often appear to emerge include:

failure or difficulties in identifying problems common with, but additional, to hearing impairment (e.g. visual defects);
difficulties in ensuring continuous effective function of devices like hearing aids — monitoring audiological and otological condition;
the individual 'integrated' person (see Dale 1984) may become an

individual isolate, relating only to the adult interpreter/tutor/care person, without opportunity, ability or skills to relate to others, feel successful, see himself as being like others and not a 'freak';

difficulties in extension of signed vocabulary (unless a close link is maintained with outside agencies/groups) particularly when relying on adult to use TC with SSE;

artificial restriction of communication to a few adults who use and 'sign';

problems in continuing communication when key personnel depart; communication with the child needing TC signs limited to sessions with adults, or when the adult is communicating directly with the child — thus isolating the child to make him appear unusual in the group;

staff failure to recognize TC (SSE or SE) as a mode of communication and not a magical solution to a complex problem — language and communication do not automatically occur when signs are used;

hesitancy from non-TC (SE/SSE) users in communicating with the child when it may be possible to communicate through gesture/mime.

Although there is a need to be cautious in generalizing from clinical and applied experience, it would appear that it is not possible to meet the complex needs and abilities of the HI, AIHI or MHHI without careful planning and a heterogeneous provision. A constancy model is not appropriate in assessment, placement, intervention or management of the AIHI or MHHI. Very significant changes (both positive and negative) may occur as a result of medical conditions or intervention, neurological change, communication and environmental intervention (see Bond 1979, 1982, 1984).

Many AIHI and MHHI individuals continue to be appropriately catered for in a heterogeneous range of facilities integrated into normal and special education. Problems of communication and learning difficulties created through combinations of handicaps need special consideration. Careful comprehensive and continuous assessment remain a constant need in every programme. It would also appear essential that the facilities and appropriately trained and qualified personnel must be available to ensure that the HI, AIHI and MHHI are not (as is possible) damaged by inappropriate assessment, or intervention.

The Organization of Educational Provision

In Chapter 14 of this book and in other articles (e.g. Bond 1982, 1984) the writer has outlined four major groups, adapted from Murphy (1977) into which the AIHI and MHHI might be grouped for treatment purposes, i.e. the AIHI or MHHI who show:

1. slight or significant additional impairments which do not significantly interfere with function or success in the environment in which they operate;
2. additional impairment by exogenous factors;
3. hidden specific learning difficulties such as aphasoid difficulties;
4. severe multiple handicaps adversely affecting learning, social communicational, behavioural and verbal educational function to such a degree that they are likely to require protected, sheltered or care-orientated environments throughout their lives.

These groups are not mutually exclusive; e.g. Groups 1 and 4 may show characteristics from Groups 2 and 3, and Group 2 characteristics from Group 3, and vice versa. The general usefulness of this grouping is to identify:

1. possible modes of function;
2. significant factors which will affect educational need, management and curricular organizations;
3. factors which are likely to be influential in decisions about assessment, diagnosis, and intervention.

At a practical level, the network of regional provision (see Jackson 1981; Reed 1984; Tucker and Nolan 1984) for pre-school and school-aged HI, AIHI and MHHI should include the following.

Multi-disciplinary Diagnostic Assessment and Management Team

This should consist of:

> Advisory Teacher of the Hearing Impaired;*
> Medical Officer;*
> Specialist Educational Psychologist.*

Specialists to whom the Team should have access should include:

> otologist — ear, nose and throat consultant;
> ophthalmic surgeon — eye specialist;
> psychiatrist;*
> other medical personnel, e.g. paediatrician, geneticist;
> speech and physiotherapists, orthoptists, etc;
> architect (with experience in acoustic assessment and treatment of environments);
> members of Educational Support Advisory Team.

Educational Support Team

This should consist of:

Advisory Teachers of the Deaf* including Educational Audiologist(s);
Peripatetic Teachers/Tutors;
Audiological Technician(s);
support where necessary from other advisory staff in the Educational
Services (e.g. psychologists, advisory teachers on visually, physically
and learning impaired, specialist curricular advisers).

In general, as more HI children are integrated into other areas of education, there should be more demands on and proportionately increasing numbers of the Educational Support Team. This increase should occur both to support, advise, guide and educate pupils, teachers, parents and others, and to ensure that placement and treatment is appropriate.

Integrated Provision for the Hearing Impaired

Mainstream schools and Special Education (e.g. special schools for learning difficulties, physically handicapped, etc.) should provide for children with the following needs:

no need for additional assistance;
regular additional specialist assistance (e.g. remedial teacher, speech
therapist, teacher of the deaf);
individual tutor/translator/teacher (see Dale 1984);
a special class or resource unit (in mainstream or Special Education);
Specialist Teacher of the deaf (from occasional or individual small group
tutoring to occasional 'integration' with mainstream;
see Jackson 1981; Dale 1984; Reid 1984)

Specialist Provision for the Hearing Impaired

Special arrangements could take the following forms:

1. Classes or units
   where mode of communication is different from that used with
   others (e.g. signs or tactile signs or symbolics or kinaesthetic —
   braille, etc.);
   where needs of group are significantly different and special management techniques are necessary, e.g. behaviourally emotionally
   disturbed, special care groups, etc.
2. Special Schools for the Hearing Impaired
   for HI with special abilities
   for aural/oral HI
   for visual/spatial HI — Total Communication (Signed English, etc).

---

*Whenever possible these members of the multi-disciplinary Assessment and Management Team, and the Educational Support Team should have additional specialist qualifications in the field of hearing impairment. It is assumed that advisory and peripatetic teachers of the deaf also hold a specialist qualification in education of the hearing impaired.

Both integrated and specialist provision should have access to services available through the educational support team or their equivalent e.g. in some specialist schools for the deaf there is additional provision for access to the whole range of medical specialists, physiotherapists, speech therapists, psychologists, audiologists, educational advisory teachers (visually, physically or learning impaired), curriculum advisors, etc. In addition, integration with a variety of special and mainstream educational provision occurs in some Special Schools for the Hearing Impaired.

Educational Management

This section will be limited to those MHHI whose functional abilities are within the range of mild to severe multi-handicap, and whose behaviours include:

1. overall non-verbal cognitive function with the range of mild to severe intellectual handicap — some within extreme variations in cognitive performance (many falling into the range of additional learning difficulties — see Chapter 14, this volume)
2. functional hearing impairment of a severe or greater loss;
3. non-primary auditory–articulatory encoders, i.e. pupils who rely primarily on visual information supporting auditory–articulatory information and need Total Communication where signs are used simultaneously to support spoken English.
4. a variety of additional handicapping conditions (usually as a result of the cause of hearing loss), including one or more of:

> a variety of disturbed and disturbing behaviour patterns (mild to severe);
> learning difficulties including specific learning difficulties (mild to severe) and intellectual impairment;
> visual impairments (mild to light–dark awareness) only;
> physical handicaps;
> neuro-muscular and involuntary hyperkinetic difficulties, epilepsy, etc.;
> exogenous factors, e.g. environmental cultural and communicational deprivation (usually in conjunction with behavioural, learning and/or other impairments and handicaps).

The majority of these pupils will require protected living and occupational environments when they leave school. Some may manage in sheltered open employment, but most have the potential to function successfully within sheltered environments, at home or sheltered accommodation (sheltered housing to sheltered hostel), and within sheltered workshop or day-training centre environments. (Provision for the severely to profoundly handicapped will not be included in this chapter.)

Given appropriate environmental conditions, some pupils (usually some of those with exogenous handicaps) should be able to progress to classes within a Special School for the Deaf or other suitable educational provision and eventually to more independent functions in open society. Conversely, damaging or inadequate environmental conditions may result in many of these youngsters becoming more dependent, eventually needing more costly special care environments.

Criteria Affecting Management of the MHHI

For the group of MHHI who function within the range described above, and who also need specialist provision (in units for deaf/MHHI or schools for deaf), the following management and environmental programming factors appear to contribute to positive changes in behaviour and function (see Bond 1982, 1984; Nolan and Tucker 1984).

1. There should be adequate staff–pupil ratios, both within the class and out of school environment, staffing at ratios of 2:3 to 2:5 depending on the needs of pupils (teacher and classroom assistant).
2. Staffing should be at a level which enables staff to work preventatively and to be able to cope with crises whilst leaving adequate cover for other pupils.
3. To ensure effective use of high staff–pupil ratio, it would also appear essential to work in small manageable departments in which all staff share ideas on child management, work out consistent methods to overcome problems, and develop problem-solving versus problem-orientated strategies. There should also be regular in-service training programmes for all staff, to cover:
   (i) behaviour analysis, observation skills and strategies; problem identification and simple problem solving strategies;
   (ii) simple behaviour management training (but *not* to be used in place of good curriculum and programming);
   (iii) communication (e.g. consistent Signs Supporting English) with emphasis on levels of difficulty;
   (iv) developmental psychology — language development, etc.
4. Staff should attend external courses, and make contact with others. Professional reading for stimulation and exchange of ideas is to be recommended. Staff should be encouraged to take responsibilities for different areas of development, curriculum or

special needs (e.g. audiometry and audiological aids or visual conditions and low-vision aids).

5.   A support service should be provided through head, deputies, educational psychologist, medical and other staff. Staff should be encouraged and supported to develop their own skills in methods, programmes and apparatus to solve problems rather than relying on outside expertise. Staff should be encouraged to use, adapt and modify advice and ideas to treat problems.

6.   Unit should be equipped with suitable and adequate material to enable *all* staff to work effectively encouraging appropriate work, social and other skills. This may involve considerable expenditure even on materials or apparatus which may be used less than 10 per cent of the time, but may be crucial to an intervention programme.

7.   Good liaison between home and school is vital, particularly on communication skills and experience programmes, and behaviour management. Where residential placement is involved, accommodation for parents would appear important to assist parent guidance and co-operative liaison. Parents can be trained in behaviour management through e.g. Portage-type programmes (Bluma, Shearer, Frohman and Hilliard 1976).

8.   Alternative strategies should be investigated to change behaviour; e.g. in 1980 a young pupil who had severe behavioural problems, psoriasis, eczema and severe asthma was placed on a goat's milk diet. When given cow's milk (owing to non-availability of goat's milk) on one occasion, there was an immediate deterioration in skin condition (he was reported to have started scratching almost immediately) and an increase in asthma. In May 1982 a trial period on an additive-free diet was broken on one occasion — an asthmatic attack followed almost immediately. Whilst the effects of special dieting *must* be treated and interpreted with caution, diet has *assisted* an improvement in behaviour and in health, in this case. Other forms of diet have assisted in approximately 30 per cent of selected cases.

9.   Consistency and constancy of staff would appear to be extremely important factors, particularly with the more dependent pupils. As pupils become more skilled and more independent, programmes should be organized or designed to ensure contact with an increasing variety of persons (i.e. in keeping with the model of mainstream education) where pupils start with one teacher but eventually move from one teacher to another for more specialized tuition or activities.

10. It would appear essential that tasks are structured to ensure a high level of occupation and success (i.e. 80 per cent plus through a carefully organized curriculum.)

Curriculum

The primary goal in education of the MHHI cannot realistically be 'to develop the ability to read and write the common language of the general society' as 'most deaf students ... do not attain even adequate ability to read and write English' (Quigley and Kretschmer 1982, pp. 65-6). For the MHHI, the primary education goal needs to be literally 'preparation for life' and optimum independence in life. The areas for development which contribute directly to the primary goal would appear to be:

communication;
independence in self-help skills;
behaviour and adjustment;
social interaction;
work and leisure skills and behaviour.

Developmental skills must play an important part in the curriculum, but only when incorporated into a comprehensive structured developmental programme of normatively based real-life experiences with sufficient flexibility for adaptation and inclusion of new or day-to-day conditions and developments. Adherence to rigid curricular outlines based solely on skill development may lead to stereotypic teaching strategies and style. This may affect awareness of environmental stimuli and pupil needs and motivators. For example, some years ago the writer visited a special class for mild to moderate intellectually impaired, behaviourally difficult students. The teacher was taking an extremely well-prepared, well-thought-out lesson based on the structured-skills-based curriculum. In view from the classroom a crane with steel ball was demolishing a building in spectacular style. It does not take much imagination to guess where pupil motivation and interest lay, or from where useful meaningful language and experience may have come!

Some Principles for Curriculum Development

Principles of curriculum development which the writer has found useful include:

1. The curriculum should be a positive, usable, useful, working guide which facilitates the work of teaching and other staff. It should positively help staff in planning more detailed individual and group programmes to meet the needs of pupils.
2. The curriculum for the MHHI should be structured and based on a balance of developmental skills and experiences from the normal range of development and relevant to the community and environments in which the MHHI exist. It should focus on, and be relevant to, pupil interest, motivation and level of function.

3. Context and structure of the curriculum should ensure that long-term and short-term programmes inter-relate and consistently reinforce and overlap with both future and past learning, providing opportunity for teachers to structure detailed programmes to ensure a high level of individual success.

4. The curriculum should be a flexible, developing, growing structure, both to meet changes within the environment and to meet changing pupil needs.

   In addition the writer has previously suggested (see Bond 1982, 1984) that, as part of the curriculum development and establishment, the following stages would appear appropriate to both structuring and evaluating intervention and should assist planning and development of curriculum and criterion-referenced assessment:

   > identify the specific goals to be taught — a broad statement of objectives and testable aims;
   > identify the specific skills to be taught;
   > sequence skills in order of difficulty or in other order in which the tasks should be taught;
   > break sets of skills into a structured developmental hierarchy of small bits with which the child can cope (task analysis);
   > teach building/linking sub-skills to skills;
   > analyse/assess/test effectiveness of tuition/intervention;
   > during intervention, observe regularly (e.g. hourly, daily, weekly) to test results of intervention and to indicate levels of competence reached in new skills or in the behaviours being modified.

   Some form of learning hierarchy should also be incorporated into the objectives-based curriculum, e.g. Haring and Eaton (1978):

   > acquire the behaviour
   > achieve fluency of response
   > demonstrate generalization in classroom
   > adapt learning to novel situations outside classroom.

5. The curriculum and its foundations must be understood by the teachers using it. Involvement of all staff in curricular development, evaluation and modification would appear essential to both effective development and application of a curriculum.

6. Developmental language and communication should be linked to all aspects of the curriculum. Utilization of all sensory channels is essential, e.g. auditory aids to assist and encourage use of residual hearing, visual, vibratory (tactual) and other aids which may assist in communication, understanding, and improving function in the

environment. Communication and language experience and thus the mode of communication for the MHHI must be a useful, meaningful continuous and consistent process both in and out of the classroom environment. It would appear that the most valuable communication systems or modes to use with the MHHI are those which are at least compatible if not the same as those which they are likely to use most of their lives. The native sign language (British or American Sign Language) used by the deaf, or derivatives from the language which are designed for educational purposes (e.g. Total Communication, Signed English, Signs Supporting English; see Clare 1984) or for those in more limited environments (e.g. Makaton; see Walker 1980) would appear relevant to the needs of the MHHI, particularly those who are likely to have contact with other HI people.

7. For most MHHI individuals the language curriculum needs to have structure in view of learning and specific learning difficulties (see Chapter 14). As learning difficulties often include short-term memory, sequencing difficulties, visual attentional problems and limitations in vocabulary, developmentally based language and communication programmes should be usefully incorporated with the overall curriculum.

8. Wherever possible it is both useful and time-saving to incorporate the works of others into an overall curriculum. This should include specific skills, training programmes, material from psycho-educational assessment (see Chapter 14, this volume) and more general material:

> developmental guides and checklists (Gesell 1954; Bluma *et al.* 1976; Jeffree and McConkey 1976; Cunningham and Sloper 1978);
>
> language (Crystal, Fletcher and Garman 1976; Masidlover and Knowles 1982);
>
> visual–perceptual (Frostig 1972);
>
> books which have invaluable teaching suggestions, e.g. developmental ideas (Clure 1972; Freeman 1975);
>
> curricular development e.g. *In Search of a Curriculum* by Staff of Rectory Paddock School (1983) is an invaluable reference; borrow curriculum from other schools or units who have similar MHHI students;
>
> behaviour management (e.g. Westmacott and Cameron 1981; Ferster and Culbertson 1982).

Development of a Curriculum for the MHHI

In general it is rare that curriculum development should have to start without useful ideas from previous curricula or programmes. Care should be taken to ensure preservation of useful ideas, as there is a danger where new or different ideas are seen to offer a solution to educational problems that new ideas are sometimes used at the expense of previously useful techniques and proven theoretical approaches. Curricula would appear to have more validity where practice is linked to theories and the reality of proven practical application. The development of a curriculum should be a scientific process in which programmes, goals and new ideas are systematically applied and tested, then retained, modified or rejected, depending on the results.

A programme toward developing a curriculum might include some of the following stages:

1. Prepare a programme involving staff in individual and group assessments, case discussions, in-service training of staff; send staff on courses, establishing links with facilities where there are useful curriculum ideas, and highlighting areas where the current curriculum needs further development.

2. Work to evaluate or establish key areas of the curriculum for specific skill development, e.g. in previous exercises of this nature teachers of the MHHI have listed:

> language and communication including total communication, reading, other symbolic systems, speech and speech reading;
> behaviour including interaction, interpersonal relationships, self-understanding and relation to self, work behaviours, on-task, attention to task;
> social skills, e.g. self-help (eating, dressing, toileting) independence, adaptability, ability to choose and make decisions;
> cognitive–intellectual, e.g. memory, sequencing, visual discrimination, analogous and associative reasoning;
> locomotor, gross motor and mobility skills;
> verbal educational skills, e.g. measurement, number, knowledge about environment;
> leisure, free time, occupation;
> practical constructive skills as applied to work tasks, e.g. woodwork, cooking.

Choose topics around which the curriculum might be based; e.g. topics listed by staff working with the MHHI have included:

> health education;
> home care;
> environmental studies;
> gardening;
> practical work — woodwork, metal work;
> art and craft;

verbal educational;
number and reading work, often linked to environmental studies and other areas.

Specific topics related to, e.g. environmental studies, can include 'myself', home, 'people who help me', school, transport, things we eat, growing things, animals, animal care, farms, seasons.

3. Staff working in small groups can then develop areas of the curriculum in which they are interested, e.g.

assess needs and current levels of pupils in specific area;
decide skills and knowledge necessary; check other material which might be incorporated, e.g. specific skill training;
extrapolate from current level of function to projected level in, e.g. five years;
arrange skills and experiences/topics in hierarchical order over, e.g. one- and five-year spans (five-year more general);
discuss with other groups and inter-link relevant areas of the curriculum.

4. Plan guides over a period in detailed form for short-term use. Sample guides are available in, e.g., *In Search of a Curriculum* (Rectory Paddock School 1983). These guides should give an indication of information which should be included in curricular guides.

5. Develop checklists, tests and skill tasks which can be used as a criterion-referenced method of evaluating acquisition of knowledge, curriculum. Then apply and test.

Summary

There are problems in defining the MHHI. It would appear that a definition based on functional level (i.e. severity of impairment) of hearing impairment, behaviour, independence, social relationships, communication, cognitive skills, mobility and projected level of independence post-school should form a useful basis for grouping for overall management.

Owing to difficulties in defining the MHHI, it would not appear to be valid to suggest that one curriculum would be appropriate to meet the needs of all. As the MHHI have fairly heterogeneous needs, more specific curricular programmes are probably best designed within individual schools, departments or units with the functional skills, activities, needs and guesstimated potentials in mind. There is a wide variety of published training programmes, and publications which can contribute to development of a more specific curriculum. *In Search of a Curriculum* (Rectory Paddock School 1983) is a particularly useful resource guide, and there are others.

Successful implementation of a curriculum would appear dependent on a number of factors, including staff, staff commitment, relevance of curriculum to needs and abilities, adequate staffing ratios, and staff support and guidance systems including both in-service and external specialist training. Curricular organization should be part of an overall problem-solving orientated environment in which the whole system is directed toward provision of opportunity for structured progressive success.

In development of curriculum management, organization and other techniques, care should be taken to ensure that an objective systematic and scientific approach is taken toward improving educational resources designed to meet the needs of the MHHI. New or different methods rarely provide miraculous universal solutions and, although new methods and ideas are vital to continued improvements, there is often a danger that rejection of existing organization, curriculum and method may result in existing positive aspects being lost.

References

Bluma, S., Shearer, M., Frohman, A. and Hilliard, J. (1976) *Portage Guide to Early Education* C.E.S.A., 12 Box 564 Portage, Wisconsin

Bond, D.E. (1979) 'Aspects of Psycho-Educational Assessment of Hearing Impaired Children with Additional Handicaps', *Journal, British Association Teachers of the Deaf* (3)

—— (1982) 'Management of Hearing Impaired Children who have additional learning and behavioural difficulties', paper presented to Heads of Services and Schools for Hearing Impaired, Conference, University of Manchester 1982; published in proceedings of that conference, Manchester University Press 1983

—— (1983) 'Hearing impaired and deaf, the psychology and education' in R. Harre and R. Lamb (eds.), *The Encyclopaedic Dictionary of Psychology*, Blackwell Reference, Oxford

—— (1984) 'Hearing Impaired Children. Some aspects of additional impairment and multiple handicap' in D.E. Bond and R. Reid (eds.), Special Edition on Hearing Impairment, *Journal of the Association of Educational Psychologists*

Clare, M. (1985) 'An Introduction to Manual Communication Systems in Educational Psychology in Practice' in P.C. Love (ed), *Journal of the Association of Educational Psychologists*, *1*(1), 33-6

Clure, M. (1972) *Why didn't I think of that?* Bowmar Publications

Conrad, R. (1979) *The Deaf School Child: Language and Cognitive Function*, Harper and Row, London

Crystal, D., Fletcher, P. and Garman, M. (1976) *The Grammatical Analysis of Language Disability: A Procedure for Assessment and Remediation*, Studies in language Disability and Rehabilitation. Edward Arnold, London

Cunningham, C. and Sloper, P. (1978) *Helping Your Handicapped Baby*, Souvenir Press, London

Dale, D.M.C. (1984) *Individualised Integration: Studies of deaf and partially hearing children and students in ordinary schools and colleges*, Hodder and Stoughton, London

Ferster, C.B. and Culbertson, S.A. (1982) *Behaviour Principles*, Prentice-Hall, New Jersey

Freeman P. (1975) *Understanding the Deaf–Blind Child*, Heineman Health Books; London

Frostig, M. (1972) *Pictures and Patterns. The Developmental Program in Visual Perception*, Teachers Guide (Beginning) Follett, Chicago

Gessell, A. (1954) *The First Five Years of Life*, Methuen and Co., London

Haring N. and Eaton, M. (1978) 'Systematic Instructional Procedures: An Instructional Hierarchy' in N. Haring, T. Lovitt and M. Eaton (eds.), *The Fourth R: Research in the*

Classroom Columbia, Merrill

Jackson, A. (1981) (ed.) *Ways and Means III. Hearing Impairment*, Globe Educational Publishers, Basingstoke

Jeffree, D.M. and McConkey, R. (1976) *Parental Involvement Project Development Charts*, Hodder and Stoughton, London

Kropka, B. and Williams, C. (1980) 'The Deaf and Partially Hearing in Mental Handicap Hospitals. The Disadvantaged Minority', *British Journal Mental Subnormality*, 26, 89-93

Masidlover, M. and Knowles, W. (1982) *Derbyshire Language Scheme*, Educational Psychology Service, Derbyshire.

Murphy, L.J. (1977) 'The Multihandicapped Child' in *Proceedings N.Z. Conference of Teachers of the Deaf*, Kelston, NZ

Quigley, S.P. and Kretschmer, R.E. (1982) *The Education of Deaf Children*, University Park Press, Baltimore

—— and Paul, P.V. (1984) *Language and Deafness* Croom Helm, London, and College Hill Press, San Diego

Rectory Paddock School (1983) *In Search of a Curriculum* Robin Wren Publications (2nd Edn. revised), Kent

Reed, M. (1984) *Educating Hearing Impaired Children*, Children with Special Needs Series, Open University Press, Milton Keynes

Tucker, I.G. and Nolan, M. (1984) *Educational Audiology*, Croom Helm, London

Walker, M. (1980) *Revised Makaton vocabulary*, Makaton Development Project, Camberley, Surrey

Westmacott, E.V.S. and Cameron, R.J. (1981) *Behaviour can Change*, Globe Education (Macmillan), Basingstoke

18 AN EDUCATIONAL CURRICULUM FOR DEAF–BLIND MULTI-HANDICAPPED PERSONS

Jan van Dijk

The Target Population

It is my intention in this contribution to write an outline of a curriculum for severely sensorily deprived children, i.e. deaf–blind children. 'Curriculum' means a specific course of study (Webster, New Twentieth Century Dictionary). In order to make this course of study meaningful, I should first try to describe the population which has to be educated by means of it. In my long career in the field of the education of the severely handicapped child I became very aware of the unique status of the child who is deprived of hearing and sight, from birth.

An organism so deprived of the main natural channels of stimulation, responds to such a condition in a very strong way. One can observe how such children try to overcome their loss of vision by pushing on their eyeballs, by staring into the sun or another strong source of light, while moving their hands in front of their eyes. I have explained these stereotyped behaviour patterns as a reaction to sensory loss (van Dijk 1982).

It is noticeable that when these children meet a person, they try to climb on his body and they want to be carried around. When nobody is around it is sometimes observed that a child makes 'jumping' movements on a windowsill or similar objects. From the deprivation theory I have developed, this behaviour might be explained in terms of lack of mothering. When given an unknown object it is quite possible that the child hardly explores it, but either uses it as an extension of his/her body (e.g. by moving it in front of his/her eyes) or throws it away. This child is not curious and not aroused by the novelty of the new toy.

In developing a curriculum along gross lines, the type of child on whom I focus is one who is sensorily, emotionally and intellectually deprived of all adequate stimulation.

The aetiology of the children I have in mind is mainly congenital Rubella, but professionals dealing with children who have suffered a multiple sensory loss because of Cytomegalovirus infection (Hanshaw and Dudgeon 1978) or other types of infection in early pre-natal development, may find similar behaviour in these youngsters.

Our Educational Approach

If my deprivation theory is accepted, the educational approach we have employed during the past two decades becomes rather plausible.

374

Descriptions of this theory can be found in Tervoort, van de Geest, Hubers, Prins and Snow (1972), Robbins (1977), Cardineaux, Cardineaux and Löwe (1981), Hammer (1982), Hewitt (1982), Coll, Dumoulin and Sourion (1983) and Cardineaux (1983).

A child deprived from birth of his senses of hearing and sight, however partially this might be, tries to make up for his sensory loss and, in order to keep his damaged organism in balance with the environment, exhibits the types of stereotypic behaviour I have described. This balance is very delicate between the child and his environment. When there are minor changes, the child might be already very upset or over-aroused (Berlyne 1960; Hutt and Hutt 1965). This may lead to headbanging, biting own lips and fingers, or hours of endless crying.

The first demand of an educational programme is, therefore, that all people in the child's environment try to understand, i.e. try to 'read', the child's behaviour. This requires that only people who are familiar with the child's behaviour and who are very sensitive towards his needs will be able to accomplish something positive. When the child bites his fingers one day more than he did the previous one, this behaviour might be interpreted as due to lack of attention given to the child on that particular day. When the child cries for a long time, he might be suffering from his separation from home. When the child pokes his eyes more often than normally, his environment might be too complex for him. By means of his behaviour, however difficult it might be to interpret it, the child signals his needs. The steps the teacher should take depend a great deal on a child's temperament. When the child is over-excited, the teacher might give him a bath where he can relax. When the child is in a state of under-stimulation, the teacher might decide to give him a massage with bodycream or carry him around and soothe him.

In the educational atmosphere I describe, the child holds the central position, the teacher 'follows' the child and, when the child responds, the teacher is present to answer the child's request. In terms of 'learning theory' (Bandura 1969), I am more in favour of a curriculum based on the principles of operant conditioning than on a strict S–R model. In the latter it is always the teacher who wants the child to carry out activities, which often the child does not like. I refer to activities such as matching exercises, pegboards, stringing beads, etc. In responding to the child, we aim to develop in the child the very important feeling of mastery and competence. The child should feel that he is not at the mercy of his environment, but that he is able to control it, to influence it. It has been shown (Stephans and Delys 1973) that the expectation of a child that he can influence his situation leads to more interesting learning. By the same token, if the teacher responds appropriately to the child (response-contingent stimulation, Main 1975), the child will not only show more pleasure in his activities, but will also attach himself to that person (Ainsworth and Bell 1974; Bowlby 1979).

In our ideas on the education of severely sensorily impaired children, development of attachment has become a more and more vital issue. We consider it as the basis for learning. In the process of bonding, vision plays a dominant role, as can be clearly observed in attachment characteristics such as smiling, stretching out the arms when a familiar person approaches the child, and eye contact (Tait 1972; Fraiberg 1975). It is logical to assume that this process develops much more slowly in a completely deaf–blind child than in the child with residual vision.

Attachment

Our program of stimulation of attachment can be divided into three steps (see van den Tillaart 1985).

Co-active Movements and Responsiveness

Co-active movement means that the teacher 'joins-in' with the activity of the child, e.g. if the child wants to jump, the teacher jumps with him. Daily living activities, especially, give ample opportunity for doing things together (washing the face, brushing teeth, pulling on the socks, etc.). By adequate reaction to the child's co-operation, however minor this can be, an atmosphere of security and confidence will grow. This procedure has been nicely described as our 'hands-on' method because often one has to lead the child's hands through all these activities. The child will become more active himself, when the same activity is repeated day after day, in the same situation, by the same person. We call this:

Structuring the Child's Daily Routine

It has proven a fruitful approach when the day of a multiple sensorily impaired child is built around some important activities, such as taking a bath, mealtime, preparing a snack, going to the swimming pool, preparation for going to bed, etc. By structuring these daily living routines, one builds up a 'chain of expectancies' (Vygotsky 1983). After such a chain is established (e.g. taking the toothbrush, putting paste on the brush, etc.), one leaves out a vital element (e.g. the cup of water). At that moment it is quite possible that an orienting reflex will arise (Berlyne 1960; Mescheriakov 1962). The child will look for the cup, and lead the teacher's hand to the shelf where the cups are kept. Responding to this may establish the bond between child and teacher.

Characterization

Another important element in the bonding proces is that a person who is assigned to the child comes to be recognized by a special characteristic. This can be, for instance, the teacher's ear-ring.

When that particular person comes on duty she refers to her body, leading the child's hand over her face, arms and legs, but finally she leads the child to her ear-ring. Immediately after this, they carry out a favourite activity, e.g. jumping on the bed. After this association is established, the ear-ring might be used as an indicator for that particular person. She announces herself by placing the ear-ring in the child's hands. Using this procedure in characterizing special persons, we were able to help the children to differentiate between people. Using a pipe, a particular child got to know his father, a scarf indicated the mother, a small bowl the young sister. These transitional objects are very important in helping the child to overcome separation anxiety, e.g. if he has to live in residence. After the child has associated 'scarf' with his mother, we use this object in preparation for going home. We have made the following arrangements for this system: every day of the week is indicated by a special box. In the box the 'highlight' of that day is indicated by an object. (When there is swimming on Tuesday, the trunks will be in the 'Tuesday' box. When the child goes home on Friday, he will find mother's scarf and father's pipe in that box.) The boxes (called memory boxes, see Jurgens 1977) are lined up and, by referring every day to the 'Friday' box with the parents' attributes, one is able to maintain the child's memories of his parents during the weekdays. We have found this a very good method of stimulating attachment behaviour. In order to be successful, however, one should take the child's developmental level into consideration. A child who has not reached the level of object and/or personal permanence is not ready yet for this type of work.

When the child has residual vision, as many of the so-called deaf–blind children have, one can use drawings of the favourite persons, or photographs as 'objects of reference'. We have found that drawings are often more valuable, because this activity can be carried out together with the child and the characteristic element, e.g. an ear-ring, freckle on the nose, can be emphasized.

Development of Communication

In the educational approach to severely sensorily impaired children described above, the development of a relationship between teacher and child is essential (see also Stillman and Battle 1984); the context in which communication takes place is constructed in the following ways.

Anticipation

By means of structuring the daily activities around 'highlights', the child may anticipate the coming events. In this anticipatory situation the child might initiate a signal himself, e.g. if he wants water in the bathtub he might touch the faucet. This touching movement is reinforced by turning on the water. From that moment the teacher accepts the child's signal. At the next bathtime the teacher first waits to see whether the child will make the signal again. If the child does not produce the signal, the teacher may initiate it by taking the child's hand.

There are some children who will hardly ever take the initiative for making a signal to satisfy certain needs. In these cases the teacher has to invent a signal and lead the child. The most effective signals are those which are centred around the body. We have found that tapping on the mouth for food is an 'easy to learn' signal; so are: tapping on the breast for going out (buttoning the coat); moving both hands vertically down the body (taking off pants); horizontal movements in the mouth (brushing teeth); vertical movements on the child's body (washing).

It is important that for this type of child the gestures are easy to execute. Therefore it is more appropriate to start with the communication gestures within the motoric competence of the individual child. The objection that different gestures are used in each unit, ward or home is not relevant. The number of gestures in the initial stage are so limited that they can easily be learned by the staff. More important is that the child gets the notion that with relatively little effort he is able to signal his basic needs to his environment.

In the development from signal to symbol it is important that the child discovers the similarity between the gesture and what it depicts, e.g. between 'hands making a sliding movement' and the activity of playing on the slide. Whether or not the child discovers this similarity is largely dependent on his intelligence.

The basic steps in the development of communication as described above are in line with the levels in the evolution of the human forebrain. In human ontogeny the first signals are manual gestures, which the infant makes to satisfy affective needs. Gestures develop first because neo-cortical components of the pyramidal motor systems that control hand–arm activity, mature first (Lamendella 1977, p. 195).

Use of Drawings

The development of these signals can be stimulated by drawings in the case of residual vision. Some visually deprived children seek visual stimulation continuously. To watch the drawing activity can be a rewarding experience. Making a drawing of an activity for which the child already has a sign, often helps the child to memorize the sign better. It has been found that even for severely intellectually retarded sensorily impaired children ($<$ IQ 50) these drawings can be schematized, e.g. for indicating an eating situation one does not need to draw a plate, sandwich and cup, but only a circle for a plate, or a rectangle indicating a sandwich. This is an important step, because if the child understands these schematized drawings, they can be used to explain more complex situations, such as the number of events which take place on a particular day (see Leygraaf 1985). For a totally blind child a number of schematized objects can serve the same purpose (see Jansen 1985). With the introduction of schematized pictures we come very close to Bliss symbols (Bliss 1965) and Rebus Reading and Premack symbols (Clark and Woodcock 1976). However in our system the picture and its schematization (until it becomes a pictogramme) is a process which is led by the child. For example a picture of a slice of bread

meaning breakfast, is reduced by the child to

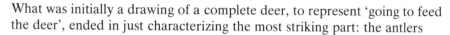

What was initially a drawing of a complete deer, to represent 'going to feed the deer', ended in just characterizing the most striking part: the antlers

(Leygraaf 1985).

Picture language is often conceptually simpler than signs (Murphy, Steele, Gulligan, Ycow and Spare 1977; Lancioni 1983) with which many children have difficulty, because of severe motor problems; we have called this 'dyspraxia' (van Dijk 1982; van Uden 1983). The pictures do not have to replace the signs, but can be used together with them. We have evidence that pictures support the recall of the signs. For some children also, a particular colour of the drawing can be helpful, as can adding the written word to it. We do not know to which stimulus a child responds, but the impression is that the different representations (sign, picture, written word) have different origins and course of development (see also Stillman, Chapter 15, this volume). By the same token we add the spoken word as well in case the child has useful residual hearing. In some instances even vibro-tactile stimulation, the so-called Tadoma-method, can be added. We consider the information coming from the different sources to be additive, i.e. the information coming from different sources is processed independently from each other (Morton 1969). The ideas, wishes and needs the child expresses during interaction are 'written' down in a special book, in which the day of the week on which the conversation took place, might have a particular colour. This entry is an extremely important source for the child as a reference book allowing past and present experiences to be linked together. For a completely deaf–blind child, books in which the schematized objects are fixed can have the same purpose.

Imitation

To facilitate the use of gestures by the child, emphasis should be placed on imitation, especially of body movements. This process originates in the so-called resonance phenomenon. This is that 'sub-consciously' the child joins in with the movements the teacher initiates, such as tapping on the table, clapping hands, opening and closing of the mouth, etc. Sometimes one has to lead the child's hands in order to get any response at all. This stage leads to the use of co-active movements, an important step in the education of this type of child (van Dijk 1966).

The attention of the child is directed towards the movements the teacher makes. Very often this can be done by the teacher imitating the spontaneous (including stereotyped) movements of the child. Suppose a child likes to swing his body from left to right. When the child initiates this, the teacher stands or sits in front of the child and imitates what the child is doing. If teacher and child also hold each other, a fine interactive play might be elicited. The teacher joins in with the child and the child with the teacher. They can jump, swing, roll on the floor, pull each other, etc., all co-actively. The teacher's responsiveness gives the child a feeling of security. After this is established, both can venture into more complex situations. In our programme we have chosen 'circuit-training'. A number of interesting objects are placed in a fixed order in a special room, such as slide, swing and trampoline. Both child and teacher move along these objects and experience the pleasure of sliding down, sitting on the swing, jumping on the trampoline. By carrying out such a training programme everyday, the child might remember the sequence of the movements. When this occurs, he will anticipate the next activity. This is a very good situation for eliciting signs from the child (Mescheriakov 1962; Ward 1981; Hammer 1982).

Imitation can be stimulated, too, by using pictures and dolls. Certain body positions can be drawn or shown by means of a doll. This has proved to be a useful procedure even for very low-functioning children (Lancioni, Smeets and Oliva 1984). This approach helps the child to become more aware of his body, and to learn how to use his hands and legs and how to manipulate objects. Needless to say, this is of enormous importance also for training of self-help skills. Together with the development of communication and physical activities, we consider this training essential in the curriculum for these children (see also McInnes and Treffry 1982).

Behaviourists have shown us how good results can be obtained in this area through careful task analysis and step-by-step procedures (Mahoney and Mahoney 1973; Finny 1981; Singer and Yarnall 1981; Walsh 1981; McInnes and Treffry 1982).

The basis of a successful programme, however, is rooted in the motivation of the child. Then he has the feeling that he is capable of coping with the world around him, despite his multiple handicaps. We think that the curriculum sketched here gives the multiply sensorily impaired child the best chances to become such a person.

References

Ainsworth, M.S.D. and Bell, S.M. (1974) 'Mother infant interaction and development of competence' in K. Connolly and J. Bruner (eds.), *The Growth of Competence*, Academic Press, New York

Bandura, A. (1969) *Principles of Behavior Modification*, Holt, Rinehart and Winston, New York

Berlyne, D.E. (1960) *Conflict, Arousal and Curiousity*, McGraw Hill, New York

Bliss, C. (1965) *Semantography*, Semantography Publications, Sydney

Bowlby, J. (1979) *The Making and Breaking of Affectional Bonds*, Tavistock Publications, London

Cardineaux, V., Cardineaux, H. and Löwe, A. (1981) *Nehmt mich an. Die Erziehung Taubblinder Kinder*, Julius Groos Verlag, Heidelberg

Cardineaux, H. (1983) *Weit ist der Weg*, Deutsches Taubblindeswerk, Hanover

Clark, C.R. and Woodcock, R.W. (1976) 'Graphic systems in communication' in L. Lloyd (ed.), *Communication, Assessment and Intervention Strategies*, University Park Press, Baltimore

Coll, J., Dumoulin, M. and Sourion, J., (1983) 'L'Examen auditif et les moyens de communication chez le sourd-aveugle', *Bulletin d'audiophonologie*, *1*, 16-52

Finny, N.R. (1981) *Handling the young cerebral palsied child at home*, William Heinemann Medical Books, London

Fraiberg S. (1975) 'The development of human attachments in infants blind from birth', *Merrill-Palmer Quarterly*, *21* (4), 315-34

Hammer, E. (1982) 'The development of human attachments in infants blind from birth', *Merrill Palmer Quarterly*, *21*, 315

Hanshaw, J.B. and Dudgeon, J.A. (1978) *Viral Disease of the Fetus and Newborn*, Major Problems in Clinical Paediatrics, *17*, Saunders Company, London, Toronto and Philadelphia

Hewitt, H. (1982) *Diagnostic Questions*, Proceedings 7th International Conference on the Deaf–Blind, Hanover

Hutt, C. and Hutt, S.J. (1965) 'Effects of environmental complexity on stereotyped behaviour of children', *Animal Behaviour*, *13*, 1-4

Janssen, M. (1985 in press) 'Objects of reference', in *Proceedings of the 8th conference on Deaf–Blind Education*, New York Institute for the Blind

Jürgens, M. (1977) *Confrontation Between the Young Deaf–Blind Child and the Outer World*, Swets and Zeitlinger, Lisse

Lamendella, J.T. (1977) 'The Limbic system in human communication' in Haiganoosh Whitaker and Harry Whitaker (eds.) *Studies in Neurolinguistics*, Academic Press, New York

Lancioni, G.E. (1983) 'Using pictorial representation as communication means with low functioning children, *Journal of Autism and Developmental disorders*, *14*, 87-105

Lancioni, G.E., Smeets, P.M. and Oliva, D.S. (1984) 'Teaching severely handicapped adolescents to follow instructions conveyed by means of three-dimensional stimulus configurations', *Applied Research in Journal Mental Retardation*, *5*, 107-23

Leygraaf, M. (1985, in press) 'Communication development in a deaf–blind girl' in *Proceedings of the 8th Conference on Deaf–Blind Education*, New York Institute for the Blind

Main, M. (1975) 'Exploration, play, cognitive functioning and the mother–child relationship', Paper presented at the bi-annual meeting of the Soc. for Research in child development, Denver

Mahoney, M.J. and Mahoney, F.E. (1973) 'A residential program in behaviour modification' in R. Rubin, S. Body and J. Henderson (eds.), *Advances in Behaviour Ther.*, Vol. I, Academic Press, New York, pp. 93-102

McInnis, J.M. and Treffry, J.A. (1982) *Deaf–Blind Infants and Children: a Developmental Guide*, University of Toronto Press, Toronto

Mescheriakov, A. (1962) *Forming of Image by Blind and Deaf and Dumb Children and the Structure of Image*, Report of a seminar on the teaching of deaf–blind children at Condover Hall

Morton, J. (1969) 'Interaction of information in word recognition' *Psychological Review*, *76*, 165-78

Murphy, G., Steele, K., Gulligan, T., Ycow, J. and Spare, D. (1977) 'Teaching a picture language to a non-speaking retarded boy', *Behav. Res. and Therapy, 15*, 198-201

Premack, D. (1970) 'A functional analysis of language', *Journal exp. Anal. Behav., 14*, 107–125

Robbins, N. (1977) 'Educational assessment of deaf–blind and auditorily-visually impaired children' in E.L. Lowell and C.C. Rouin (eds.), *State of the Art. Perspectives in serving deaf-blind children*, California State Department of Education

Singer, L. and Yarnall, G. (1981) 'Teaching a mentally retarded, deaf–blind adult to follow commands in his living environment', *Journal Vis. Imp. and Blindness*, January, 17-19

Stephans, S.M. and Delys, P. (1973) 'External control expectancies among disadvantaged children at preschool age', *Child Dev., 44*, 670-4

Stillman, R.D. and Battle, C.W. (1984) 'Developing Pre-language communication in the severely handicapped: An interpretation of the van Dijk Method', *Seminars in Speech and Language, 5* (3), 159-70

Tait, P. (1972) 'The Effect of Circumstantial Rejection on Infant Behaviour', *The New Outlook, 66* (5), 139-50

Tervoort, B., Van de Geest, A.J.M., Hubers, G.A.C., Prins, R.S., and Snow, C.E. (1972) *Psycholinguistiek*, Prisma, Utrecht

van den Tillaart, B. (1985 in press) 'Development of attachment-behaviour' in *Proceedings of the 8th Conference on Deaf–Blind Education*, New York Institute for the Blind

van Dijk, J. (1966) 'The first steps of the deaf–blind child towards language', *Journal of the Education of the Blind*, pp. 114-22

—— (1982) *Rubella Handicapped Children. The effects of bi-lateral cataract and/or hearing impairment on behaviour and learning*, Swets and Zeitlinger, Lisse

van Uden, A. (1983) *Diagnostic Testing of Deaf Children. The Syndrome of Dyspraxia*, Swets and Zeitlinger, Lisse

Vygotsky, L.S. (1983) *Sobranie socineij V. Osnovy defektologü*, Pedagogika, Moskow

Walsh, S.R. (1981) 'The educational implications of deaf–blindness' in S. Walsh and R. Holzberg (eds.), *Understanding and Educating the Deaf–blind/Severely and Profoundly Handicapped*, Ch. C. Thomas Publ., Springfield, Ill.

Ward, M. (1981) 'An overview of motor development: implication for educational programming' in S. Walsh and R. Holzberg (eds.), *Understanding and Educating the Deaf–blind/Severely and Profoundly Handicapped*, Ch. C. Thomas Publ., Springfield, Ill.

19 CONSIDERATIONS IN SELECTION OF SIGN SYSTEMS AND INITIAL LEXICA

Gwendolyn Pennington, George R. Karlan and Lyle L. Lloyd

Introduction

Assuming that the use of manual or (unaided non-speech) communication has been established as the appropriate approach for sensorily-impaired severely handicapped individuals, this chapter will present:

1. A brief overview of gesture and manual sign systems with additional references to more detailed information that might be required by the clinician attempting to use one or more of these systems.
2. General considerations summarized from available approaches for selection of an initial sign lexicon for mentally retarded non-speakers.
3. Gesture and manual sign systems used with mentally retarded adults and children.
4. Considerations pertaining to: (i) specific handicaps among mentally retarded individuals and in particular those identified as autistic-like, deaf–blind, hearing impaired or physically disabled; (ii) sign/gesture systems and lexica used with these populations; (iii) programme results; and (iv) specific considerations in programming for each group.

OVERVIEW OF GESTURE AND MANUAL SIGN SYSTEMS

Two approaches to manual communication have been used successfully with mentally retarded persons who have not learned to speak: gesture and manual sign systems (Fristoe and Lloyd 1979a, b). Gesture systems refer to relatively concrete movements which usually represent the action or object that they symbolize. Hence, the meaning of a gesture usually can be guessed easily. Gestures typically involve more total body movement than sign and tend not to have the linguistic constraints that signs do, although they may have cultural constraints. Gestures are a part of communicative interaction used by both normal speakers and those with severe communication problems. Examples of gesture systems used with severely handicapped non-speakers include mime (Levett 1969, 1971; Balick, Spiegel and Green 1976), generally understood gestures (Hamre-Nietupski, Stoll, Holtz, Fullerton, Flottum-Ryan and Brown 1977; Karlan and Fiocca 1982); and Amer-Ind, based on American Indian Hand Talk

(Skelly, Schinsky, Smith, Donaldson and Griffin 1975; Topper 1975; Skelly, 1979; Daniloff and Shafer 1981; Lloyd and Daniloff 1983).

Sign systems are gestures that are more conventionalized and conform to certain language rules (Lloyd and Karlan 1984). True natural sign languages have their own grammatical rules and, therefore, are not easily translated directly into spoken languages, e.g. American Sign Language (ASL) and British Sign Language (BSL) do not parallel spoken English (Bellugi and Klima 1975; Wilbur 1976, 1979). Although ASL and BSL signs have frequently been used with the mentally retarded, they typically have been used in an English word order. That is, the word order used parallels reasonably well that of English structure, in what might be referred to as Manually Coded English (e.g. Signed English and other pedagogical systems that will be discussed later). These signs have also been used to support English, only the key or major words in a sentence being signed while the rest of the sentence is spoken (e.g. the Makaton approach which tends to sign only part of the spoken utterance).

The Paget–Gorman Sign System (PGSS) was one of the first pedagogical systems to be used with mentally retarded non-speakers in the United Kingdom, although it was originally developed for the hearing impaired (Paget 1971; Craig 1978). Other sign systems used with mentally retarded non-speakers include Signed English (Bornstein and Hamilton 1978), Signing Exact English (Gustason, Pfetzing and Zawolkow 1972) and Signing Essential English (Anthony 1971). Currently in the United Kingdom other Manually Coded English approaches are being used as well. Signed English is being developed by the Working Party on Signed English (Sayer 1984) and one-handed finger spelling and British Signs with speech are being used at the Northern County School for the Deaf (Savage, Evans and Savage 1981; Evans 1982). A third system, that of Signs Supporting English (Sutcliffe 1983), is being developed by the Makaton Vocabulary Development Project (Walker 1973, 1978). Approximately 350 BSL signs comprise the system, none having been made up or contrived for use in this system. There is no English marking system, although signs are used in spoken English word order to represent some but not all spoken words. These manual and gesture systems will be discussed in more detail in a later part of the chapter.

General Considerations in Selection of a Gesture or Manual System

When selecting a sign system, especially for multiply handicapped non-speakers, the following system characteristics are important to consider:

Iconicity. This refers to the resemblance of a manual sign (or other symbol) to its referent or to part of its referent including 'distinctive actions performed by or upon a referent that can be imitated with the hands well enough to bring the referent to mind' (Brown 1978, p. 29). Bellugi and Klima (1975) define iconicity as 'the degree to which the elements of a sign are related to visual aspects of what is denoted'. The more iconic a sign, the easier it is to learn (Fristoe and Lloyd 1979a, b, 1980; Lloyd 1982; Karlan and Lloyd 1983, 1985; Lloyd and Karlan 1984). Iconicity can also include an association made by the learner which is not necessarily based on physical resemblance between a sign and its meaning (Griffith, Robinson and Panagos 1982).

Motoric Characteristics. The motoric characteristics of a sign language determine how easily a sign can be produced. Manual signs containing motor movements that the individual has in his motor repertoire should be developed first; this is an important consideration for a population where physical disability or motoric delays are often present. Previous research would suggest that 'touch' signs (one hand comes in contact with the signer's other hand, e.g. BALL, or another part of the signer's body, e.g. COAT) should be taught before non-touch signs (Stremel-Campbell, Cantrell and Halle 1977; Kohl 1981; Bornstein and Jordan 1982; Doherty and Lloyd 1983; Lloyd and Doherty 1983). It has been suggested that reducing the number of topographically similar items in an initial lexicon would also appear appropriate, although no studies have been conducted on this issue. It has also been recommended that the first signs taught be clearly visible (Stremel-Campbell *et al.* 1977; Goosens and Lloyd 1981; Lloyd, 1982; Karlan and Lloyd 1985), e.g. signs produced in front of the individual should be taught before those produced over the individual's head (Stremel-Campbell *et al.* 1977; Blau 1983).

Efficiency. Blau (1983) has suggested that efficiency of production should be considered, noting that handicapped persons often cannot pro-duce complete signs due to physical limitations. Because normal children produce immature vocalizations and words, and hearing-impaired children produce 'baby signs' which are practised and later refined into more mature forms, sign approximations by severely handicapped persons should also be accepted either as a transitional form in the case of a young child or, in the case of an adult, as the best that they can produce (Bornstein and Jordan 1982).

Flexibility. Flexibility, or the ability of the system to accommodate change, is an important consideration when selecting a manual or gestural system. One must be able to add new items as they become relevant for the individual. Just as normal children move from the production of sounds to single and then multiple word utterances in transition from early childhood to adult language, non-speaking persons must be provided with the means of moving from rather simple gestural communication to more sophisticated linguistic manual signing. Such was the case at Meldreth School (Levett 1969, 1971) where, after introducing mime, it was felt years later that a more formal sign system which allowed for more language growth could be learned by the residents.

Specific criteria for selecting a sign system will not be addressed in this paper; however, Carlson (1982), Blau (1983) and Lloyd and Karlan (1983, 1984) each present specific considerations for selection of symbol systems.

GENERAL CONSIDERATIONS IN SELECTION OF AN INITIAL SIGN LEXICON

Although the selection of an initial vocabulary set or lexicon for the handicapped individual must take into account the person's needs, life experiences and living/working environments, certain general considerations pertain to this overall process for any person with a handicap. There have been a number of approaches presented for selecting initial lexicons (Miller and Yoder 1974; Schiefelbusch and Lloyd 1974; Holland 1975; Lahey and Bloom 1977; Guess, Sailor and Baer 1977). The general considerations listed below are consistent with these various models in that they are based upon the normal language development and behavioural-remedial approaches.

Functional Utility.   Select items that have functional utility for the non-speaker. Because non-speakers live in a yes/no world (Blau 1983), initial items may be those that merely code yes/no. Other items, such as 'eat', 'drink', 'toilet', 'cold' to indicate needs, are more functional than teaching the non-speakers to label pictures (Miller and Yoder 1974; Holland 1975; Guess *et al.* 1977; Lahey and Bloom 1977; Fristoe and Lloyd 1980; Wilson 1980; Blau 1983; Karlan and Lloyd 1983). Karlan and Lloyd (1983) stressed the importance of functionality for these initial items as the non-speaker will be using them longer than normal children would. That is, the time span between the acquisition of single word utterances and the development of multiple phrases will be greater for handicapped children, in most cases, than for the normal child. Fristoe and Lloyd (1980) also indicated that using one sign to represent several concepts rather than a single concept (e.g. using the sign EAT to represent 'food' and 'drink' as well as 'eat') may be more functional for the individual because the number of signs that can be taught is often limited by the person's physical and cognitive abilities. Blau (1983) also stressed choosing items which can convey the *most* amount of information. Functional items can be selected from activity-based inventories, direct observation and informant information. Most important, these items should be selected with the assistance of the non-speaker. For specific inventories used to select initial lexical items, see papers by Guess *et al.* (1977), Carlson (1982) and Blau (1983).

Personal Preferences. Select items that are *important* to the individual (Holland 1975; Blau 1983), that are *preferred* by the individual (Guess *et al.* 1977) or that have the highest *interest value* for the individual (Blau 1983). Items that are high in both interest value and reinforcement value are also important to include in the initial lexicon, even if the items do not occur with high frequency. An inventory of preferred activities can be taken using the non-speaker as the primary source of information. Preferred items are easiest to select if the individual can indicate preferences non-verbally. Preferences can also be noted by observing spontaneous choices made by the individual (Karlan 1980) or by recording the amount of time spent participating in or observing the activity (Carlson 1982). Items can then be rank-ordered for preference on the basis of the amount of time spent with the activity. Items of importance to the individual also may be taken from events in the non-speaker's daily 'routine' such as mealtimes, bathing and dressing. Carlson (1982) and Blau (1983) agreed that the non-speaker should participate in the initial selection of items, even if it is only on the basis of preoccupation with an object by a severely/profoundly retarded individual. Input of parent/care-givers is also important (Carlson 1982; Blau 1983) as is that of parents, siblings and related professionals (e.g. teachers, therapists, psychologists).

Frequency of Occurrence. Choosing lexical items according to their frequency of occurrence or the opportunity to use the item is also important. The lexical items should reflect the frequency with which the individual comes into contact with an object or event, how often an activity occurs, and how often there is an opportunity to use the item (Guess *et al.* 1977). The experiences that an institutionalized individual has are very different from those of a non-institutionalized handicapped person. Often communication opportunities within a residential facility are limited due to the structure or routine of the person's daily schedule. It is, therefore, critical for staff to create such communication opportunities, even at the expense of disrupting schedules. It is important that opportunities exist for a word and/or sign to be used, so that the individual can learn the word/sign or, if already learned, so that maintenance and generalization can be established (Miller and Yoder 1974).

Flexibility. Flexibility, or the ability of an item to communicate several functions, is an important consideration when selecting initial lexical items. For example, using 'more' to indicate several different functions or the use of any other single lexical item which may have multiple meanings or multiple grammatical functions (Fristoe and Lloyd 1979a; Leonard 1984).

Opportunity for Use.   Equally important is selection of items that are *generative.* That is, select items which eventually can be combined into longer utterances (Miller and Yoder 1974; Holland 1975; Wilson 1980). It has been observed that 35 to 50 words are acquired by the normally developing child before he or she begins to combine them into two-word utterances (Nelson 1974). However, for the handicapped child, the initial lexicon may need to be larger before single words and/or signs are combined. For instance, if retarded individuals are taught a good balance of substantive and relational terms, they may produce two word/sign utterances once 50 to 80 single items have been acquired. For other severely handicapped non-speakers, however, only a few lexical items will be learned; hence, selection of those items must be carefully planned.

Immediacy.   Vocabulary items should be chosen on the basis of reflecting the *here* and *now* of ongoing activities and events (Holland 1975; Lahey and Bloom, 1977; Fristoe and Lloyd 1980). However, Blau (1983) notes that severely physically handicapped individuals who cannot act immediately upon their environment may not talk about what they are doing, but rather what they have done or are expected to do.

Age-appropriateness.   Selecting items on the basis of being age-appropriate is another consideration. Karlan (1980) addressed the importance of selecting items that are age-appropriate for older clients. Items for adult clients often have been selected on the basis of their mental age rather than chronological age. This may reinforce infantile interests and behaviours. Teaching more age-appropriate vocabulary and using more age-appropriate and functional items is encouraged. However, one must still consider the clients' interests even if they are to play with a toy (doll) as opposed to a more age-appropriate item (radio). The point is to make more age-appropriate and interesting activities available within the experience of adult handicapped persons. Fostering a sense of immediate, active participation in their own life (by folding towels or assisting in table setting) is important for the older individual, as well as the younger individual, regardless of the severity of the handicap. Good judgement on the part of the teacher is in order when selecting age-appropriate items.

Efficiency and Effectiveness.   Blau (1983) cautioned against selecting items that the individual can already produce no matter how idiosyncratically, using their residual oral skills or non-verbal signals and gestures. So, for example, one would not teach the sign DRINK as an initial lexical item if the person already had an idiosyncratic gesture for it. Blau (1983) recommended focusing instead upon efficiency and effectiveness of the initial lexicon. Idiosyncratic symbols (e.g. eye movements, wiggling toes, specific facial gestures, body movements) have often been used by handicapped individuals to convey needs (Carlson 1982); they are interpreted by their care-givers in much the same manner as normal infants' gestures and vocalizations are interpreted by their mothers. These types of idiosyncratic 'indicators' have not been conventionalized into a formal system. Unfortunately, this can result in a situation in which gestures are misinterpreted and are 'difficult to explain to new people entering into the nonspeakers' community' (Carlson 1982). After a number of conventional words/signs are mastered, the idiosyncratic symbols can be modified to or replaced by more conventional symbols.

Communicative Intent.   Initial lexical items should be selected for their ability to increase the expression of communicative intent (or communicative competence) and to enhance existing or emerging pre-linguistic communicative skills. In the past, concern for communication intervention with the mentally handicapped non-speaker has focused upon the acquisition of language skills which would allow the non-speaker to manipulate his environment (Rees 1978; Karlan 1980; Karlan and Lloyd 1985, in press). The use of manual communication has facilitated the language gains of these persons. However, less attention has been given to enable the non-speaker to initiate conversations or greetings, to draw attention and make requests, to give or share information, to refuse or protest, to control conversations by turntaking, or to ask questions and express feelings (Karlan 1980; McShane 1980; Leudar 1981; Karlan and Lloyd 1985, in press). With normal children, language develops from the infant's attempts to manipulate the environment. Thus, a speaking child typically has a history of functional pre-linguistic communication to bring to the language learning process (e.g. pointing). The person with multiple handicaps, however, has cognitive, motor and sensory deficits which have inhibited this pre-linguistic development (Carlson 1982). Hence, training that emphasizes pre-linguistic communication skills is essential.

Communicative functions expressed most frequently in lexical form by young children are requesting, naming and answering (Leonard 1984). Leonard noted that lexical items also are used to (1) secure attention, (2) describe, (3) inform, (4) indicate giving, (5) indicate doing, (6) initiate interaction and (7) solicit information. His findings suggest that young children use their relatively limited lexicons to convey a variety of communicative intentions that were developed through pre-linguistic communication interactions. Leonard also indicated that some lexical items should be chosen for comprehension training while the greater proportion of lexical items are chosen for production training; this would certainly be an appropriate strategy for teaching handicapped non-speakers. Finally, associating new words/signs with more than one communicative function has also been emphasized as a training strategy (Fristoe and Lloyd 1979a; Leonard 1984).

For the handicapped non-speaker functioning at a pre-linguistic level of communication, the acquisition of any form of 'index' (e.g. pointing, eye focus on the referent, or a specific body movement) shows an increase in pragmatic development (Leonard 1984). For persons who will not develop speech as a communication mode, such non-verbal indicators should be strengthened if they already exist in their repertoire, or should be taught directly if they are not already used (Arwood 1984). Initial items might include a generalized request signal (e.g. a wave, meaning 'I need you' or 'Please pay attention'), a request for a person to do something for the non-speaker, or a request for a person to get something (i.e. an object or substance). The object request might be pointing, an open palm reach, or an idiosyncratic indication gesture using the hand, arm, eyes, or head movement. Pointing is clearly a form of communication in young children and should not be overlooked as a pre-signing gesture in handicapped non-speakers. Body positioning of the non-speaker may also be indicative of communicative intent, e.g. 'I want to say something' or 'I need you to notice me'. On the other hand, other mentally retarded or autistic-like non-speakers may not be willing or capable of signalling by eye contact, pointing or body positioning. Finally, where conventional or idiosyncratic gestures are within the repertoire of the non-speaking individual, their response time might be significantly slower than that which occurs within normal interactions. This may require that the listener be aware not only of the presence of the non-verbal communication behaviour but also of the longer response production time. Hence, there is a need for the listener to learn to wait long enough for the non-speaker to communicate.

Additional Considerations Once the Initial Sign Lexicon Has Been Chosen

A Non-speech Environment. This needs to be created in order to familiarize others in the non-speakers' surroundings with the advantages of the gesture or sign system selected. Hopefully this will lead to acceptance and use of the sign mode to communicate with the non-speaker (Kopchick, Rombach and Smilovitz 1975; Kopchick and Lloyd 1976; Johnson and Bloomberg 1983), which will in turn provide the non-speaker with experience in using signs to communicate with others. Providing the institutionalized non-speakers with an opportunity to communicate would provide inherent rewards to reinforce this communication. This would require consistency in using sign or gesture systems once they have been introduced (Kopchick *et al.* 1975; Mayberry 1978; Blau 1983). A willingness by staff to participate with the non-speaker, no matter how difficult the client, is critical for a successful non-speech environment. The non-speech environment must provide opportunities for communicative interaction during mealtimes, bathing, dressing and leisure time, as well as during therapy and school, in order to foster the communicative use of signs.

Non-speech Models.   In addition to providing a non-speech environment, there is a need for non-speech models in the environment other than the therapists and teachers who do the initial training; hence, parents, professional staff and non-professional staff all must be taught to sign. Non-speech models will motivate and reinforce the non-speaker to sign (Kopchick and Lloyd 1976; Mayberry 1978; Blau 1983). Watching others sign can help the non-speaker develop the concept of non-speech as an 'accepted, valued communication method' (Kopchick and Lloyd 1976; Carlson 1982).

Combined Symbol Approaches.   Not only can manual signs be combined with speech (simultaneous or Total Communication), but graphic symbol systems can also be combined with speech and/or signs as combined symbol approaches. There has been an increase in such a multimodal approach using manual, graphic and spoken symbols. One of the first attempts to use signs in conjunction with graphic symbols was the Minnesota Early Language Development (MELDS), or the later Clark Early Language Program Symbols, which combine signs with AGS-type rebuses (Clark and Greco 1973; Clark and Moores 1973, 1983). A number of clinicians have been combining graphic systems such as pictograms (Johnson 1981; Walker 1984) and Blissymbols (Silverman, McNaughton and Kates 1978) with signs. A creative innovation of combining graphic symbols with manual signs are the Sigsymbols developed by Cregan (1980, 1982, 1984; Cregan and Lloyd, 1984). Sigsymbols actually integrate hand-shape, location and motion features of signs into some of the graphic symbols. Although this chapter will not go into detail concerning the integrated use of manual signs and graphic symbols, these approaches are mentioned as other possible considerations in the selection of manual signs and lexica for work with severely handicapped non-speakers. Some individuals may be confused by, or may not be able fully to utilize, all modes in a multimodal approach. However, for many severely handicapped non-speakers a multimodal approach will probably be of benefit in language and communication training, just as various modes are effectively used by normally speaking individuals.

GESTURE AND MANUAL SIGN SYSTEMS AND THE MENTALLY RETARDED

Language training for mentally retarded non-speakers has typically focused upon teaching oral speech and language. In the 1960s, manual signs were reintroduced as an educational medium for the severely hearing impaired. In the 1960s and 1970s, they were also used as an alternative mode of communication for autistic children and for the non-hearing-impaired mentally retarded, especially those who had made little or no progress with oral language training. Many of these persons resided in institutions and exhibited multiple disabilities in addition to their mental retardation (Bricker and Bricker 1970; Hall and Talkington 1970; Hoffmeister and Farmer 1972; Creedon 1973; Walker 1973; Topper 1975; Kopchick and Lloyd 1976; Kiernan 1977; Fristoe and Lloyd 1979; McDade, Simpson and Booth, 1980; Lloyd and Karlan 1984). Signs were found to improve communication abilities and social behaviour in many of these persons, although language gains varied across individuals.

The following gesture and sign systems have been used with non-speaking mentally retarded adults and children (for more information about these systems see Kopchick and Lloyd 1976; Wilbur 1976, 1979; Kiernan 1977; Mayberry 1978; Kiernan, Reid and Jones 1979, 1982; Musselwhite and St Louis 1982; Karlan and Lloyd 1985, in press).

Mime.   Mime is an example of a gesture system and is defined as the use of gross motor movements, frequently involving full-body as well as hand and facial movements and expressions. Levett (1969, 1971) introduced mime to mentally handicapped persons in the United Kingdom after having unsuccessfully tried communication boards and orthographic methods. She selected approximately 50 items and taught them with some success using an oral and mime approach (simultaneous communication) in the natural environment. Vocabulary items were selected by observing the children, school staff and the school psychologist. More than one meaning was often attached to a single mime. In addition to the students, staff were trained in the use of the mime gestures, and, in a follow-up programme, gesture training for parents was initiated. The gestures were chosen from the spontaneous gestures already used by the children and from the book, *Language of the Silent Word* by Frank Goodridge (cited in Levett 1969). Results of this programme showed that the children used mime with the trainer as well as with other students using mime. Levett eventually introduced a more formal sign system and felt that mime might be considered an appropriate transitional approach before introducing a systematic sign system. Fenn and Rowe (1975) presented a similar project.

Generally Understood Gestures.   These have been defined as simple body movements that convey information (Hamre-Nietupski *et al.* 1977). Generally understood gestures include arm or hand signals, facial expressions, mime or imitation of the movement of a referent, pointing, drawing objects or aspects of objects in the air or shaping hands into the representation of an object. Since many of these gestures frequently can be interpreted by people without specialized training, they often have the advantage of a more extensive communication audience than formal sign (Doherty, Karlan and Lloyd 1982; Karlan and Fiocca, 1982). Hamre-Nietupski *et al.* (1977) and Hobson and Duncan (1979) used a simultaneous communication approach with gestures to teach the mentally handicapped. Procedures included modelling and handshaping, and items trained were chosen for being functional and offering the most meaning to the non-speaker.

Amer-Ind (or American Indian Hand Talk).   This is another example of a gesture system used with handicapped non-speakers based upon the hand signals used by American Indian tribes to cross language barriers. A modern version has been further developed and revised by Madge Skelly *et al.* (1975) for use with non-speaking adult patients. It has also been used in the United States to teach severely retarded non-speakers to communicate (Daniloff and Shafer 1981). Skelly *et al.* (1975) modified the Amer-Ind gestures for non-speaking individuals by creating new signals as necessary and by deleting those gestures that were specific to the Indian culture. Amer-Ind has been designed to be learned easily and to be understood by a naïve viewer, but it is not a true language because it does not have its own grammatical rules. An important feature of Amer-Ind is that, as well as being simple and concrete, it also contains many one-handed signs benefiting persons with physical impairments (Daniloff and Vergara 1984).

American Sign Language.   (ASL or Ameslan). This is the language of the deaf and is a true language with its own grammar which does not parallel spoken or written English (Bellugi and Klima, 1975). ASL, although having a high communicative value, may not be appropriate for use with the mentally retarded due to the need to understand its language structure. This would require an understanding of grammar, syntax and morphology. When used with mentally retarded non-speakers, ASL signs have been used with English syntax (Wilbur, 1976; Siple (ed.) 1978); and have frequently been shortened and/or modified.

Signed English.   This is a contrived or 'pedagogical' (or instructional) system (Bornstein and Hamilton, 1978; Bornstein, Hamilton, Saulnier and Roy 1983) used to represent spoken English. It was initially constructed for use with young, hearing-impaired schoolchildren (Bornstein and Hamilton 1978), using signs primarily taken from ASL but placed into the order of spoken English. Additional signs were created to represent 14 grammatical morphemes (e.g. /ed/or/ing/) found in spoken English. It is not a true language, however, but a manual coding of English. Bornstein *et al.* (1983) provided suggestions for modifying their system for mentally retarded non-speakers and included 'aids' in the programme for parent education. Signed English was used in a Total Communication approach to develop verbal skills of mentally retarded adolescents (Linville 1977). The non-speaking students worked their way from single-sign production to two- and three-sign combinations as a result of their training. They also used signs at home due to parent participation in the programme. Linville (1977) also reported positive behavioural changes as a result of the sign training, including being 'more friendly' and 'more responsive', and an 'increased willingness to interact with classmates'.

British Sign Language (BSL).   This is the natural sign language of the deaf community in Great Britain (Woll, Kyle and Deuchar, 1981). A vocabulary of BSL signs has been developed by Margaret Walker for use with the mentally handicapped. The MAKATON approach, or BSL(M) as it is called, is described as a sign lexicon divided into eight sequenced stages. BSL(M) is used by the majority of day schools and hospitals serving the mentally handicapped in the United Kingdom (Kiernan 1977). A study reported by Bailey and Tait (1979) used Makaton with five severely-retarded, non-speaking adults which resulted in an overall improvement in their language functioning. Signs were selected on the basis of daily needs.

Paget–Gorman Sign System.   Another important sign system used in the United Kingdom is the Paget–Gorman Sign System (PGSS). It was created by Sir Richard Paget as a contrived sign system (not using BSL signs) with English word order to be used specifically with the deaf and mentally handicapped. Each category of items (e.g. food, animals) has a basic or root sign to identify that word in the group. (See Introduction to PGSS, 1971 for a further description.) Fenn and Rowe (1975) discussed using PGSS as a means of providing a systematic approach to language development after initially using Meldreth mime. In their work, a Total Communication approach was used, although only essential words in the spoken sentences were 'highlighted' with signs. Nouns were taught first, followed by two-sign structures. This programme also included staff training.

CONSIDERATIONS FOR THE SELECTION OF SIGN SYSTEMS AND LEXICA FOR THE MENTALLY RETARDED

Autistic-like Mentally Retarded Non-Speakers

Initially, the focus of treatment for autistic children was not upon speech, but upon central information processing (Konstantareas, Oxman and Webster 1978). In the early 1970s, after Hewitt and Lovaas made a systematic effort to improve the communication skills of autistic children, early language programmes for autistic mentally retarded children became behavioural in nature and focused upon oral speech (Konstantareas *et al.* 1978; Carr 1979). However, these oral language programmes were not universally effective and did not always promote acquisition of spontaneous speech. At that point, manual signs were examined as an alternative mode of communication which appeared to be successful in many cases (Creedon 1973; Bonvillian and Nelson 1978; Konstantareas *et al.* 1978; Carr 1979; Cohen 1981).

Little information has been available on the language acquisition of autistic children, perhaps because it is only recently that their language deficits have been viewed as central to their problem (Konstantareas *et al.* 1978). Language impairments in this population typically include delayed onset of speech, echolalia and mutism with severe comprehension deficits (Bonvillian and Nelson 1978; Konstantareas *et al.* 1978). Little, if any, communication competency in the form of initiation of speech (e.g. pointing, nodding the head for yes/no) is evident; hence, it usually has to be trained with this group of non-speakers (Alpert 1980). In addition, this group exhibits deficits processing auditory information and may not respond to noise (Alpert 1980). Visual and motor responses tend to be similar to those of normal children, whereas auditory and vocal skills are more deviant (Bonvillian and Nelson 1978). Autistic children may over-select a modality and tend to rely upon visual cues (Konstantareas *et al.* 1978). These individuals tend to function in a more concrete manner with limited symbolic representation. A visual–motor symbol system such as sign might then take advantage of underlying skills that are relatively unimpaired in contrast to speech and language handicaps. Unusual behaviours are also exhibited by these individuals which include ritualized body, head and hand movements, and impaired (often non-existent) social relationships.

In reviewing studies which discuss the use of sign with autistic-like mentally retarded children or adults, it is not always apparent which sign system is used and often there is no information comparing the sign systems (Leslie, Layton and Helmer 1982). In general, modifications of sign systems are not discussed although Layton and Helmer (1981) have addressed this issue.

ASL signs have been taught using behaviour modification techniques (i.e. modelling, differential reinforcement, shaping, facilitation, time out for errors and misbehaviour and stimulus control) in conjunction with a Total Communication environment using ASL signs plus speech. This approach was reported as a successful means of decreasing echolalia in a four-year-old autistic child (Cohen 1981). Bonvillian and Nelson (1978) cited a successful study using both Signing Exact English (SEE) signs and ASL signs to teach an autistic non-speaker to produce one- to three-word sign utterances and 19 individual words.

Signed English has also been used with verbal speech to train language in severely retarded non-speakers who exhibited infrequent vocalizations. A behaviour modification approach with high positive reinforcement (first edibles, then peer social reinforcement) and chaining procedure was used to teach pivot words and phrases. As a result, the non-speakers learned to sign two-word sentences. Parent participation was also utilized in this project with positive results (Creedon 1973).

Most mentally retarded non-speakers are taught sign using a simultaneous communication approach; that is, speaking plus signing at the same time or 'highlighting' by signing certain words in sentences. In the case of autistic-like mentally retarded non-speakers, there is some controversy as to whether or not using two modalities is beneficial. Bonvillian and Nelson (1978) and Carr (1979) felt that a Total Communication approach using the bimodal method of speech (auditory) plus visual (sign) is confusing, because the tendency for this group is to attend to the visual. See Creekmore (1982) and Schaeffer (1980) for further information on this issue.

Initial lexical items have been selected for autistic non-speakers based upon items such as 'tickle' or 'hug' that were naturally reinforcing (Alpert 1980; Leslie *et al.* 1982). Alpert suggested that this information can be gained from parents and teachers as well as by observing the children play. She also suggested that items be chosen according to the language structure to be taught (Alpert 1980). Most authors agree that signs taught first should be iconic (e.g. Bonvillian and Nelson, 1978; Konstantareas *et al.* 1978; Fristoe and Lloyd, 1979b, 1980; Leslie *et al.* 1982), and functional or useful (Leslie *et al.* 1982).

Also noted in studies teaching sign to autistic-like non-speakers were such positive behavioural changes as an increase in social activity and a decrease in self-stimulation (Creedon 1973; Leslie *et al.* 1982). Although communication training results vary, Carr (1979) indicated that gains appeared to be most prominent in the area of noun usage (i.e. labelling and requesting food). Increases in the acquisition of vocabulary and production of vocalizations, reduction of echolalic responses, and increases in unprompted vocal labelling have also been noted by Bonvillian and Nelson (1978) and Cohen (1981). Although it has been shown that autistic children show deficits in *creative* and *generative* aspects of language, Creedon (1973) found some autistic-like children were able to generate creative responses using signs. However, problems continued to exist in mastering abstract concepts and complex language skills.

Deaf–Blind Mentally Retarded Non-speakers

Of the approximately 6,000 deaf–blind persons (Gold and Rittenhouse 1978) in the United States, Jensema (1981) estimated that about 60-75 per cent were severely to profoundly retarded. Although the terms 'deaf' and 'blind' are used, most individuals may have less severe hearing and/or visual impairment than the terms indicate but are classified as deaf-blind because of the severity of the problem resulting from the combination of the two impairments. Language abilities of these persons are limited. The methods used for communication tend to be gesture and mime (with very little oral language), although a sign/oral approach is generally used for teaching. Communication abilities are affected by the degree of hearing and visual losses, the age of onset, the severity of behavioural problems, and the presence of additional handicaps (Griffith *et al.* 1982). The signing approach used with these individuals has been Signed English; teachers of this population have indicated that they preferred adopting methods which could be used to express Standard English rather than teaching another language (Jensema 1981). Given the complexity of the problems of these non-speakers, Jensema (1981) noted that teachers of the deaf–blind used a variety of communication methods to get concepts across; they did not limit themselves to one system. She also noted a willingness among these teachers to experiment with techniques until comprehension by the child was achieved.

Manual Communications for Deaf–Blind Non-speakers

Signs are one of the most frequently used forms of communication with deaf–blind children. Considerations for teaching sign to this population include emphasizing the tactile channel by placing the non-speaker's hands on those of the speaker to 'feel' the sign and thereby enhance feedback. Gauging an appropriate distance for the 'speaker' to stand, based on the nature of the deaf–blind person's visual losses, is important. Other considerations include: (1) modifying the scope of the sign by making it more spatially compact; (2) altering the production rate of the sign when teaching by slowing it down; (3) accepting crude gesture/sign approximations; and (4) using speech and sign together to provide redundant information to facilitate comprehension. The methods to be discussed in detail below are those most appropriate for severely handicapped deaf–blind non-speakers. Jensema (1981) has described other modes, such as fingerspelling and palm writing (using the index finger to draw the letters of the alphabet in the palm of the deaf–blind person to spell out the word), which will not be reviewed in this discussion.

The Paget–Gorman Sign System (PGSS) has been used with the deaf–blind in the United Kingdom with some success (Craig 1978).

Gold and Rittenhouse (1978) also presented a programme to teach the deaf–blind that included eight practical signs, but the sign system used was not noted. The criterion for selection of the eight signs was based upon communication need. Signs were reported to have been taught in a natural setting as opposed to an 'artificial training environment'. The technique of handshaping, plus reinforcement of sign production by the activity (e.g. signing 'eat', then sitting down to a meal) was used. The following manually based systems were designed for deaf–blind non-speakers.

The Tadoma Method.   This is a method of receiving spoken communication through the sense of touch. Developed by Sylvia Alcorn (Jensema 1981), the procedure is as follows: the deaf–blind person places a hand on the face of the speaker, the thumb covers the mouth and feels the lips, jaw and tongue movements and the other fingers are spread over the cheek, jaw and throat to detect vibrations. Children with limited vision use this form of oral communication, but it can also be an effective supplementary tool for a child who normally uses visually-processed speechreading. Although this is considered by Jensema (1981) to be more of an oral communication method rather than a manual system, it seems important to include this as a method for the deaf–blind.

Cross Code.   This is a signal system initially developed by a deaf–blind man to communicate with his family. The code is based on the position of contact on the back of the hand. The communicator taps the alphabet positions to spell words (Jensema 1981). Obviously, using an alphabet is not appropriate for a severely mentally handicapped person, but the system could be modified to include associating a specific request with a touch to the hand, arm or shoulder.

Braille Hand Speech.   This is a method of holding the initial, middle and ring fingers of both hands in such a position on the receiver's body that the tips represent the six dots of the braille cell. Braille hand speech is especially useful for people who are blind from early childhood and subsequently lose their hearing. Modifications of this technique for the severely physically handicapped might include less specific finger positions (Jensema 1981). Even though alphabet coding is a difficult task for the severely handicapped non-speaker, Thorley, Watkins and Binepal (1984) in Australia have had some success in teaching a totally blind–deaf mentally retarded person to use braille.

Vocabulary Items for Deaf–Blind Non-speakers

Griffith *et al.* (1982) felt the criteria suggested by Holland (1975), Lahey and Bloom (1977) and Fristoe and Lloyd (1980) are appropriate for selecting initial lexical items for deaf–blind children, regardless of age. They suggested emphasizing the following criteria for the selection of initial items for deaf–blind non-speakers: (1) focus upon highly familiar items; (2) focus upon manipulatives whose whole design can be perceived tactilely (spoon, drink/cup), and (3) choose action signs that are meaningful to the person ('eat', 'swing', 'rock'). Griffith *et al.* (1982) also indicated that most of these items will be iconic, but those which are the *most* iconic and meet other criteria (e.g. developmental) as well should be the easiest for these non-speakers to learn. Griffith's study provides a rating of tactile iconicity for signs that also have been rated for visual iconicity. Her findings showed that tactile iconicity was similar to visual iconicity for signs suggested for an initial lexicon by Fristoe and Lloyd (1980).

Hearing-impaired Mentally Retarded Non-speakers

Programmes for normal hearing-impaired individuals have often excluded hearing-impaired non-speakers who are mentally retarded. In addition to the hearing impairment and the fact that these individuals must learn through a visual medium, cognitively these persons are at a disadvantage. Pointing has often been used as a mode of communication, although several individuals (Hall and Talkington 1970; Hoffmeister and Farmer 1972; Walker 1973; Kopchick *et al.* 1975) have presented signing programmes specifically designed for hearing-impaired mentally retarded non-speakers.

In 1970, Hall and Talkington presented an approach to teaching hearing-impaired mentally retarded non-speakers which 'was suited both to their hearing handicap and the lowered level of comprehension and ability'. Although the authors did not indicate which sign system was used, we know from personal communication that the signs were taken from ASL. The language programme was designed to be part of an education programme that focused upon three areas: (1) vocabulary building; (2) language stimulation, and (3) acquisition of independent living skills. The vocabulary was taught by categories (e.g. vegetables, transportation). It appeared that 'most' of their subjects demonstrated rapid comprehension and functional use of the manual sign system. The authors indicated that 'academic skills and interests developed' as well, after four hours of daily instruction over a six-month period of time (Hall and Talkington, 1970). They also grouped the individuals in one residence to facilitate the communicative use of signs outside the classroom.

Hoffmeister and Farmer (1972) also taught signs to institutionalized hearing-impaired mentally retarded non-speakers who ranged from 12 to 62 years of age. These authors stressed that the signs chosen were iconic and that individual items were chosen from the person's daily programming needs. All but two of the fourteen persons in the programme increased both receptive and expressive vocabulary. Kòpchick *et al.* (1975) initiated a 24-hour approach to teach sign language to hearing-impaired severely retarded individuals by creating a non-speech environment. The programme came about as a result of realizing that the students were not using sign outside of the classroom but were 'withdrawing and using esoteric gestures instead' (Kopchick *et al.* 1975). The non-speakers were trained for a period of six months using a simultaneous signing and speaking approach. During training, the rate of presenting sign was slowed down. Staff were also included in the training programme. Although most of the clients had been institutionalized for more than 20 years, almost all 'made some type of progress' with this programme. This programme was further developed and generalized for use with other retarded persons (Kopchick and Lloyd 1976).

In the United Kingdom Makaton (BSL(M)) was developed as a result of a project exploring the use of sign language with hearing-impaired mentally handicapped adults. The Makaton Vocabulary comprises 350 or so English-word translations of British Sign Language (BSL) signs. Modifications that were made by Margaret Walker included replacing a few BSL signs which appeared too complex for mentally handicapped persons with more simple 'standardized' BSL signs (Walker 1973, 1978). The authors of this programme initially devised a vocabulary which could be used in a hospital setting; in 1976, an expanded version was produced for school/ home settings.

Mentally Retarded Non-speakers With Severe Physical Disabilities

Many mentally retarded non-speakers may also exhibit severe physical disabilities. Hence, oral language acquisition and communication skills may present a problem for these individuals as a result of physical as well as cognitive deficits. In addition, there may be accompanying visual, auditory and sensory deficits that prevent normal exploration, movement and discovery of the environment. This is turn may result in deficits in perceptual and conceptual skills thought to be prerequisites for language learning. Cognitive and physical limitations which typically confine these individuals to wheelchairs, mats or beds also inhibit their ability to initiate interactions with other people. Informal modes of communication for this population have included the use of idiosyncratic signals (using eyes and/or face, hands, arms) and vocalizations. Formal language training has focused upon oral language or non-speech modes such as the use of communication boards and electronic communication devices; however, the use of gestures, signs or gestural approximations should not be ruled out as a method of communication.

These non-speakers often have a rich repertoire of idiosyncratic signals, gestures, or vocalizations. These include eye gazes, facial expressions, hand, arm and body movements as well as distinctive vocalizations which are often well known by dormitory staff but not by therapists, teachers or other professionals. One suggestion is to build upon the previously mentioned movements and refine them into more conventional movements, if feasible. Also, one should educate staff working with the non-speaker to increase their sensitivity of what is being communicated. This can lead to an awareness by staff members that the non-speaker can indeed communicate and that communication is not limited to oral speech. Increased staff responsiveness to communication attempts will facilitate further communication development. With this group of non-speakers, a combination of systems is often efficient and appropriate. Since motoric deficits may limit the use of refined sign systems, gesture or sign approximations (e.g. gross approximations, single-handed signs) can be used instead, and others can be taught to understand them (Stremel-Campbell *et al.* 1977; Kiernan *et al.* 1979). The following gesture and sign systems have been used with these persons:

Mime.   Van Mierlo (1975) used Dominolan mime language with non-speaking severely motorically handicapped individuals because he found 'gesture language too abstract and difficult'. Van Mierlo felt a sign system used with these persons should be simple, no more than two gestures per idea; in contrast, Dutch sign traditionally used three signs per idea. Van Mierlo also believed the system should be concrete, and it should incorporate use of spontaneous gestures. Motoric constraints also required one-handed gestures to be located on 'reachable' parts of the body (e.g. head, chest, arm). Van Mierlo selected vocabulary items according to the daily needs of the child. He also mentioned the use of Pedomilan, a foot-gesture system for non-speakers who could not use their hands.

Paget–Gorman Sign System (PGSS).   Its use has also been reported with severely physically handicapped children in the United Kingdom. Kiernan's survey of sign and symbol usage in schools in the UK indicated that, although graphic symbol systems were favoured by schools for the physically handicapped, PGSS and other signs (BSL and BSL(M)) were also used. However, his study did not specifically address what percentage of the physically handicapped children were also mentally retarded (Kiernan, Reid and Jones 1979, 1982).

Amer-Ind.   This could be considered for this group of non-speakers as it contains more one-handed signs than does ASL (Daniloff and Vergara 1984). The study by Daniloff and Vergara (1984) demonstrated that Amer-Ind compared to ASL is less complex, especially in terms of movement and that there are fewer handshapes to be learned.

SUMMARY AND CONCLUSION

This chapter has presented a brief overview of sign systems used with mentally handicapped persons and considerations for selecting an initial sign lexicon. These considerations have been summarized from several sources and include some specific lexicon selection information for autistic-like, deaf–blind, deaf and physically disabled mentally retarded persons. It is clear that selection of an initial sign lexicon involves not only choosing the system to be used but also considering the individual and his communication needs. Given this information, when selecting the first 2 to 5 symbols, certain of the discussed considerations may have an even stronger influence. The first and foremost consideration for selecting initial lexical items to be taught is that they fulfil important communicative functions (e.g. requesting, recurrence, rejecting, or terminating an activity). This will provide the non-speaker with the fundamental skill to facilitating reciprocal action for the purposes of communication. Research has shown that an item with high iconic value is easier to learn and is a very important consideration when selecting the first 2 to 5 items. Clinical recommendations to exclude topographically dissimilar and conceptually dissimilar items are also important considerations. The other considerations discussed in the chapter, such as selecting items that are age-appropriate or that communicate more than one function, would assume a more general relevance as the individual's vocabulary grows.

Acknowledgements

The authors wish to thank K. Bloomberg, J. Byler and J. Doherty for their comments and suggestions on earlier drafts of this manuscript. However, the authors take full responsibility for the contents of this paper. The preparation of this chapter was supported in part by a pre-doctoral personnel preparation grant in the area of Nonspeech Communication from the Office of Special Education Rehabilitative Services, US Department of Education (G00830068) and by a Fulbright Senior Research Scholarship awarded to the third author for the Spring and Summer 1984. The contents, however, do not necessarily represent the policies of the supporting agencies and the endorsement of the federal government should not be assumed.

References

Alpert, C. (1980) 'Procedures for determining the optimal nonspeech mode with the autistic child' in R.L. Schiefelbusch (ed.), *Nonspeech Language and Communication Analysis and Intervention*, University Park Press, Baltimore *16*, 389-420

Anthony, D. (1971) *Signing Essential English*, Vols. 1 & 2, Educational Services Division, Anaheim Union School District, Anaheim, California

Arwood, E.L. (1984) *Pragmaticism: Treatment for language disorders*. The Interstate Printers and Publishers, Inc., Danville, Illinois

Bailey, R.D. and Tait, E. (1979) 'Knowing, but not doing, Makaton', *Apex*, *7* (2), 65-7

Balick, S., Spiegel, D. and Green, G. (1976) 'Mime in language therapy and clinician training', *Archives of Physical Medicine and Rehabilitation*, *57*, 35-8

Bellugi, U. and Klima, E. (1975) 'Aspects of sign language and its structure', in J.K. Kavanagh and J.E. Cutting (eds.), *The Role of Speech in Language*. The MIT Press, Cambridge, Mass.

Blau, A.F. (1983) 'Vocabulary selection in augmentative communication: Where do we begin?' in H. Winitz (ed.), *Treating Language Disorders: For Clinicians by Clinicians*, University Park Press, Baltimore *12*, 205-33

Bonvillian, J. and Nelson, K.E. (1978) 'Development of sign language in autistic children and other language-handicapped individuals' in P. Siple (ed.), *Understanding Language Through Sign Language Research*, Academic Press, New York, pp. 187-209

Bornstein, H. and Hamilton, L. (1978) 'Signed English', in T. Tebbs (Co-ordinator), *Ways and Means*, Globe Education, Basingstoke

—, ——, Saulnier, K. and Roy, H. (1983) *The Signed English Dictionary for preschool and elementary levels*, Gallaudet College Press, Washington DC

—— and Jordan, I.K. (1982) 'The relationship between sign characteristics and understandability of simple sign forms' in J.M. Berg (ed.), *Proceedings of the VIth Congress of the International Association for the Scientific Study of Mental Deficiency*, University Park Press, Baltimore

——, Saulnier, K.L. and Hamilton, L.B. (1983). *Comprehensive signed English Dictionary*, Gallaudet College Press, Washington DC

Bricker, W.A. and Bricker, D.D. (1970) 'A program of language training for the severely language handicapped child', *Exceptional Children, 1*, 101-10

Brown, R. (1978) 'Why are signed languages easier to learn than spoken languages?' Part Two, *Bulletin The American Academy of Arts and Sciences, 32* (3), 25-44

Carlson, F. (1982) *Alternate Methods of Communication*, Interstate Printers and Publishers, Danville, Illinois

—— and James, C.A. (1980) 'Picsyms symbol system' Unpublished paper, Meyer Children's Rehabilitation Institution of the University of Nebraska Medical Center, Omaha, Nebraska

Carr, E.G. (1979) 'Teaching autistic children to use sign language: Some research issues' *Journal of Autism Developmental Disorders, 9* (4), 345-59

Clark, C.R. and Greco, J.A. (1973) *MELDS glossary of rebuses and signs*, Research, Development and Demonstration Center in Education of Handicapped Children, University of Minnesota, Minneapolis

—— and Moores, D.F. (1973) *Minnesota Early Language Development Sequence (MELDS)*, Report of the proceedings of the 46th Meeting of the Convention of American Instructors of the Deaf

—— and —— (1983) *Clark Early Language Program*, DLM Teaching Resources, Allen, TX

Cohen, M. (1981) 'Development of language behavior in an autistic child using total communication', *Exceptional Children, 27* (5), 379-81

Craig, E. (1978) 'Introducing the Paget–Gorman Sign System' in T. Tebbs (Co-ordinator) *Ways and Means*, Globe Education, Houndmills, Basingstoke, Hampshire, pp. 162-3

Creedon, M. (1973) 'Language development in nonverbal autistic children using a simultaneous communication system', Paper presented at the Society for Research at Child Development Meeting, Philadelphia

Creekmore, N. (1982) 'Use of sign alone and sign plus speech in language training of nonverbal autistic children', *The Journal for the Association for Severely Handicapped, 6*, 45-55

Cregan, A. (1980) 'Sigsymbols — a nonvocal aid to communication and language development', Long study submitted in partial fulfillment of the Advanced Diploma in Education of children with Special Needs, Cambridge Institute of Education

—— (1982) *Sigsymbols Dictionary*. LDA Cambridge (obtain from A. Cregan, 76 Wood Close, Hatfield, Herts AL10 8TX England)

—— (1984) 'Sigsymbols — A graphic aid to communication and language development', A paper presented at the Curriculum Conference, Cambridge Institute of Education

—— and Lloyd, L.L. (1984) 'Sigsymbols: Graphic symbols conceptually linked with manual signs', *Proceedings of the Third International Conference on Nonspeech Communication*, International Society for Augmentative and Alternative Communication, Boston

Daniloff, J., Fristoe, M. and Lloyd, L. (1980) 'Amer-Ind recognition in aphasic subjects', *ASHA, 22*, 711

—— and Lloyd, L. (1983) 'Amer-Ind transparency', *Journal of Speech and Hearing Disorders, 48*, 103-10

—— and Shafer, A. (1981) 'A gestural communication program for severely and profoundly handicapped children', *Language Speech and Hearing Services in Schools, 12*, 258-67

—— and Vergara, D. (1984) 'Comparison between the motoric constraints for Amer-Ind and ASL sign formation', *Journal of Speech and Hearing Research, 27* (1), 76-88

Doherty, J.E. (1983) 'The effects of sign characteristics on sign acquisition and retention: An integrative review of the literature', Unpublished manuscript, Purdue University

——, Karlan, G.R. and Lloyd, L.L. (1982) 'Establishing the transparency of two gestural systems', ASHA Abstract, p. 834

—— and Lloyd, L.L. (1983) 'The effects of production mode, translucency and manuality on sign acquisition by retarded adults', Paper presented at the convention of The American Association of Mental Deficiency, Minneapolis (manuscript in preparation for journal publication)

Evans, L. (1982) *Total Communication: Structure and strategy*, Gallaudet College Press, Washington DC

Fenn, G. and Rowe, J. (1975) 'An experiment in manual communication', *British Journal of Disorders of Communication*, *10*, 3-16

Fristoe, M. and Lloyd, L. (1979a) 'Nonspeech communication' in N.R. Ellis (ed.), *Handbook of Mental Deficiency: Psychological therapy and research*, Lawrence Erlbaum Associates, New York

—— and —— (1979b) 'Signs used in manual communication training with persons having severe communication impairment', *AAESPH Review*, *4* (4), 364-73

—— and —— (1980) 'Planning an initial expressive sign lexicon for persons with severe communication impairment', *Journal of Speech and Hearing Disorders*, *45* (2), 170-80

Gold, M. and Rittenhouse, R.K. (1978) 'Task analysis for teaching eight practical signs to deaf–blind individuals', *Teaching Exceptional Children*, *10*, 34-7

Goodman, L., Wilson, P. and Bornstein, H. (1978) 'Results of a national survey of sign language programs in Special Education', *Mental Retardation*, April, 104-6

Goosens, C. and Lloyd, L.L. (1981) 'Clinical experience and research: Implication for teaching nonspeech communication', A short course presented at the Annual Convention of the American Speech–Language–Hearing Association in Los Angeles on 20 November

Griffith, P., Robinson, J. and Panagos, J. (1982) 'Tactile iconicity: Signs rated for use with deaf–blind children', A paper presented at AAMD, Boston, Massachusetts (available from Kent State University, Kent, Ohio, 44242).

Guess, D., Sailor, W. and Baer, D. (1977) 'A behavioral–remedial approach to language training for the severely handicapped individual' in E. Sontag (ed.), *Education Programming for the Severely and Profoundly Handicapped*, pp. 360-77, Division on Mental Retardation, Council for Exceptional Children, Reston, Virginia

Gustason, G., Pfetzing, D. and Zawoklow, E. (1972) *Signing Exact English*, Modern Signs Press, Rossmoor, California

Hall, S.M. and Talkington, L. (1970) *Learning by doing: A unit approach for deaf–retarded*, Mental Retardation Research Series, No. 18, Austin State School

Hamre-Nietupski, S., Stoll, A., Holtz, K., Fullerton, P., Flottum-Ryan, M. and Brown, L. (1977) 'Curricular strategies for teaching selected nonverbal communication skills to verbal and nonverbal severely handicapped students' in L. Brown, J. Nietupski, S. Lyon, S. Hamre-Nietupski, T. Crowner and L. Gruenewals (eds.), *Curricular Strategies for Teaching Functional Object Use, Nonverbal Communication and Problem solving and Mealtime Skills to Severely Handicapped Students, Vol. VII, Part 1*. University of Wisconsin–Madison and Madison Metropolitan School District, Madison, WI

Hobson, P. and Duncan, P. (1979). 'Sign learning and profoundly retarded people', *Mental Retardation*, *17* (1), 33-7

Hoffmeister, R.J. and Farmer, A. (1972) 'Development of manual sign language in mentally retarded individuals', *Journal Rehabilitation of the Deaf*, *6*, 19-26

Holland, A. (1975) 'Language therapy for children: Some thought on context and content', *Journal of Speech and Hearing Disorders*, *60*, 514-23

Jensema, C.K. (1981) 'A review of communication systems used by deaf–blind people', Part 1, *Deaf–Blind News*, A.A.D., October, 720-5

Johnson, H., and Bloomberg, K. (1983). 'The development and application of nonspeech systems', unpublished paper, Victoria, Australia

Johnson, R. (1981) *The Picture Communication Symbols*, Mayer–Johnson Co., Solana Beach, California

Kahn, J.V. (1981) 'A comparison of sign and verbal language training with nonverbal retarded children', *Journal of Speech and Hearing Research*, *46*, 113-19

Karlan, G.R. (1980) 'Issue in communication research related to integration of developmentally disabled individuals' in A.R. Novak and L.W. Heal (eds.), *Integration of Developmentally Disabled Individuals into the Community*, Paul H. Brookes, Baltimore, Maryland *9*

—— and Fiocca, G.A. (1982) 'Generally Understood Gestures: An approach communication for mentally retarded language impaired individuals', unpublished manuscript, Purdue University

—— and Lloyd, L. (1983) 'Considerations in the planning of communication intervention: I. Selecting a lexicon', unpublished manuscript, Purdue University

—— and —— (1985) *Communication Intervention for the Moderately and Severely Handicapped*, University Park Press, Baltimore, Maryland (in press)

Kiernan, C. (1977) 'Alternatives to speech: A review of research on manual and other forms of communication with the mentally handicapped and other noncommunicating populations', *British Journal of Mental Subnormality, 23*, 6-28

——, Reid, B. and Jones, L. (1979) 'Signs and symbols — who uses what?' *Special Education Forward Trends, 6* (4), 32-4

——, —— and —— (1982) *Signs and Symbols: A Review of Literature and Survey of the Use of Non-Vocal Communication*, Heinemann Educational Books, London

Kohl, F. (1981) 'Effects of motoric requirements of the acquisition of manual sign responses by severely handicapped students', *American Journal of Mental Deficiency, 85* (4), 396-403

Konstantareas, M.M., Oxman, J. and Webster, C.D. (1978) 'Iconicity: Effects on the acquisition of sign language by autistic and other severely dysfunctional children' in P. Siple (ed.), *Understanding language through sign language research*, Academic Press, New York pp. 213-35

Kopchick, G.A. and Lloyd, L.L. (1976) 'Total communication programming for the severely language impaired' in L. Lloyd (ed.), *Communication Assessment and Intervention Strategies*, University Park Press, Baltimore

——, Rombach, D.W. and Smilovitz, R. (1975) 'A total communication environment in an institution', *Mental Retardation*, June, 22-3

Lahey, M. and Bloom, L. (1977) 'Planning a first lexicon: Which words to teach first', *Journal of Speech and Hearing Disorders, 42*, 340-9

Layton, T.L. and Helmer, S.H. (1981) 'Initial language program for autistic and developmentally disordered children', Paper presented at AMMD Convention, Detroit

Leonard, L.B. (1984) 'Normal language acquisition: Some recent findings and clinical implications' in A. Holland (ed.), *Language Disorders in Children*, College-Hill Press, San Diego, pp. 1-36

Leslie, C.M., Layton, T.L. and Helmer, S.H. (1982) 'A critical review pertaining to sign language acquisition in autistic children', Paper presented at 15th Annual Gatlinburg Conference, April, Gatlinburg, Tennessee

Leudar, I. (1981) 'Strategic communication in mental retardation' in W.I. Fraser and R. Grieve (eds.), *Communication with Normal and Retarded Children*, John Wright and Sons Ltd., Bristol

Levett, L.M. (1969) 'A method of communication for nonspeaking severely subnormal children', *British Journal of Communication Disorders, 4*, 64-6

—— (1971) 'A method of communication for nonspeaking severely subnormal children — trial results', *British Journal of Disorders of Communication, 6*, 125-8

Linville, S.E. (1977) 'Signed English: A language teaching technique with totally nonverbal, severely mentally retarded adolescents', *Language, Speech and Hearing Services in Schools, 8*, 170-5

Lloyd, L.L. (1982) 'Symbol and initial lexica selection', A paper presented at the Second International Conference on Nonspeech communication, Toronto

—— and Daniloff, J. (1983) 'Issues in using Amer-Ind code with retarded persons' in T.M. Gallagher and C.A. Prutting (eds.), *Pragmatic Assessment and Intervention Issues in Language*. College-Hill Press Inc., San Diego, California pp. 171-92

—— and Doherty, J.E. (1983) 'The influence of production mode on recall of signs in normal adult subjects', *Journal of Speech and Hearing Research, 26*, 591-600

—— and Karlan, G.R. (1983) 'Symbol selection considerations', *Proceedings of the XIX World Congress of Logopodics and Phoniatrics* (Vol. III), Edinburgh pp. 1155-60

—— and —— (1984) 'Nonspeech communication symbols and systems: Where have we been and where are we going?' *Journal of Mental Deficiency Research, 28*, 3-20

Mayberry, R.I. (1978) 'Manual communication' in H. Davis and S.R. Silverman (eds.), *Hearing and Deafness* (4th edn.), Holt, Rinehart and Winston, New York

McDade, H.L., Simpson, M.A. and Booth, C. (1980) 'The use of sign language with handicapped, normal-hearing infants', *Journal of Childhood Communication Disorders, 4*, 82-9

McShane, J. (1980) *Learning to Talk*, Cambridge University Press, Cambridge, England

Miller, J.F. and Yoder, D.E. (1974) 'An ontogenetic language teaching strategy for retarded children' in R.L. Schiefelbusch and L.L. Lloyd (eds.), *Language Perspectives: Acquisition, Retardation and Intervention*, University Park Press, Baltimore

Moores, D.F. (1981) 'Issues in the modification of American Sign Language for instructional purposes', *Journal of Autism and Developmental Disorders, 11* (1), 153-62

Musselwhite, C.R. and St. Louis, K.W. (1982) *Communication programming for the severely handicapped: Vocal and non-vocal strategies*, College-Hill Press, San Diego, CA

Nelson, K. (1974) 'Concept, word and sentence: Interrelations in acquisition and development', *Psychological Review, 81* (4), 267-85

Orlansky, M.D. and Bonvillian, J.D. (1984) 'Recent research on sign language acquisition: Implications for multihandicapped hearing-impaired children', *Journal of National Student Speech, Language and Hearing Association*, 72-87

Paget, R. (1971) 'An introduction to the Paget–Gorman Sign System with examples', AEDE pamphlet

Rees, N. (1974) 'Pragmatics of language: Applications to normal and disordered language development' in R.L. Schiefelbusch and L.L. Lloyd (eds.), *Language Perspectives: Acquisitions, Retardation and Intervention*. University Park Press, Baltimore

Richardson, T. (1975) 'Sign language for the SMR and PMR', *Mental Retardation, 13*, 17

Savage, R.D., Evans, L. and Savage, B. (1981) *Psychology and Communication in Deaf Children*, Grune and Stratton, London

Sayer, D.J. (1984) Personal communication about the development of signed English in the UK and the future publication of a book titled *Signed English for Schools*: Vol 1 Structural Language (Feb. and April, 1984)

Schaeffer, B. (1980) 'Teaching signed speech to nonverbal children: Theory and method', *Sign Language Studies, 26*, 29-63

Schiefelbusch, R.L. and Lloyd, L.L. (1974). *Language Perspectives: Acquisition, Retardation and Intervention*, University Park Press, Baltimore

Silverman, H., McNaughton, S. and Kates, B. (1978) *Handbook of Blissymbols*, Blissymbols Communication Institute, Toronto

Siple, P. (ed.), (1978) *Understanding Language Through Sign Language Research*. Academic Press, New York

Skelly, M. (1979) *Amer-Ind Gestural Code: A simplified Communication system based on universal hand talk*, Elsevier North Holland, Inc., New York

—— Schinsky, L., Smith, R., Donaldson, R. and Griffin, J. (1975) 'American Indian Sign: A gestural communication system for the speechless', *Archives of Physical Medicine and Rehabilitation, 56*, 156-60

Stremel-Campbell, K., Cantrell, D. and Halle, J. (1977) 'Manual signing as a language system and as a speech initiator for the nonverbal severely handicapped student' in E. Sontag, J. Smith and N. Certo (eds.), *Educational programming for the severely and profoundly handicapped*, Division on Mental Retardation, Council for Exceptional Children, Reston, Virginia

Sutcliffe, B.M. (1983) '"Total Communication" or total confusion', *Journal of the British Teachers of the Deaf, J* (7), 134-6

Thorley B.J. and Jardine, J. (1983) 'The use of printed language stimuli with severely handicapped deaf/blind child', unpublished (draft) paper Macquarie University North Rocks Project, Sydney, Australia, January 1983

——, Watkins, E. and Binepal, T. (1984) 'Teaching a severely intellectually retarded deaf–blind child to use Braille stimuli: a two-year project', manuscript in preparation

Topper, S.T. (1975) 'Gesture language for a nonverbal severely retarded male', *Mental Retardation, 13*, 30-1

Van Mierlo, J.M.A. (1975) 'Communicatology. A new technical approach to communicational problem-solving', Mimeographed copy

Walker, M. (1973). 'An experimental evaluation of the success of a system of communication for the deaf mentally handicapped', unpublished M.Sc. Thesis, Human Communication Studies, University of London

—— (1978) 'The Makaton Vocabulary' in T. Tebbs (ed.), *Ways and Means*, Globe Education, Basingstoke

—— (1984) Personal Communication

Wilbur, R.B. (1976) 'The linguistics of manual language and manual systems' in L.L. Lloyd (ed.), *Communication Assessment and Intervention Strategies*, University Park Press, Baltimore

—— (1979) *American Sign Language and Sign Systems*, University Park Press, Baltimore

Wilson, K.D. (1980) 'Selection of a core lexicon for use with graphic communication systems', *Journal of Childhood Communication Disorders*, *4*, 111-23

Woll, B., Kyle, J. and Deuchar, M. (1981) *Perspectives on British Sign Language and Deafness*, Croom Helm Ltd., London

20 MOBILITY TRAINING FOR VISUALLY IMPAIRED MENTALLY HANDICAPPED PERSONS

Randall K. Harley and Mary-Maureen Hill

Introduction

Goal

According to Hill and Ponder (1976), the eventual goal of orientation and mobility (O&M) is 'to enable the student to enter any environment, familiar or unfamiliar, and to function safely, efficiently, gracefully, and independently by utilizing a combination of these two skills' (p. 1). With regard to the visually impaired mentally handicapped population, one must consider if this goal is, in fact, feasible. One must determine if the visually impaired mentally handicapped are capable of independent travel and, if so, to what extent.

Philosophy

For visually impaired mentally handicapped persons, individualized experiences must be provided which facilitate the gratification of their own needs and desires, thereby making movement a rewarding experience. The acquisition of O&M skills may be limited to immediate environmental travel in order to fulfil basic needs. For some visually impaired mentally handicapped persons extensive outdoor travel may be unreasonable; however, the individual may become a proficient indoor traveller, relying on a sighted guide when venturing outdoors. Others may be able to learn a specific route to a bus stop, take the bus to a different neighbourhood, and walk a number of blocks to a specific destination. Some may be capable of travelling several blocks in a business area, whether to places of employment, sheltered workshops, health clinics, and recreational and commercial facilities.

Murphy (1964) provided O&M training to a 20-year-old visually impaired mentally handicapped man which enabled him to follow instructions, utilize landmarks constructively, utilize public transportation, and to maintain his orientation consistently. McDade (1969) directed a three-year federally sponsored project to teach institutionalized visually impaired mentally handicapped persons and concluded that systematic and sequential O&M programming could benefit from 20 to 40 per cent of the visually impaired mentally handicapped population in most states. Johnston and Corbett (1973) maintained that emphasis on fundamental pre-cane skills and a breakdown of standard teaching techniques would facilitate the acquisition of O&M skills by visually impaired mentally handicapped persons.

Independent travel for multiply handicapped visually impaired persons was demonstrated through the implementation of specific goals using behaviour modification techniques (Gallagher and Heim 1974). Harley, Merble and Wood (1975b) studied the feasibility of providing pro- grammed instruction in O&M to multiply handicapped visually impaired children and developed the Peabody Mobility Scale for identifying requisite skills in the development of a systematic programme of instruction.

Cratty (1980) maintained that 'the quality of instruction that can be imparted to a retarded child is partly dependent on the degree and causes of the retardation' (p. 221). Consequently, some visually impaired mentally handicapped persons may learn very little, and others may conceptualize and utilize many of the techniques in everyday travel. Geruschat (1980) stressed the importance of taking into account both the long-range goal, i.e. preparation for sheltered workshop or the acquisition of daily living skills, and the living arrangement anticipated. In other words, is the O&M skill functional and does its acquisition apply within the context of the indi- vidual's environment? Are routes applicable? Does learning how to travel a route actually increase the individual's independence? Before these questions can appropriately be answered, it is first necessary to evaluate the individual's needs and capabilities. Interaction with other professionals is imperative in developing the requisite perspective for designing realistic goals and adapting procedures. Traditionally, individuals receiving O&M training participated in every phase of instruction. Our perceptions of O&M training programmes must be modified to provide instruction in those areas in which the visually impaired mentally handicapped person can achieve success and the greatest possible degree of normalization within society. Rather than being inclusive, programmes can be designed to offer only that training which can assist the individual in becoming a viable part of the environment. Independent travel for visually impaired mentally handicapped persons entails more than just the physical act of moving and walking; it also encompasses their awareness of the environment from day to day.

Assessment in Orientation and Mobility

Comprehensive Assessment

A comprehensive assessment in O&M with visually impaired mentally handicapped children and adults must involve specialists in a team approach because of the complexity caused by multiple impairments. Bourgeault, Harley, DuBose and Langley (1977) described an assessment programme for severely handicapped visually impaired children which included a diagnostic team approach with special teachers, psychologists and ancillary paediatric, orthopaedic and ophthalmological personnel as needed. The assessment process included parent intervention, measure- ment of mental abilities, and a detailed educational prescriptive programme in the areas of motor, language, cognitive-adaptive and social self-care skills. Reassessment occurred after six months.

In order to determine the nature and extent of O&M training for visually impaired mentally handicapped persons, a comprehensive evaluation is needed to determine the person's abilities and need for training. Many kinds of information are needed, such as medical reports, psychological reports, eye reports, parent or family conference reports and educational reports. In addition, a report from an O&M specialist is critical to make a decision in regard to starting a training programme.

Geruschat (1980) suggested a thorough evaluation of each child before starting O&M services for deaf–blind children. The areas to consider include the following:

> visual evaluation;
> medications and restrictions;
> evaluation from other specialists;
> mode of communication;
> body awareness/environmental awareness;
> description of child's movement.

Characteristics of Trainees

The characteristics of individuals who can profit from O&M instruction are variable according to age, intelligence, types of additional handicapping conditions, degree of vision and experience. The nature of the travel task can vary widely, but the aforementioned variables seem to be the most important factors to consider in most situations.

Although age is an important factor, individuals from all age groups have been shown to profit from O&M instruction. Multiply handicapped visually impaired pre-school children can benefit from O&M training (Moore 1970). School-age multiply handicapped children also can profit from O&M training (Harley, Wood and Merbler 1980). Hill and Harley (1984) suggested modifications in O&M for aged visually impaired persons with additional disabilities.

Intelligence is also considered as an important factor in teaching O&M skills necessary for independent travel. Higher intelligence may be a prerequisite for following the more complex routes that a visually impaired person might need to travel in going to work in a large city. Travelling to the bathroom within a home would probably require much less ability, but it would be an important goal in making the mentally handicapped visually impaired person more independent. Cortazzo and Sansone (1969) found that social maturity, emotional stability and parent co-operation were the most important criteria in choosing successful trainees in a travel programme for severely mentally handicapped adults who demonstrated IQ scores in the low profound–severe handicapped range. Intelligence was felt to be of much less importance than when they first started the programme.

Boe and Zubrycki (1976) found that two individuals who had tested IQs within the 50-80 range and had been institutionalized for 35 years could learn to use dog guides successfully.

Physically handicapped visually impaired persons have learned O&M techniques that enabled them to become more independent in travel. Seelye and Thomas (1966) described successful O&M training for a twelve-year-old girl with cerebral palsy (spastic quadriplegia), double knee-caps and total blindness, and an eight-year-old deaf–blind girl. Enzinna (1975) described an O&M programme for a totally blind, bilateral amputee which included use of the long cane. Morse (1980) taught cane travel to a 14-year-old deaf–blind girl with a physical problem that pre-vented her from moving the cane right and left or from lifting it or sliding it on the floor. A wide variety of adaptations can be made for many different kinds of physical handicaps by the resourceful O&M instructor for mentally handicapped visually impaired persons.

Degree of vision is another important factor to consider in learning O&M skills. Harley and Merbler (1980) found that low-vision multi-handicapped children could profit from instruction in O&M, and Harley *et al.* (1980) found that visually impaired multiply handicapped children could profit from O&M instruction. Much more emphasis is now being made on O&M for low-vision persons. Better optical aids and more know-ledge about optical-aids training have helped to improve instruction in O&M for low-vision persons. Likewise, the development of electronic travel aids has helped to improve travel skills of totally blind persons.

The experience of the visually impaired mentally handicapped person in various types of environments is also an important characteristic to consider. McDade (1969), Johnston and Corbett (1973) and Uslan (1979) found that institutionalized visually impaired mentally handicapped persons could profit from O&M instruction. Seelye and Thomas (1966) and Murphy (1964) showed that visually impaired mentally handicapped persons could profit from O&M training in becoming more independent in their neigh-bourhoods and communities. Freedom to move about is an important factor to consider. Orientation and mobility training in institutions where 'herding' or moving by groups is practised does not give the mentally handicapped visually impaired person the opportunities to improve in the development of O&M skills that a less restrictive environment would pro-vide.

Assessment of Orientation and Mobility Skills

A review of the literature indicates that several instruments have been developed to assess skills needed by low-functioning visually impaired children in O&M training. Eichorn and McDade (1969) designed an evalu-ation instrument for visually impaired mentally handicapped persons from ages 10 to 59. The instrument was developed with 120 items grouped in twelve units in such areas as body concepts, textures and dimensions, environmental patterns and positions, sighted guide techniques, and geographical relationships. They concluded that the same basic skills needed by the 'normal' visually impaired population are applicable to this population with some needed adaptations. The most important difference was the level and method of presentation and the time needed to learn the skills.

Laus (1977) listed four requisites for mentally handicapped candidates for O&M instruction. These requisites included: (1) demonstration of social emotional readiness; (2) ability to learn basic routines; (3) ability to distinguish a particular bus from a set of others, and (4) ability to make decisions and to initiate movement. More specifically, he used a series of questions to evaluate the O&M readiness of a candidate. Examples of these questions included the following. Does pupil get along with his/her peers? With familiar and unfamiliar adults? Does pupil deal appropriately with new and unexpected situations? How long a time-period can pupil attend to a task in a group setting? In a one-to-one situation? Does pupil follow directions? Can you rely on pupil to complete a task once it is begun? Is pupil able to communicate orally his/her home address and phone number? Does pupil initiate movement within classroom or building or does he/she wait for directions (pp. 43-5).

In the assessment of a visually impaired person for a dog guide, several factors must be taken into account. These factors include: orientation skills, safety, personal preference, life circumstances, activity level, amount of remaining vision, age and physical condition (Whitstock 1980). Of these factors, orientation skills and safety are problems for many mentally handicapped persons. In orientation, a trainee with inadequate concepts about objects in the environment may have difficulty making intelligent decisions about travel. The trainee may have difficulty recalling descriptions or instructions, or understanding complex spatial relationships, such as irregular placement of driveways, walks and buildings. Remembering directions or the route from his/her home to the workshop or recreational centre may be difficult. Using models or graphic aids, such as maps and diagrams, may be problematic. The dog guide can help in many aspects of travel, but it must be given intelligent directions.

The Use of Orientation and Mobility Scales in Assessment

Some special developmental scales have been written in criterion-referenced format to be used in the assessment of O&M skills for mentally handicapped visually impaired children and youth. Harley *et al.* (1975a) used a scale (Lord 1969) with multiply handicapped visually impaired children which was designed to measure O&M skills in pre-school visually impaired children. This scale incorporated a developmental task approach using child development data and lists of skills compiled fom experienced teachers. The subscales included self-help skills, movement in space, sensory cues in travel and directions, and turns in travel.

Harley *et al.* (1980) developed the Peabody Mobility Scale which was designed specifically for measuring O&M skills in multi-handicapped visually impaired children. The scale was later revised and adapted for multi-handicapped low-vision children (Harley and Merbler 1980). The guidelines for selection of subjects included the following: (1) functions non-visually in the environment (or for low-vision scale possesses a visual acuity of 6/200 light projection); (2) possesses at least one additional handicap to blindness; (3) makes positive responses to simple commands, and (4) functions at the pre-school level.

The Peabody Mobility Scale is divided into four major areas: motor development, sensory training, concept development and mobility skills. The sensory training scale for the low-vision children emphasized visual tasks and the sensory training for the visually impaired children emphasized sound localization, and tactual and olfactory discrimination.

An advantage of using the Peabody Mobility Scale is that there are training activities designed in an easy-to-follow step-by-step programmed instruction for each scale item. Another advantage is that the scale and training materials were validated with 40 multi-handicapped visually impaired and low-vision children and youth in nine facilities in a 16-week field test. The experimental group, using the programmed instructional materials, demonstrated significant overall performance gains over a control group.

Assessment of Vision

Assessment of vision in low-vision mentally handicapped children can be accomplished by using the Functional Vision Inventory (Langley 1980). This teacher-administered scale can be used to assess the child's vision to determine whether a visual impairment is causing a visual problem which interferes with the child's learning process or to plan intervention strategies that will help the child to use his/her vision more efficiently. This inventory, which was designed for multi-handicapped children, provides assessment data in the areas of structural defects, reflexive reaction, eye movements, near and distance vision, visual field preference and visual perception. An advantage of this scale is that prescription lessons are outlined at the following levels:

awareness of visual stimuli;
fixation, convergence, shift, or gaze;
tracking;
near distance;
scanning;
peripheral field vision;
eye—hand integration;
form and colour description;
visual perceptual skills.

An added feature of the Functional Vision Inventory is a short visual screening test that can be used to determine if visual problems are present.

The Diagnostic Assessment Procedure (DAP) (Barraga and Morris 1980) may be appropriate for some of the higher functioning multiply impaired low-vision children who function at a kindergarten level. One of the major advantages of this assessment kit is the observational checklist which can be used to assess functional use of vision in travel. The DAP also has lessons that match the assessment items. These lessons are carefully sequenced and outlined in a format that can be easily adapted into a child's Individual Educational Program (IEP) giving objective, visual task, materials, procedure, response, procedural notes, and additional auditory, kinaesthetic and tactile activities.

Assessment of Non-Visual Sensory Skills

The Peabody Mobility Kit (Harley *et al.* 1975a) has sensory assessment scales that have been used successfully with multi-handicapped visually impaired children (including mentally handicapped children). These scales include sound localization, tactual discrimination with hands, tactual discrimination with feet, and olfactory discrimination. Lord (1969) developed three scales designed to measure sensory skills used in localization, identification and travel. If in doubt about the person's level of auditory functioning, a pure-tone audiometer may be used to measure sensitivity to sound. Similarly, if in doubt about the individual's tactual sensitivity, a modified Optacon may be used to measure finger sensitivity to vibration (Harley, Pichert and Morrison, 1985).

Assessment of Concept Skills

MacWilliam (1977) suggested prerequisite concepts to O&M training which include knowledge of basic spatial concepts, such as in-out and up-down, demonstration of impulse control, and adequate physical condition. Boe and Zubrycki (1976) listed use of sensory cues, concept development, body awareness and spatial orientation as areas of prerequisite training before training in the use of sighted guides with mentally handicapped visually impaired adults.

Several instruments have been utilized to assess concepts needed by visually impaired mentally handicapped children in O&M. Cratty and Sams (1968) developed an instrument, Body Image of Blind Children, which is designed to assess the child's ability to identify body planes and body parts, and to demonstrate various body movements, such as laterality and directionality. Guldager (1970) designed a body image scale for pre-school multi-handicapped Rubella children based on the child's ability to initiate body movement and to demonstrate object concepts based on the theories and observations of Jean Piaget. Hill (1981) designed a performance test, Hill Performance Test of Selected Positional Concepts, which was developed to assess spatial concepts needed in O&M by visually impaired children from ages six to ten inclusive. The Tactile Analog to the Boehm Test of Basic Concepts (Caton 1977) is designed to identify children whose overall level of concepts, such as 'between', 'around', 'over', 'forward' and 'through' are among the concepts considered in this assessment which has been adapted for visually handicapped persons.

Assessment of Motor Development

Motor scales for visually impaired children can be found in the Peabody Mobility Kit and several more general developmental checklists. However, special motor scales can also be utilized. Scales with which to assess motor and sensory functions of mentally handicapped visually impaired, low-vision or visually impaired children include *AMMP* (awareness, movement, manipulation of environment, and posture and locomotion) (Webb 1969), the Peabody Development Motor Scales, and Activity Cards (Folio and Fewell 1983). The Peabody Developmental Motor Scales are especially suited for mentally handicapped visually impaired children. These gross and fine motor scales were designed for children with developmental delays and, in the early stages of development, the items were administered to visually handicapped children.

Assessment of Emotional and Social Development

The importance of diagnosis and consideration of emotional and social development is emphasized by O&M specialists. Mentally handicapped low-vision and visually impaired children are often rejected or over-protected by their parents. Many of them have spent extensive periods of time in hospitals, institutions or in beds at home. Lack of independent travel often leads to increased dependency and a negative self-concept. The California Personality Inventory (Gough 1956) is an example of a personality inventory which has been adapted for use with the visually impaired, especially adolescent visually impaired. The Adolescent Emotional Factors Inventory (Bauman 1964) is a personality inventory which has been designed specifically for use with visually impaired adolescents. In addition to these inventories, teacher or parent observation of day-to-day activities is a simple procedure to obtain valuable information on personal–social problems. An advantage of this procedure is that it provides continuous data over a long period of time. A disadvantage is that the teacher or parent may be too biased to note the really important characteristics of the child's day-to-day behaviour.

The following checklist (Harley, Henderson and Truan 1979) can be used to indicate presence of emotional–social problems:

low interest;
poor rapport with other pupils;
fear of failure;
inability to sit quietly;

hostility;
withdrawal symptoms;
nervousness;
mannerisms;
excessive attention-getting behaviour;
low self-concept;
preference for routine over new activities;
excessive bragging;
low initiative;
compulsiveness in activities;
refusal to participate.

In using this checklist or other similar lists, precautions should be taken to make any referrals for psychological assistance on the observation of a cluster of characteristics rather than on observation of only one or two items.

Evaluation of attitudes of parents and professionals who come into contact with the visually impaired mentally handicapped person is extremely important. Some parents and professionals may be over-zealous in their attempts to protect or keep the multi-handicapped child from anticipated dangers from moving about in his/her environment. Samuel Gridley Howe, the founder of the Perkins School for the Blind, said that it was better to get a few injuries from an active life than to let the child rust through inactivity (Buell 1966). Robert Perske (1972) agreed with giving pupils opportunity for risk-taking, saying:

> Many who work with the handicapped, impaired, disadvantaged, and aged tend to be over zealous in their attempts to 'protect', 'comfort', 'keep safe', 'take care' and 'watch'. Acting on these impulses at the right time can be benevolent, helpful and developmental. But, if they are acted upon exclusively or excessively without allowing for each client's individuality and growth potential, they will overprotect and emotionally smother the intended beneficiary. In fact, such overprotection endangers the client's human dignity, and tends to keep him from experiencing the risk-taking of ordinary life which is necessary for normal human growth and development (p. 195).

Since work with multi-handicapped visually impaired children may cause inhibitions on the part of parents and teachers, it is essential that good communication be established between the O&M instructor and the other adults who work with the child. A thorough evaluation of the child's abilities and needs is necessary before starting the instruction.

Programming

Factors to Consider in Orientation and Mobility

Whatever the goal of the individualized O&M training programme, early intervention is critical and must be considered an integral part of any instructional programme, whether in schools, sheltered workshops, residential facilities, rehabilitation and/or activity centres, or in the home. Everyone who interacts consistently with these individuals should be active participants in the learning process and reinforce appropriate techniques. Parents and families are an important component of the training programme. Uslan (1979) discussed the need for professional interdependence among teachers of the visually impaired and of the mentally handicapped, emphasizing that the 'exchange of practical and theoretical resources among professionals ... is ... essential' (p. 54). A team approach is necessary in the delivery of O&M services to ensure utilization of the new knowledge and skills in a variety of settings.

An O&M training programme for the mentally handicapped visually impaired person must be functional, realistic and purposeful with an emphasis on movement for a reason. The learning process should be developmental, incorporating both formal and informal, structured and unstructured instruction. Instructions should be offered in simple, direct and frequently repeated language. Presentation of skills should remain consistent.

'Because many retarded blind have lived very sheltered lives and exhibit difficulty remembering instructions and following directions, the training programme should "distinguish between incapacity that results from inadequate training, from specific prohibitions, or from mental deficiency"' (Laus 1974, p. 36). Training should incorporate instructions to be followed sequentially in preparation for future travel which could conceivably involve remembering a somewhat complicated route. To facilitate learning, O&M instruction should be provided within the context of the actual task to be performed, i.e. learning a specific route is best communicated if instruction is offered at the appropriate time in the individual's daily routine. Furthermore, in order for significant learning to occur, the individual must interact successfully with the environment in a meaningful way (Hill, personal communication, 1982). Skills should be incorporated which the individual already knows and, where feasible, the mentally handicapped visually impaired person should have the opportunity to make choices and/or decisions regarding the training programme.

Several factors are critical in the success of any O&M training programme. A one-to-one relationship for all travel skills is essential for safety reasons and to ensure continuity of instruction throughout the entire learning experience. This consistency allows the O&M specialist to make an informed judgement of each individual's mastery of travel skills. The close working relationship also enables the O&M specialist to recognize the visually impaired mentally handicapped individual's saturation point, at which time additional information can no longer be absorbed. A rest period may be necessary before new material can be introduced.

Group lessons can be incorporated into the training programme to teach gross motor movements, concept development, basics of orientation, and body and sensory awareness. Classroom teachers can enhance the utilization and reinforcement of these concepts and participate in an ongoing evaluation and assessment of their student's O&M skills. How well the teachers understand the principles of O&M and how actively involved they are in the actual implementation of the training programme facilitate an ideal sequential O&M programme for the visually impaired mentally handicapped.

Designing a Programme and Components

When developing an individualized O&M programme for visually impaired mentally handicapped persons, several factors must be considered. When should intervention begin? What selection criteria should be established? Are some O&M skills optional? If so, which ones? In what sequence are skills to be presented? What pre- and requisite skills are necessary for independent travel? How is independent travel defined? Is there a basic minimum of pre- and requisite skills for independent travel? How are social maturity and emotional readiness for travel training measured? How long should training continue? Should training be ongoing? What does the future hold for the individual? What skills are necessary to prepare a visually impaired mentally handicapped individual for the future? With these questions in mind, the O&M specialist must decide upon an appropriate curriculum for teaching O&M skills. Because of the various deficiencies in concept development, environmental experiences, and cognitive abilities exhibited by many visually impaired mentally handicapped persons, the typical O&M programme for non-mentally handicapped visually impaired can be modified and applied with visually impaired mentally handicapped. Components from many O&M training programmes have been revised and incorporated within the following suggested curricular areas (McDade 1969; Thomas 1972; Harley *et al.* 1975b; Hill and Ponder 1976):

Pre-cane Skills: non-cane skills which allow safe and independent indoor travel/orientation; body concepts, body relationships involving gross body movements, balance, posture, gait, co-ordination; environmental concepts, including texture, dimensions, temperature, patterns, geographical relationships; auditory perceptual skills, including sound identification, localization, tracking.

Travel Skills: skills without the use of a mobility aid/sighted guide, self-protective techniques allowing independent travel, including forearm techniques, trailing, object location; long cane — diagonal technique indoors, modified diagonal technique outdoors, touch technique indoors and outdoors; residential, semi-business, business.

However the O&M specialist chooses to design the O&M programme, interim periods of independent travel should be provided in the appropriate setting after each stage of instruction. This process allows for evaluating the individual's performance, instils confidence, and ensures overlearning before progressing to a higher level task. The acquisition of travel skills should be coupled with community experiences to facilitate the acquisition of social, communication, self-help, monetary and temporal skills. Community experiences might involve role-playing so the visually impaired mentally handicapped person learns how to solicit aid from the appropriate individual, i.e. adult vs. child.

The instructor/client relationship is an important facet of the training programme. During the initial travel experience, the instructor remains physically close to the client in order to offer support and instructions. As training progresses, the instructor gradually withdraws to allow the client to demonstrate confidence in each newly learned skill. A greater distance is maintained after several successful repeated objectives are demonstrated in order to measure the amount of independence exhibited by the visually impaired mentally handicapped individual. Only after successive appropriate demonstrations of route mastery is unsupervised travel allowed.

The O&M specialist can also serve as a facilitator in group follow-up counselling sessions in which individuals share information and experiences encountered during independent travel. Clients and instructors can discuss problems, concerns, methodologies and behaviour guidelines related to travel experiences.

Modifications in Training

Many of the basic O&M skills important to non-mentally handicapped visually impaired are also applicable, with some modifications, to the visually impaired mentally handicapped person. Most teachers of the visually impaired and mentally handicapped visually impaired agree that the major learning differences between the two populations involve the level and methods of presentation of information and the amount of time necessary for learning the skill. Cratty and Sams (1968) maintained that the gross aspects of one's body must be understood by low-functioning individuals before being able to conceptualize and demonstrate higher level skills, such as cane travel.

Often, visually impaired mentally handicapped persons exhibit a lack of basic concept development and body awareness due to a general lack of environmental experiences. Consequently, gait and posture are adversely affected. Much of this aberrant behaviour could conceivably be prevented if positive activities, such as O&M techniques, were introduced very early in the training process. This premiss is supported by McDade's (1969) contention, that 'orientation and mobility training should be a means to an end and not an end in itself' (p. 317).

With visually impaired mentally handicapped persons it is often necessary to reduce the process of learning O&M into very small steps, teaching only the requisite behaviour for mastery of a specific skill before proceeding to the next skill. Behaviour modification principles, such as backward chaining, may be systematically applied. The O&M specialist must remember to work with the individual's instructional level and couple all instructions with simple, concrete objects or concepts. Simpler instructions than *parallel* and *adjacent*, for example, are probably necessary. Since most visually impaired mentally handicapped persons are capable of remembering only a few details at a time, each day's lesson must be presented in the same way, adding only as much information daily as the individual can conceptualize. Depending on the individual's frustration tolerance, lessons may initially be limited to 15 minutes. The O&M specialist may have to designate concrete landmarks to facilitate the individual's orientation instead of the person utilizing independent self-familiarization techniques. Emphasis may be placed upon using the person's residual travel vision as efficiently as possible if motor co-ordination precludes use of the long cane.

Modification in Techniques

Traditionally, instruction in touch technique with the long cane has been provided to normally functioning visually impaired persons (see Figure 20.1). Safety and seeking information remain critical components of long-cane travel; yet, functional and structural modifications are being developed to meet individual needs. These modifications must be tailored to accommodate the specific strengths and weaknesses of each mentally handicapped visually impaired individual. Uslan (1979) attributed the lack of attention directed towards providing O&M instruction to severe/profound mentally handicapped visually impaired persons to the fact that the conventional meaning of O&M is irrelevant to their needs. Therefore, cane travel has historically been offered to only those mentally handicapped visually impaired individuals demonstrating the requisite intellectual and motor functioning for independent travel to familiar destinations (Uslan 1979). Mentally handicapped visually impaired individuals, however, are now carrying the long cane for identification purposes only. Uslan (1979) proposed the use of the long cane as a simple walking aid for the severely mentally handicapped visually impaired, because balance is improved, advanced warning of danger is provided, and changes in terrain along the travel path are identified. All that is required to learn the basic diagonal technique is the ability to grip the cane without exhibiting behaviour problems, making use of the cane dangerous (see Figure 20.2). Uslan (1979) does suggest, however, that 'cane travel must

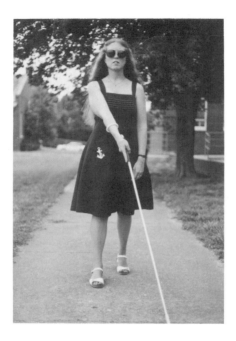

Figure 20.1: Touch Technique

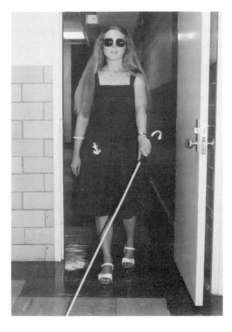

Figure 20.2: Diagonal Technique

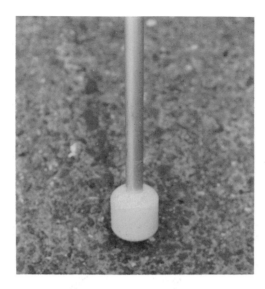

Figure 20.3: Large Marshmallow Tip

be considered as a supervised leisure time activity if it is to benefit the blind retarded individual' (p. 58).

Berdell Warzburger (personal communication, 1982) trained institutionalized visually impaired mentally handicapped persons with a large marshmallow tip on the end of the long cane to facilitate independent travel (see Figure 20.3). Residents either pushed the cane tip along the ground straight out in front of them or maintained constant touch to the ground with a sweeping motion back and forth. The modified tip prevented continual snags in the concrete or grass walking surfaces.

With multi-handicapped visually impaired persons, crutches can serve as a mobility aid by facilitating trailing, providing protection from obstacles, and promoting good balance (Hill, personal communication, 1983). Because crutches would impede travel with a sighted guide, voice cues and footsteps can indicate directions. To check straight line of travel, the individual can walk a few feet with the crutches, then check with one to locate the wall. Routes can be devised so that he stays in contact with the wall or landmark as much as possible. Although this technique is slower than conventional methods, it is equally efficient.

Structural modifications in the long cane are becoming increasingly more acceptable for those individuals incapable of maintaining continual arc motion with a conventional long cane, whether for intellectual or physical reasons. Morse (1980) attached a diagonal section to a primary cane less than half-way from the floor so the secondary cane tip touched on the opposite side where the primary cane tip arc would normally touch, thus providing body-width protection (see Figure 20.4). The constant

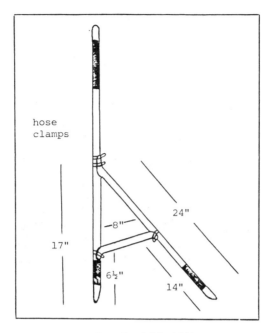

Figure 20.4: Modified Cane for Use By a Deaf–Blind Girl

position of both tips allowed adequate reaction time to stop for obstacles encountered between the two shafts. A brace positioned between the two lower shafts strengthened the structure and allowed additional reaction time by blocking narrow obstacles even sooner.

Aids

The major communication modes for visually impaired mentally handicapped are tactile and kinaesthetic. Tactile demonstrations should be provided, as well as ample opportunities to touch objects and demonstrate O&M movements to facilitate concrete and experiential learning. Tactile aids should incorporate identifiable and grossly different cues. Varying textures can be affixed to the walking surface or to the walls in facilitating preliminary route travel. A potential problem with prolonged use of runners or strips on the floor is the development of everting feet. Edges and corners of tables or other obstacles should be rounded to prevent bumps and encourage independent exploration. Environmental concepts can be introduced and reinforced, using tactual maps and aids. Mannequins and the bodies of the individual and the O&M specialist can be employed in teaching basic body concepts and the movement of body parts. Environmental concepts of shape, form, dimension and texture are reinforced with concrete aids and through repeated experience. Trainees incapable of speech should utilize hand signs and demonstrate their understanding of directions through movements. Cards with both printed and brailled instructions on the front and a corresponding photograph on the back, i.e. a picture of the bus the trainee needs to board, facilitate independent travel. The cards are also used to solicit aid from passers-by for deaf–blind mentally handicapped individuals who are incapable of making independent street crossings.

To facilitate the training of street traffic and the arrangement of blocks and buildings in residential and business areas, either the Chang Mobility Kit* or your own model can be utilized. Traffic flow along the streets is conceptualized by moving little toy cars around corners and through intersections. Blocks, sidewalks, corners and alternative routes are conceptualized by moving toy figures about the model. Travel lessons should be conducted immediately after the initial exposure to the model to reinforce concepts introduced. Many trainees benefit from additional experience with the model in the actual outdoor training area.

Auditory cues, coupled with signals emitted by photoelectric sensors, facilitate straight-line travel. Simple auditory maps can be recorded on cassettes. The use of simple taped instructions facilitates the ability to follow sequential directions and provides a level of consistency and smooth transition between each instructional phase.

Consequences of Orientation and Mobility Training

Increased mobility offers a whole new range of activities for the visually impaired mentally handicapped person. Independent travel facilitates the acquisition of new skills that are used in the performance of other daily tasks. Many individuals demonstrate an improved self-concept as evidenced in improved posture, motivation and self-confidence. Trainees develop the responsibility for being on time and dressing appropriately for the weather.

Additional advantages of O&M training for mentally handicapped visually impaired persons include reduced dependency, increased opportunities for normal societal interactions, an increased awareness of self and of the environment, increased ability to follow directions, and the opportunity to function as normally as possible, and to function more independently as an adult. A greater range and variety of experiences are more available.

Parents and families also benefit from O&M training for their visually impaired mentally handicapped family members. Parents view their children as capable of learning, and may become actively involved in assisting their children to learn to function independently. Perhaps for the first time they feel a sense of pride in their children's accomplishments.

Logistically speaking, institutions can realize a saving through reducing their staff. School systems can also realize significant monetary savings through the use of public bus transportation rather than contracting with cab companies or private transportation systems.

---

*The Chang Mobility Kit is available from: American Printing House for the Blind, PO Box 6085, 1839 Frankfort Avenue, Louisville, Kentucky 40206, USA.

Future Trends

The future teaching of O&M skills to the mentally handicapped visually impaired and low-vision population appears very promising. There appear to be a number of trends which will impact on the fundamental right to an appropriate education, which includes O&M, for every visually impaired and low-vision mentally handicapped individual. The following are 10 major trends in philosophy, services, assessment and training which point in this direction:

1. Visually impaired mentally handicapped youth and adults will be allowed more freedom to travel and will receive more encouragement to develop independent travel skills in their homes and neighbourhood environments.
2. Early intervention will be more prevalent with visually impaired mentally handicapped children.
3. Training of O&M instructors will incorporate more skills acquisition and experience with visually impaired mentally handicapped children and adults.
4. Increased services will be available. More teachers with multiple competencies will be prepared to teach O&M to visually impaired mentally handicapped children and youth.
5. Schools will provide more adequate service delivery. Visually impaired mentally handicapped children will receive more services and the teachers will receive better training. Training materials will be more comprehensive and available in greater abundance.
6. Low-vision mentally handicapped children and adults will receive more services from professional O&M instructors, as well as from teachers and paraprofessionals.
7. Special teachers' aides and parents will be incorporated in a co-operative effort to provide O&M instruction to visually impaired mentally handicapped children.
8. More adequate assessment scales will be developed that can be used with visually impaired mentally handicapped children, especially in the birth-to-toddler developmental ages.
9. More research will be undertaken to develop teaching methods, aids and materials for use with visually impaired mentally handicapped persons.
10. Traditional ideas, such as taboos for dog guides and canes for visually impaired mentally handicapped youth and adults, will be changed to a more flexible and experimental approach.

Formal O&M training has come a long way in the last 40 years, from the training of visually impaired war veterans to some of the lowest functioning mentally handicapped visually impaired persons. As attitudes have improved in our society, the home, school, agencies and communities have recognized the importance of helping these persons to function more independently in their environments. We are just beginning to scratch the surface on how best to provide the skills that are needed to develop these skills most effectively. Hopefully, in the next 40 years much new knowledge will be developed that will enable visually impaired mentally handicapped persons to reach levels of travel that have never been reached before.

References

Aitken, S. and Bower, T.G. (1982) 'The use of the Sonicguide in infancy', *Journal of Visual Impairment and Blindness, 76*, 91-100

Barraga, N.C. and Morris, J.E. (1980) *Programs to develop efficiency in visual functioning,* American Printing House for the Blind, Louisville

Bauman, M.K. (1964) 'Group differences disclosed by inventory items', *International Journal for the Education of the Blind, 13*, 101-6

Boe, E.N. and Zubrycki, J.H. (1976) 'Dog guide training for the mentally handicapped: An interagency approach', *New Outlook for the Blind, 70* (8), 326-8

Bourgeault, S.E., Harley, R.K., DuBose, R.R. and Langley, M.B. (1977) 'Assessment and programming for blind children with severely handicapped conditions', *Journal of Visual Impairment and Blindness, 71*, 49-53

Bower, T.G.R. (1982) *Development in infancy,* W.H. Freeman Company, San Francisco

Buell, C.E. (1966) *Physical education for blind children.* Charles C. Thomas, Springfield, pp. 3-4

Caton, H.R. (1977) 'The development of a tactile analog to the Boehm test of basic concepts, form A', *Journal of Visual Impairments and Blindness, 71*, 382-6

Cortazzo, H.C. and Sansone, R. (1969) 'Travel training', *Teaching Exceptional Children, 3*, 67-82

Cratty, B. and Sams, T. (1968) *Body-image of blind children,* American Foundation for the Blind, New York

Cratty, B.J. (1980) *Adapted physical education for handicapped children and youth,* Love Publishing Company, Denver

Croft, N.B. and Robinson, L.W. (1975) *Project vision-up curriculum: A training program for preschool visually impaired children,* Idaho State School for the Deaf and Blind, Gooding, Idaho

Eichorn, J.R. and McDade, P.R. (1969) *Teaching orientation and mobility to the mentally retarded blind,* Report to Division of Research and Demonstration Service, Department of Health, Education and Welfare Grant No. RD2065-5. Boston College, Chestnut Hill, Maryland

Enzinna, A.J. (1975) 'Orientation and mobility for a totally blind, bilateral hand amputee', *New Outlook for the Blind, 69*, 103-8

Felix, L. and Spungin, S.J. (1978) 'Preschool services for the visually handicapped: A national survey', *Journal of Visual Impairment and Blindness, 72*, 59-66

Finestone, S., Lukoff, I. and Whitman, M. (1960) *The demand for dog guides and the travel adjustment of blind persons,* Research Center New York School of Social Workers, Columbia University, New York

Folio, M.R. and Fewell, R.R. (1983) *Peabody developmental motor scales and activity cards,* Teaching Resources Corporation, Hengham, Maryland

Fraiberg, S. (1977) *Insights from the blind,* Basic Books, New York

Gallagher, P.A. and Heim, R.E. (1974). 'The classroom application of behavior modification principles for multiply handicapped blind students', *New Outlook for the Blind, 68*, 447-53

Geruschat, D.R. (1980) 'Orientation and mobility for the low functioning deaf–blind child', *Journal of Visual Impairment and Blindness, 74*, 29-33

Gough, H.G. (1956) *California Psychological inventory,* Consulting Psychologists' Press,

Palo Alto

Guldager, V. (1970) *Body image and the severely handicapped rubella child*, Perkins Publication, No. 27, Perkins School for the Blind, Watertown, Maryland

Harley, R.K., Henderson, F.M. and Truan, M.B. (1979) *Teaching of braille reading*, Charles C. Thomas, Springfield

—— and Merbler, J.B. (1980) 'Development of an orientation and mobility program for multiply impaired low vision children', *Journal of Visual Impairment and Blindness, 74*, 9-14

——, —— and Wood, T.A. (1975a) 'The development of a scale in orientation and mobility for multiply impaired blind children', *Education of the Visually Handicapped, 7*, 1-5

——, —— and —— (1975b) 'Programmed instruction in orientation and mobility for multiply impaired blind children', *New Outlook for the Blind, 69* (9), 418-23

——, Wood, T.A. and Merbler, J.B. (1980) 'An orientation and mobility program for multiply impaired children', *Exceptional Children, 46*, 326-31

——, Pichert J.W. and Morrison M.B. (1985) 'Braille instruction for blind diabetic adults with decreased tactile sensitivity', *Journal of Visual Impairment and Blindness, 79* (1), 12-17

——, Pichert, J.W. and Morrison, M.B. (1985) 'Braille instruction for blind diabetic adults with decreased tactile sensitivity', *Journal of Visual Impairment and Blindness, 79*(1), 12-17

Hill, E.W. (1981) *The Hill performance test of selected positional concepts*, Stoelting Company, Chicago

—— and Ponder, P. (1976) *Orientation and mobility: A guide for the practitioner*, American Foundation for the Blind, New York

Hill, M.M. and Harley, R.K. (1984) 'Orientation and mobility for aged visually impaired persons', *Journal of Visual Impairment and Blindness, 78* (2), 49-54

Johnston, B.C. and Corbett, M.C. (1973) 'Orientation and mobility instruction for blind individuals functioning on a retarded level', *New Outlook for the Blind, 67*, 27-31

Langley, M.B. (1980) *Functional vision inventory*, Stoelting Company, Chicago

Laus, M.D. (1974) 'Classroom techniques: Orientation and mobility instruction for the sighted trainable mentally retarded', *Education and Training of the Mentally Retarded, 9*, 70-3

—— (1977) *Travel instruction for the handicapped*, Charles C. Thomas, Springfield

Lord, F.E. (1969) 'Development of scales for the measurement of orientation and mobility of young blind children', *Exceptional Children, 36*, 77-81

MacWilliam, L.J. (1977) 'You can get from there to here', *Teaching Exceptional Children, 9*, 69-71

McDade, P.R. (1969) 'The importance of motor development and mobility skills for the institutionalized blind mentally retarded', *New Outlook for the Blind, 63* (10), 312-17

McGlinchey, M.A. and Mitala, R.F. (1975) 'Using environmental design to teach ward layout to severely and profoundly retarded blind persons: A proposal', *Journal of Visual Impairment and Blindness, 69*, 168-71

Moore, M.E. (1970) 'Developing body image and skills of orientation, mobility, and social competence in preschool multiply handicapped blind children', Doctoral dissertation, University of Pittsburgh. Ann Arbor, MI: University Microfilms (No. 70-20, p. 338)

Mori, A.A. and Olive, J.E. (1978) 'The blind and visually handicapped mentally retarded: Suggestions for intervention in infancy', *Journal of Visual Impairment and Blindness, 78*, 273-9

Morse, K.A. (1980) 'Modifications of the long cane for use by a multiply impaired child', *Journal of Visual Impairment and Blindness, 74*, 15-18

Murphy, T.J. (1964) 'Teaching orientation and mobility to mentally retarded blind persons', *New Outlook for the Blind, 58*, 285-7

O'Brien, R. (1976) *Alive . . ., aware . . ., a person: A developmental model for early childhood services*, Montgomery County Schools, Rockville, NY

Perske, R. (1972) 'The dignity of risk', in W. Wolfensberger (ed.), *The Principal of Normalization in Human Services*, National Institute on Mental Retardation, Toronto

Seelye, W.S. and Thomas, J.E. (1966) 'Is mobility feasible with multiply handicapped blind children?' *Exceptional Children, 32*, 613-17

Smith, A.J. and Cate, K.S. (1982) *Look at me*, Pennsylvania College of Optometry Press, Philadelphia

Swallow, R.M. (1981) 'Fifty assessment instruments commonly used with blind and partially seeing individuals', *Journal of Visual Impairment and Blindness, 75*, 65-72

Thomas, J.E. (1972) 'Mobility education for multiply handicapped blind children in day schools: What it encompasses', *New Outlook for the Blind, 66* (9), 307-13

Uslan, M.M. (1979) 'Orientation and mobility for severely and profoundly retarded blind persons', *Journal of Visual Impairment and Blindness, 73*, 54-8

Webb, R.C. (1969) 'Sensory motor training of the profoundly retarded', *American Journal of Mental Deficiency, 74*, 283-95

Whitstock, R.H. (1980) 'Dog guides', in R. L. Welsch and B.B. Blasch (eds.), *Foundations of orientation and mobility*, American Foundation for the Blind, New York

INDEX

Abnormal ECG syndrome
  see also Jervell and Lange-Nielsen
    syndrome
abnormalities
  neurological 321
  physical 321
AB-O incompatibility 130
abstraction 185–7
accessibility of information 177
accommodation, visual 211
acoustic
  environment 358
  reflex 229
acquired colour vision defects 241–2
acrocephalosyndactyly 120
  see also Apert's syndrome
adaptive behaviour 36
Adaptive Performance Instrument (API)
  284–5
additional handicaps and hearing
  impairment 300–4
additionally impaired hearing impaired
  (AIHI) 358–62
adenovirus 49
Adolescent Emotional Factors Inventory
  415
Adult Training Centres 89
Advisory Teachers of the Deaf 363
aetiology of hearing loss 115–36
age-appropriate lexical items 388
aggression 25, 27–8
  prevalence of 28
  'the triad' and 29
'air-bone gap' 116
air conduction audiometry 223–4
alcoholics 242
Alport's syndrome 120
Alstrom's syndrome 159
Alzheimer-type dementia 15
amblyopia 11
American Sign Language (ASL) 384, 393,
  401
Amer-Ind 383, 393, 401
AMMP 415
amniocentesis 154, 161, 164
ampicillin 132
amplification 115
  see also hearing aids
anisometropia 211–12
anomaloscopes 243
anophthalmos 110
  see also malformations of the eye
anoxia 298, 303
  hearing loss and 130
anticipation 377–8

anti-depressants 242
anti-epileptic drugs 241
Apert's syndrome 120
  see also acrocephalosyndactyly
aptitudes and interests 315
areas for assessment 306–7
Arthur point scale of performance tests
  308
artificial light and colour vision 244
ascertainment procedures 88
Ashkenazi Jews *see* gangliosidoses
assessment
  battery 259–65
  of concept skills 414–15
  curriculum-related 67
  of emotional and social development
    415–16
  environment and equipment 256–8
  of hearing impairment; principles
    297–9; purposes 299
  of vision 94
  of motor development 415
  of non-visual sensory skills 414
  of vision 413
astigmatism 8, 10–11, 211
  prevalence of and racial difference in
    10
attachment 376–7
audiogram 136, 140
  'left hand corner' 122
audiological
  screening in institutions 56–7
  services 218–19
  technicians 236
Auditory Assessment of Deaf–Blind
  Multi-Handicapped Children 267
auditory cues 424
Auditory Response Cradle (ARC) 231
AuroPalpebral Reflex (APR) 232
Australia 398
autism 29, 172, 321
  hearing loss and 140
autistic 29, 191–2, 195
  children 391, 394–6
autistic-like 383, 390
  mentally retarded non-speakers 394–6
autosomal
  dominant gene and deafness 119–21
  dominant syndromes 119–21
  recessive deafness 117
  recessive syndromes 117–18

backward chaining 420
  see also behaviour modification